Renal Imaging

Editors

STEVEN C. EBERHARDT
STEVEN S. RAMAN

RADIOLOGIC CLINICS
OF NORTH AMERICA

www.radiologic.theclinics.com

Consulting Editor
FRANK H. MILLER

September 2020 • Volume 58 • Number 5

ELSEVIER

1600 John F. Kennedy Boulevard • Suite 1800 • Philadelphia, Pennsylvania, 19103-2899

http://www.theclinics.com

RADIOLOGIC CLINICS OF NORTH AMERICA Volume 58, Number 5
September 2020 ISSN 0033-8389, ISBN 13: 978-0-323-79116-8

Editor: John Vassallo (j.vassallo@elsevier.com)
Developmental Editor: Donald Mumford

Radiologic Clinics of North America (ISSN 0033-8389) is published bimonthly by Elsevier Inc., 360 Park Avenue South, New York, NY 10010-1710. Months of issue are January, March, May, July, September, and November. Periodicals postage paid at New York, NY and additional mailing offices. Subscription prices are USD 513 per year for US individuals, USD 980 per year for US institutions, USD 100 per year for US students and residents, USD 594 per year for Canadian individuals, USD 1253 per year for Canadian institutions, USD 703 per year for international individuals, USD 1253 per year for international institutions, USD 100 per year for Canadian students/residents, and USD 315 per year for international students/residents. To receive student and resident rate, orders must be accompanied by name of affiliated institution, date of term and the signature of program/residency coordinatior on institution letterhead. Orders will be billed at individual rate until proof of status is received. Foreign air speed delivery is included in all *Clinics* subscription prices. All prices are subject to change without notice. **POSTMASTER:** Send address changes to *Radiologic Clinics of North America*, Elsevier Health Sciences Division, Subscription Customer Service, 3251 Riverport Lane, Maryland Heights, MO63043. **Customer Service: Telephone: 1-800-654-2452** (U.S. and Canada); **1-314-447-8871** (outside U.S. and Canada). **Fax: 1-314-447-8029. E-mail: journalscustomerservice-usa@elsevier.com (for print support); journalsonlinesupport-usa@elsevier.com (for online support).**

Reprints. For copies of 100 or more of articles in this publication, please contact the Commercial Reprints Department, Elsevier Inc., 360 Park Avenue South, New York, New York 10010-1710. Tel.: +1-212-633-3874; Fax: +1-212-633-3820; E-mail: reprints@elsevier.com.

Radiologic Clinics of North America also published in Greek Paschalidis Medical Publications, Athens, Greece.

Radiologic Clinics of North America is covered in *MEDLINE/PubMed (Index Medicus), EMBASE/Excerpta Medica, Current Contents/Life Sciences, Current Contents/Clinical Medicine, RSNA Index to Imaging Literature, BIOSIS, Science Citation Index,* and *ISI/BIOMED.*

Contributors

CONSULTING EDITOR

FRANK H. MILLER, MD, FACR
Lee F. Rogers MD Professor of Medical
Education, Chief, Body Imaging Section and
Fellowship Program, Medical Director, MRI,
Department of Radiology, Northwestern
Memorial Hospital, Northwestern University,
Feinberg School of Medicine, Chicago, Illinois

EDITORS

STEVEN C. EBERHARDT, MD
Professor and Vice Chair of Clinical
Operations, Chief of Abdominal and
Oncology Imaging, Department of Radiology,
University of New Mexico, Albuquerque,
New Mexico

STEVEN S. RAMAN, MD, FSAR, FSIR
Professor of Radiology, Surgery and Urology,
Division of Abdominal Imaging and
Intervention, Department of Radiological
Sciences, David Geffen School of Medicine at
UCLA, Los Angeles, California

AUTHORS

ASSER ABOU ELKASSEM, MD
Department of Radiology, The University of
Alabama at Birmingham, Birmingham,
Alabama

EVAN ALLGOOD, MD
Assistant Professor, Department of Radiology,
University of Southern California, Los Angeles,
California

KRYSTAL ARCHER-ARROYO, MD
Assistant Professor, Division of Emergency
and Trauma Imaging, Department of
Radiology and Imaging Sciences, Emory
School of Medicine, Emory University, Atlanta,
Georgia

PATRICIA BALTHAZAR, MD
Diagnostic Radiology Chief Resident,
Department of Radiology and Imaging
Sciences, Emory School of Medicine, Atlanta,
Georgia

LING-CHEN CHIEN, MD
Resident in Diagnostic Radiology, Department
of Radiology and Imaging Sciences, Emory
University, Emory School of Medicine, Atlanta,
Georgia

PETER L. CHOYKE, MD
Molecular Imaging Program, National Cancer
Institute, National Institutes of Health,
Bethesda, Maryland

JASON S. CHU, MD
Department of Radiology and Biomedical
Imaging, University of California, San
Francisco, San Francisco, California

RABINDRA GAUTAM
Center for Cancer Research, National Cancer
Institute, National Institutes of Health,
Bethesda, Maryland

TAREK N. HANNA, MD
Associate Professor, Division of Emergency
and Trauma Imaging, Department of Radiology

and Imaging Sciences, Emory School of Medicine, Emory University, Atlanta, Georgia

MARTA E. HEILBRUN, MD
Vice Chair for Quality, Department of Radiology and Imaging Sciences, Emory University Healthcare, Atlanta, Georgia

KEITH D. HERR, MD
Assistant Professor, Division of Emergency and Trauma Imaging, Department of Radiology and Imaging Sciences, Emory School of Medicine, Emory University, Atlanta, Georgia

HENA JOSHI, MD
Diagnostic Radiology Resident, Department of Radiology and Imaging Sciences, Emory School of Medicine, Atlanta, Georgia

KEVIN G. KING, MD
Assistant Professor of Clinical Radiology, Keck School of Medicine of USC, University of Southern California, Norris Cancer Center, Los Angeles, California

MEGHAN G. LUBNER, MD
Associate Professor, Department of Radiology, University of Wisconsin-Madison School of Medicine and Public Health, Madison, Wisconsin

ASHKAN MALAYERI, MD
Radiology and Imaging Sciences, Clinical Center, National Institutes of Health, Bethesda, Maryland

CHRISTINE O. MENIAS, MD
Professor of Radiology, Mayo Clinic Alix School of Medicine, Mayo Clinic Hospital, Phoenix, Arizona

REFKY NICOLA, MS, DO
Division of Body Imaging, Associate Professor, Department of Radiology, Roswell Park Cancer Institute, Buffalo, New York

STEVEN S. RAMAN, MD, FSAR, FSIR
Professor of Radiology, Surgery and Urology, Division of Abdominal Imaging and Intervention, Department of Radiological Sciences, David Geffen School of Medicine at UCLA, Los Angeles, California

ERICK M. REMER, MD, FACR, FSAR
Professor of Radiology, Imaging Institute and Glickman Urological and Kidney Institute, Cleveland Clinic, Cleveland, Ohio

SEPIDEH SHAKERI, MD
Department of Radiology, David Geffen School of Medicine at UCLA, Los Angeles, California

ANDREW D. SMITH, MD, PhD
Department of Radiology, The University of Alabama at Birmingham, Birmingham, Alabama

ERIK V. SOLOFF, MD
Assistant Professor, Radiology Department, University of Washington, Seattle, Washington

BARIS TURKBEY, MD
Molecular Imaging Program, National Cancer Institute, National Institutes of Health, Bethesda, Maryland

CRISTIÁN VARELA UBILLA, MD
Chief of Body Imaging, Radiology Department, Santiago, Chile

MONA VAKIL, MD
Assistant Professor, Division of Emergency and Trauma Imaging, Department of Radiology and Imaging Sciences, Emory School of Medicine, Emory University, Atlanta, Georgia

STEPHANIE M. WALKER, BS
Molecular Imaging Program, National Cancer Institute, National Institutes of Health, Bethesda, Maryland

CAROLYN L. WANG, MD
Associate Professor, Radiology Department, University of Washington, Seattle, Washington

ZHEN J. WANG, MD
Department of Radiology and Biomedical Imaging, University of California, San Francisco, San Francisco, California

MARIA ZULFIQAR, MD
Assistant Professor of Radiology, Mallinckrodt Institute of Radiology, Washington University School of Medicine, St Louis, Missouri

Contents

> Moderate and severe contrast reactions are rare but can be life threatening. Appropriate contrast reaction management is necessary for the best patient outcome. This review summarizes the types and incidences of adverse events to contrast media, treatment algorithms, and equipment needed to treat common contrast reactions, the current status of contrast reaction management training, and preventative strategies to help mitigate adverse contrast events.

> Renal masses increasingly are found incidentally, largely due to the frequent use of medical imaging. Computed tomography (CT) and MR imaging are mainstays for renal mass characterization, presurgical planning of renal tumors, and surveillance after surgery or systemic therapy for advanced renal cell carcinomas. CT protocols should be tailored to different clinical indications, balancing diagnostic accuracy and radiation exposure. MR imaging protocols should take advantage of the improved soft tissue contrast for renal tumor diagnosis and staging. Optimized imaging protocols enable analysis of imaging features that help narrow the differential diagnoses and guide management in patients with renal masses.

> Indeterminate renal masses remain a diagnostic challenge for lesions not initially characterized as angiomyolipoma or Bosniak I/II cysts. Differential for indeterminate renal masses include oncocytoma, fat-poor angiomyolipoma, and clear cell, papillary, and chromophobe renal cell carcinoma. Qualitative and quantitative techniques using data derived from multiphase contrast-enhanced imaging have provided methods for specific differentiation and subtyping of indeterminate renal masses, with emerging applications such as radiocytogenetics. Early and accurate characterization of indeterminate renal masses by multiphase contrast-enhanced imaging will optimize triage of these lesions into surgical, ablative, and active surveillance treatment plans.

> There are several potential pitfalls that radiologists face when interpreting images of the kidneys. Some result from image acquisition and can arise from the imaging equipment or imaging technique, whereas others are patient related. Another category of pitfalls relates to image interpretation. Some difficulties stem from methods to detect enhancement after contrast administration, whereas others are benign

entities that can mimic a renal tumor. Finally, interpretation and diagnosis of fat-containing renal masses may be tricky due to the complexities discerning the pattern of fat within a mass and how that translates to an accurate diagnosis.

Most renal masses are benign cysts; a subset are malignant. Most renal masses are incidental findings. Evaluation of renal cysts has evolved with updates to the Bosniak classification system and other guidelines. The Bosniak classification provides detailed definitions and extends the system from computed tomography to MR imaging. This article provides a simple approach to the evaluation of cystic or potentially cystic renal masses. The radiologist is central to this process. Key elements include confirming that a renal lesion is cystic and not solid, determining the need for further characterization by imaging, and judicious application of the Bosniak classification system.

Acute pyelonephritis is a bacterial infection of the renal parenchyma and collecting system. Diagnosis is based on clinical findings of fever, flank pain, and urinary tract infection. Computed tomography findings include renal enlargement with wedge-shaped heterogeneous areas of decreased enhancement, known as a "striated nephrogram." Imaging is primarily used to diagnose complications such as emphysematous pyelonephritis, renal abscess, and pyonephrosis. Chronic pyelonephritis can have varying appearances on imaging ranging from xanthogranulomatous pyelonephritis or, in extreme cases, renal replacement lipomatosis.

Given the incidence of small renal masses, from benign cysts to malignancy, most radiologists encounter these lesions multiple times during their career. Radiologists have an opportunity to provide critical data that will further refine the understanding of the impact of these masses on patient outcomes. This article summarizes and describes recent updates and understanding of the critical observations and descriptors of renal masses. The templates and glossary of terms presented in this review article facilitate the radiology reporting of such data elements, giving radiologists the opportunity to improve diagnostic accuracy and influence management of small renal masses.

An introduction to the expanding modality of contrast-enhanced ultrasound is provided, along with basics on contrast agents and technique. The contrast ultrasound findings of multiple renal tumors are reviewed with examples, including clear cell renal cell carcinoma, papillary renal cell carcinoma, chromophobe renal cell carcinoma, other rare renal cell carcinoma subtypes, oncocytoma, upper tract urothelial carcinoma, lymphoma, and angiomyolipoma, followed also by brief discussions of renal infections and pseudolesions.

Up to 8% of renal cancers are thought to have a hereditary component. Several hereditary renal cancer syndromes have been identified over the last few decades. It is important for the radiologist to be aware of findings associated with hereditary renal cancer syndromes to detect tumors early, enroll patients in appropriate surveillance programs, and improve outcomes for the patient and affected family members. This review discusses from a radiologist's perspective well-known hereditary renal cancer syndromes and emerging genetic mutations associated with renal cancer that are less well characterized, focusing on imaging features and known associations.

Blunt trauma accounts for more than 95% of traumatic renal injury and results from shear forces from rapid acceleration or deceleration and/or collision against the spine or ribs. The use of multiphasic contrast-enhanced computed tomography (CT) has proven pivotal in the evaluation and management of traumatic kidney injury, and CT imaging features provide the basis for nonsurgical staging. This article describes the epidemiology and mechanisms of blunt and penetrating traumatic renal injury and reviews the range of findings from various imaging modalities, with a particular emphasis on contrast-enhanced CT.

Based on Surveillance, Epidemiology, and End Results studies, most renal cancers are low grade and slow growing. Long-term, single-center studies show excellent outcomes of percutaneous thermal ablation for T1a renal cell carcinoma (RCC), comparable to partial nephrectomy without affecting renal function and with much lower rates of complications. However, there are no multicenter randomized controlled trials of multiple ablative modalities or comparison with partial nephrectomy, and most studies are single-arm observational studies with short-term and intermediate follow-up. For treatment of stage T1a RCC, percutaneous TA is an effective alternative to surgery with preservation of renal function, low risk, and comparable overall and disease-specific survival.

Radiomics allows for high throughput extraction of quantitative data from images. This is an area of active research as groups try to capture and quantify imaging parameters and convert these into descriptive phenotypes of organs or tumors. Texture analysis is one radiomics tool that extracts information about heterogeneity within a given region of interest. This is used with or without associated machine learning classifiers or a deep learning approach is applied to similar types of data. These tools have shown utility in characterizing renal masses, renal cell carcinoma, and assessing response to targeted therapeutic agents in metastatic renal cell carcinoma.

PROGRAM OBJECTIVE

The objective of the *Radiologic Clinics of North America* is to keep practicing radiologists and radiology residents up to date with current clinical practice in radiology by providing timely articles reviewing the state of the art in patient care.

TARGET AUDIENCE

Practicing radiologists, radiology residents, and other healthcare professionals who provide patient care utilizing radiologic findings.

LEARNING OBJECTIVES

Upon completion of this activity, participants will be able to:

1. Describe the current state of the art in renal imaging with a focus on renal mass imaging and intervention, including a comprehensive review of traditional topics covering CT, MRI and US imaging as well as contrast reactions and imaging pitfalls.
2. Discuss the optimization and standardization of protocols, interpretation and reporting across radiologic practices.
3. Recognize practice changes both in imaging diagnosis and treatment, as well as technologic developments and clinical management paradigms.

ACCREDITATION

The Elsevier Office of Continuing Medical Education (EOCME) is accredited by the Accreditation Council for Continuing Medical Education (ACCME) to provide continuing medical education for physicians.

The EOCME designates this journal-based CME activity for a maximum of 12 *AMA PRA Category 1 Credit*(s)™. Physicians should claim only the credit commensurate with the extent of their participation in the activity.

All other healthcare professionals requesting continuing education credit for this enduring material will be issued a certificate of participation.

DISCLOSURE OF CONFLICTS OF INTEREST

The EOCME assesses conflict of interest with its instructors, faculty, planners, and other individuals who are in a position to control the content of CME activities. All relevant conflicts of interest that are identified are thoroughly vetted by EOCME for fair balance, scientific objectivity, and patient care recommendations. EOCME is committed to providing its learners with CME activities that promote improvements or quality in healthcare and not a specific proprietary business or a commercial interest.

The planning committee, staff, authors and editors listed below have identified no financial relationships or relationships to products or devices they or their spouse/life partner have with commercial interest related to the content of this CME activity:

Asser Abou Elkassem, MD; Evan Allgood, MD; Krystal Archer-Arroyo, MD; Patricia Balthazar, MD; Ling-Chen Chien, MD; Peter L. Choyke, MD; Jason S. Chu, MD; Steven C. Eberhardt, MD; Rabindra Gautam; Tarek N. Hanna, MD; Marta E. Heilbrun, MD; Keith D. Herr, MD; Hena Joshi, MD; Marilu Kelly, MSN, RN, CNE, CHCP; Kevin G. King, MD; Pradeep Kuttysankaran; Ashkan Malayeri, MD; Christine O. Menias, MD; Refky Nicola, MS, DO; Steven S. Raman, MD; Erick M. Remer, MD, FACR, FSAR; Sepideh Shakeri, MD; Andrew D. Smith, MD, PhD; Erik V. Soloff, MD; Baris Turkbey, MD; Cristián Varela Ubilla, MD; Mona Vakil, MD; John Vassallo; Stephanie M. Walker, BS; Carolyn L. Wang, MD; Maria Zulfiqar, MD.

The planning committee, staff, authors and editors listed below have identified financial relationships or relationships to products or devices they or their spouse/life partner have with commercial interest related to the content of this CME activity:

Meghan G. Lubner, MD: received research support from Ethicon and Koninklijke Philips N.V.; spouse is a consultant/advisor for Farcast Biosciences.

Zhen J. Wang, MD: consultant/advisor for General Electric Company and owns stock in Nextrast, Inc.

UNAPPROVED/OFF-LABEL USE DISCLOSURE

The EOCME requires CME faculty to disclose to the participants:

1. When products or procedures being discussed are off-label, unlabelled, experimental, and/or investigational (not US Food and Drug Administration [FDA] approved); and
2. Any limitations on the information presented, such as data that are preliminary or that represent ongoing research, interim analyses, and/or unsupported opinions. Faculty may discuss information about pharmaceutical agents that is outside of FDA-approved labelling. This information is intended solely for CME and is not intended to promote off-label use of these medications. If you have any questions, contact the medical affairs department of the manufacturer for the most recent prescribing information.

TO ENROLL

To enroll in the *Radiologic Clinics of North America* Continuing Medical Education program, call customer service at 1-800-654-2452 or sign up online at http://www.theclinics.com/home/cme. The CME program is available to subscribers for an additional annual fee of USD 330.00.

METHOD OF PARTICIPATION

In order to claim credit, participants must complete the following:
1. Complete enrolment as indicated above.
2. Read the activity.
3. Complete the CME Test and Evaluation. Participants must achieve a score of 70% on the test. All CME Tests and Evaluations must be completed online.

CME INQUIRIES/SPECIAL NEEDS

For all CME inquiries or special needs, please contact elsevierCME@elsevier.com.

RADIOLOGIC CLINICS OF NORTH AMERICA

RELATED SERIES

Advances in Clinical Radiology
www.advancesinclinicalradiology.com
MRI Clinics
www.mri.theclinics.com
Neuroimaging Clinics
www.neuroimaging.theclinics.com
PET Clinics
www.pet.theclinics.com

THE CLINICS ARE AVAILABLE ONLINE!
Access your subscription at:
www.theclinics.com

Preface
Contemporary Renal Imaging

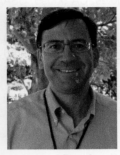   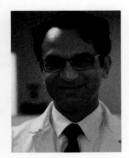

Steven C. Eberhardt, MD   Steven S. Raman, MD

Editors

This issue of *Radiologic Clinics of North America* provides a timely and practical state-of-the-art update on imaging the kidneys for the practicing radiologist. Changes in this area have occurred at a rapid pace in imaging diagnosis and treatment as well as in technologic developments and clinical management paradigms. Ongoing advances in imaging have introduced new challenges, including the optimization and standardization of protocols, interpretation, and reporting across radiologic practices. In this issue, authors provide a broad and in-depth summary of the current state-of-the-art in renal imaging with a focus on renal mass imaging and intervention by some of the leading authorities in the field today. The articles are designed as a practical and fairly comprehensive review of traditional topics covering computed tomography (CT), MR imaging, and US imaging as well as contrast reactions and imaging pitfalls. There is also an article on protocol optimization for comprehensive renal evaluation by indication and an article on renal mass reporting. Another article provides an update on solid renal mass characterization on CT and MR imaging, and one article covers renal mass biopsy and ablation. For a look into the future, additional articles focus on advances in radiomics and artificial intelligence for renal mass characterization, and a practical update on hereditary renal cell carcinoma and imaging implications. Finally, additional articles are included addressing the role of imaging in surveillance of low-risk renal masses, new thoughts on cystic renal masses, postoperative and postprocedural imaging, and imaging the kidneys in the setting of trauma.

All of the articles are designed to be highly practical in nature, focusing on that which is most relevant to radiologists' daily imaging activities. It is hoped that the reader will be able to apply insights from these articles to enhance their practice and ultimately benefit patient care.

We are delighted to have been provided the opportunity to serve as editors for this issue and extend our appreciation to Dr Frank Miller, Consulting Editor of *Radiologic Clinics of North America*, for considering us for this role. We would also like to thank the many contributing authors, without whom this work would not be possible. We are also grateful for the outstanding assistance from Donald Mumford, Developmental Editor for this issue, and John Vassallo, Associate Publisher, as well as the remainder of the Elsevier staff. We also acknowledge our colleagues, collaborators, and mentors at UCLA and the University of New

Radiol Clin N Am 58 (2020) xi–xii
https://doi.org/10.1016/j.rcl.2020.07.001
0033-8389/20/© 2020 Published by Elsevier Inc.

Mexico and our families for their continual encouragement and support.

Steven C. Eberhardt, MD
Department of Radiology
University of New Mexico
MSC10 5530, 1 University of New Mexico
Albuquerque, NM 87131, USA

Steven S. Raman, MD
Department of Radiology
UCLA Medical Center
757 Westwood Plaza, Suite 1621
Los Angeles, CA 90095, USA

E-mail addresses:
seberhardt@salud.unm.edu (S.C. Eberhardt)
SRaman@mednet.ucla.edu (S.S. Raman)

Contrast Reaction Readiness for Your Department or Facility

Carolyn L. Wang, MD*, Erik V. Soloff, MD

KEYWORDS

- Contrast reaction management • Iodinated contrast media • Gadolinium-based contrast agents
- High-fidelity simulation • Hypersensitivity reactions • Contrast extravasation
- Allergic-like reactions to contrast media

KEY POINTS

- Moderate and severe hypersensitivity reactions to iodinated contrast media and gadolinium-based contrast agents are rare but can be life threatening.
- Frequent training augmenting didactic lectures with hands-on or computer-based simulation, or educational online modules can improve knowledge and comfort at managing contrast reactions.
- Epinephrine administration errors are common and may be reduced by having autoinjectors available. However, frequent hands-on training is still required to ensure appropriate use.
- Treatment algorithms, visual aids, and safety checklists should be posted throughout radiology departments to improve team comfort at managing reactions and reduce errors.
- Appropriate screening may reduce the risk for hypersensitivity reactions and extravasations, although break-through reactions may still occur, usually of similar severity.

INTRODUCTION

Radiographic contrast agents, such as iodinated contrast media (ICM) and gadolinium-based contrast agents (GBCA), are useful for evaluating organs and identifying pathologic conditions. Their utilization has rapidly increased in the past few decades with approximately 48 million contrast-enhanced computed tomographic scans (CTs) and 17 million contrast-enhanced MR images performed annually in the United States.[1–3] However, adverse events, such as hypersensitivity reactions and extravasations can occur, and the radiology department's readiness to appropriately manage these will affect the patient's outcome.[4] The rarity of moderate and severe reactions results in few radiologists having first-hand experience at managing reactions.[5] Published survey data suggest that radiologists have knowledge gaps in appropriate contrast reaction management, particularly anaphylaxis.[6–8] Bartlett and Bynevelt[7] found that 57% of their respondents either did not know or gave incorrect dosing for the administration of epinephrine, which was more likely overdose (66%) versus underdose (33%). More recently, Nandwana and colleagues[9] surveyed radiology attendings, residents, fellows, and nurses, and only 29% of respondents correctly answered the rate, dose, and route of epinephrine administration for anaphylaxis. Several recent studies have used hands-on simulation contrast reaction scenarios as a surrogate to evaluate the incidence of treatment errors and have confirmed a high rate of management errors.[10–12] This review summarizes the types and incidence of adverse events to

Radiology Department, University of Washington, Box 357115, 1959 Northeast Pacific Street, Seattle, WA 98195, USA
* Corresponding author.
E-mail address: wangcl@uw.edu
Twitter: @CarolynLWang (C.L.W.)

Radiol Clin N Am 58 (2020) 841–850
https://doi.org/10.1016/j.rcl.2020.04.002
0033-8389/20/© 2020 Elsevier Inc. All rights reserved.

contrast media, treatment algorithms, and equipment needed to treat common contrast reactions, the current status of contrast reaction management training, and preventative strategies to help mitigate adverse contrast events. The scope of this review is limited to adult patients.

REVIEW OF THE TYPES AND INCIDENCE OF ADVERSE EVENTS
Hypersensitivity Reactions

The incidence of hypersensitivity, including both allergic and allergic-like reactions to low osmolar (LOCM) and iso-osmolar (IOCM) ICM, ranges from 0.2% to 0.6%: 0.4% to 0.5% mild, 0.04% to 0.1% moderate, 0.006% to 0.01% severe.[4,13,14] Death is extremely rare and estimated to be approximately 0.0006%.[14] The incidence of reactions is lower with GBCAs and estimated to be 0.08% to 0.2%: 0.02% to 0.1% mild, 0.01% to 0.02% moderate, and 0.006% to 0.0007% severe.[13,15,16] The mortality owing to GBCA reported to the Food and Drug Administration was 0.00008% between 2004 and 2009.[17] Some data suggest that the risk of adverse events is higher in ionic linear agents than in nonionic linear GBCA agents.[16,18]

Hypersensitivity reactions are now classified into acute and nonacute/delayed reactions. The acute or immediate reactions occur within 1 hour after contrast administration, and many are caused by mast cell activation that may or may not be caused by immunoglobulin E mechanisms, explaining why the term allergic-like reactions was previously used.[19,20] These reactions range from mild hives to anaphylaxis and are classified by their severity and morbidity by the American College of Radiology (ACR), as seen in **Table 1**.[21]

Delayed reactions are defined as reactions starting more than 1 hour after contrast administration but typically occurring more than 3 hours to 2 to 5 days after exposure and are suspected to be related to T-cell–mediated hypersensitivity.[19] These delayed reactions usually manifest as macular or maculopapular exanthema but rarely can be associated with more severe skin conditions, such as toxic epidermal necrolysis or Stevens-Johnson syndrome.[20] The exact incidence of delayed reactions is difficult to determine likely because of underreporting, but is estimated to be 0.5% to 9%.[22] Loh and colleagues[23] showed the most common delayed adverse reactions were cutaneous, such as rash, itching, skin redness, and swelling. Overall delayed reactions are commonly self-limited.

Extravasation

Contrast extravasation is another recognized adverse event related to contrast media injection and is rarely serious, although it can result in severe skin ulcerations, tissue necrosis, and compartment syndrome.[24–27] A recent systematic review of MR and CT contrast media

Table 1
Different types and severity of hypersensitivity reactions adapted from the American College of Radiology Contrast Manual

Mild	Moderate	Severe
Self-limited and no evidence of progression; treatment usually not necessary; no vital sign alterations	Symptoms may require medical treatment; however no significant vital sign alterations	Symptoms may be life threatening and require treatment to avoid morbidity or death; vital signs are abnormal
Limited hives	Diffuse hives	Diffuse hives with hypotension
Limited itchiness	Diffuse itchiness or erythema, stable vital signs	Diffuse itchiness and or erythema with hypotension
Cutaneous edema	Facial edema but no dyspnea	Diffuse edema including facial with dyspnea
Limited itchy/scratchy throat or eyes	Wheezing but no hypoxia	Wheezing with hypoxia
Nasal congestion/runny nose	Throat tightness but no dyspnea	Laryngeal edema with stridor and or hypoxia
		Anaphylactic shock (hypotension + tachycardia)

Adapted Table 1 from the 2019 Contrast Manual (categories of acute reactons); adapted information from the chapter entitled 'PATIENT SELECTION AND PREPARATION STRATEGIES BEFORE CONTRAST MEDIUM ADMINISTRATION' for the specific recommendations for premedication regimens; Adapted information from Table 4 ("EQUIPMENT FOR CONTRAST REACTION KITS IN RADIOLOGY'); with permission.

extravasations found 17 papers that reported 2191 extravasations out of 1,104,872 patients (0.2%) with a rate of 0.26% for ICM and 0.045% for GBCA.[28] The rate of extravasations is lower with gadolinium likely related to the lower volumes, lower rates of injection, and increased frequency of hand injection.

MANAGEMENT OF ADVERSE EVENTS
Acute Hypersensitivity

Appropriate management for contrast reactions varies based on the type of reaction. As a result, it is vital to have an emergency cart stocked with various supplies and medications as well as appropriate training of staff to be able to manage reactions. The management of contrast reactions is not unique to the use of iodinated contrast, and the treatment is the same, regardless of the inciting factor. Although vasovagal reactions are considered a physiologic reaction and not allergic-like hypersensitivity reaction, it is included in the treatment flowchart for completeness. It is generally considered best practice to preserve intravenous (IV) access and monitor vital signs, including pulse oximetry for all reactions, including mild reactions. **Fig. 1** provides a flowchart for managing bronchospasm versus laryngeal edema, and **Fig. 2** provides a flowchart for managing vasovagal versus anaphylaxis.

- Hives/urticaria, itchiness, or diffuse erythema
  - Mild scattered or transient hives or erythema usually does not require treatment; however, vital signs should be monitored, and IV access preserved.
  - If the hives worsen or become more numerous/widespread or bothersome, treatment with diphenhydramine 25 to 50 mg orally or fexofenadine 180 mg orally (less sedating) could be considered.
  - If the hives or diffuse erythema are accompanied by hypotension:
    - Give IV fluids normal saline 1 L bolus
    - Elevate legs ≥60°
    - Give oxygen by face mask (at least 6–10 L/min)
    - Give epinephrine (**Table 2**)
- Bronchospasm
  - Oxygen by mask, at least 6 to 10 L/min
  - Beta2 agonist inhaler 2 puffs (90 μg/puff) and can repeat up to 3 times total

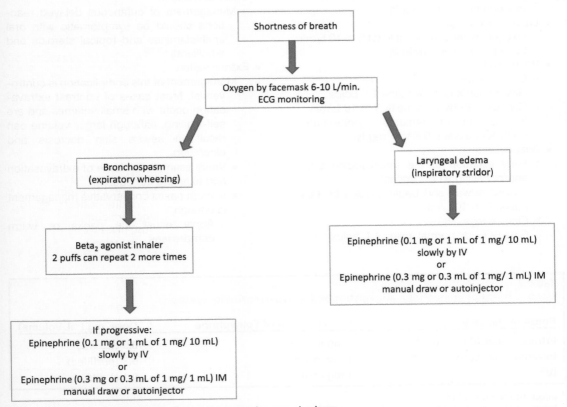

Fig. 1. The management of bronchospasm versus laryngeal edema.

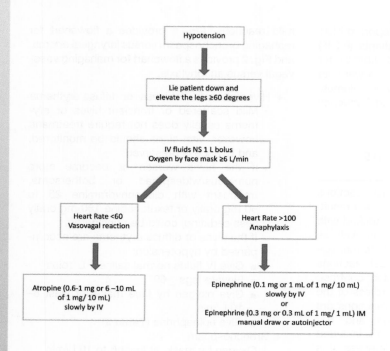

Fig. 2. The management of hypotension related to vasovagal versus anaphylaxis.

- In severe cases or if the bronchospasm is progressive or unresponsive to the inhaler, epinephrine (see **Table 2**)
- Laryngeal edema
  - Oxygen by face mask, at least 6 to 10 L/min
  - Epinephrine (see **Table 2**)
- Vasovagal
  - Elevate legs ≥60°
  - Give IV fluids normal saline 1 L bolus
  - Give oxygen by face mask 6 to 10 L/min
  - If the patient remains symptomatic, consider atropine 0.6 to 1 mg IV
- Anaphylaxis
  - Early initiation of the resuscitation team and/or calling 911 is critical
  - Assess airway and begin oxygen by face mask, 6 to 10 L/min
  - Elevate legs ≥60°
  - Give IV fluids normal saline 1 L bolus

- Give epinephrine (see **Table 2**)
- Delayed reaction
  Management of cutaneous delayed reactions should be symptomatic with oral antihistamines and topical steroids and emollients.[29,30]
- Extravasation
  Management of this complication is controversial. Most cases of contrast extravasation occur with small volumes and are self-limiting, although larger volume can result in severe skin necrosis and ulceration.
- Verify estimated volume of extravasation and examine the patient.
- In most cases conservative management is enough.
  - Apply either ice packs or warm compresses

Table 2
Various forms of epinephrine administration for hypersensitivity reactions

Route of Delivery	Concentration of Epinephrine	Dose, mg (mL Volume)
Intramuscular (IM) manual[a]	1 mg in 1 mL	0.3 (0.3 mL)
Intramuscular autoinjector[a]	1 mg in 1 mL	0.3 (prefilled)
IV[b]	1 mg in 10 mL	0.1 (1 mL)

[a] Inject into the lateral thigh.
[b] Inject slowly into an IV line with fluids running or followed by a slow flush.

- ○ Elevate the limb
- ○ Check pulses and sensory function for neurovascular compromise
- ○ Monitor patient vital signs as well as site of extravasation
- ○ Can mark skin to determine size of involvement
  - If symptoms worsen, consult a surgeon if concerned about compartment syndrome.

REQUIRED EQUIPMENT

Table 3 summarizes the suggested medications and supplies needed for managing contrast reactions. Please refer to your own radiology department's contrast management policy for the minimum equipment and medications required because these may vary depending on institutional policies and practices.

CONTRAST REACTION MANAGEMENT TRAINING

Although moderate and severe hypersensitivity reactions are rare, usually the first and potentially only responders are the radiologists and the radiology staff. Questionnaire surveys and hands-on simulation testing have demonstrated that contrast reaction management knowledge gaps exist for radiologists, radiology nurses, and technologists.[5,9,31] Trainees and radiologists in practice for less than 5 years or more than 15 years appear to benefit the most from contrast reaction management training.[32] At many academic centers, the first responders are radiology residents.[33] Several survey studies demonstrate that traditional annual didactic lecture remains the preferred format for contrast reaction management training at most US radiology residencies.[33–35] Studies have shown that online educational modules for contrast reaction management can improve knowledge and comfort at managing reactions with short-term knowledge assessment.[5,36] High-fidelity simulation training has been shown to be superior to didactic lecture alone.[37] Multiple studies have shown the value of high-fidelity simulation training for such high-acuity low-frequency scenarios at improving not only knowledge but also comfort at managing contrast reactions.[32,38,39] Ali and colleagues[40]

Table 3
Equipment and medications needed for contrast reaction management

Medications	Supplies	Advanced Life-Support Supplies[a]
Epinephrine 1 mg in 1 mL vial (for IM injections)	Needles and syringes (eg, 1 mL needle for IM administration of epinephrine with 20-G needle)	Automatic external defibrillator
Epinephrine 1 mg in 10 mL box (for IV administration)[b]	Face mask/oxygen	Oral and or nasal airways
Epinephrine autoinjectors IM (0.1 mg for infants; 0.15 mg for children; 0.3 mg for adults)[c]	Stethoscope	Suction tubing and catheters
Atropine 1 mg in 10 mL box (for IV administration)	Pulse oximetry	Protective barriers for mouth to mouth and or bag-valve-mask device
1 L normal saline IV fluid bags	Sphygmomanometer	
Beta-2 agonist inhaler	IV catheters	
H_1 antihistamine (oral or IV)		

[a] These items will likely be found on code/crash carts in hospital settings and may exceed the required equipment for limited outpatient imaging facilities.
[b] Epinephrine 1 mg in 10 mL is typically in code/crash carts in hospital settings.
[c] Epinephrine autoinjectors may not be stocked because of the high cost associated compared with manual IM epinephrine.
Adapted Table 1 from the 2019 Contrast Manual (categories of acute reactons); adapted information from the chapter entitled 'PATIENT SELECTION AND PREPARATION STRATEGIES BEFORE CONTRAST MEDIUM ADMINISTRATION' for the specific recommendations for premedication regimens; Adapted information from Table 4 ("EQUIPMENT FOR CONTRAST REACTION KITS IN RADIOLOGY'); with permission.

also expanded the hands-on simulation training to include other less common events, such as seizures, hypocalcemia, and panic attacks.

Hands-on simulation training continues to be used less commonly than didactic lecture, although the percentage of programs surveyed that use it appears to be increasing in the literature: 18% in 2010, 30% in 2013, and 37.8% in 2015.[33–35] Cost has been reported to be a limiting factor, and 1 study estimated to be around $256.76 per resident for the first year and $203.46 for each subsequent year of hands-on simulation training compared with less than $5 for didactic lecture.[41] They also noted the differences in nonmonetary costs as well, such as faculty time and effort developing and administering the program as well as trainee time away from clinical duties to participate in the course. Other published self-reported barriers to hands-on simulation training include insufficient availability, no trained faculty, and time constraints.[35] The timing and frequency of training are important because studies have shown a decline in both confidence and knowledge of managing contrast reactions by 6 to 9 months, suggesting that a 6-month refresher should be considered.[32,42] It may be more cost-effective to supplement hands-on simulation training with either traditional in-person didactic lecture, online education modules, or computer-based simulation.

It is important to train not only radiologists but also radiology nurses and technologists who are also key members of the response team. Effective teamwork and interprofessional communication are critical to ensure patient safety. High-fidelity and computer-based simulation has been shown to be useful for training interprofessional teams of radiologists, technologists, and nurses for both contrast reaction management and team communication skills as tested with a high-fidelity simulation scenario, although a single session appeared inadequate for mastery of such complex teamwork skills, suggesting refreshers are necessary.[31]

Although training is critical, it is important to have treatment algorithms posted throughout the radiology department so that no one is relying on their memories during these high-stress situations. Gardner and colleagues[12] demonstrated that fewer errors in management were committed by groups of participants who had a visual aid flowchart than those who did not during a high-fidelity severe contrast reaction scenario. Safety checklists, which are critical in the airline industry, have also been shown to be an effective tool at reducing treatment errors during testing with a high-fidelity severe contrast reaction simulation scenario.[43] These types of visual aids and checklists should be included in any contrast reaction kit box or code cart found in the radiology suites to use as reference during reaction management. It is imperative that the treating members, including radiologists, technologists, and nurses, have familiarity with and working knowledge of the checklists and visual aids to be able to use them most effectively.

Several studies have demonstrated that the most common errors made during high-fidelity simulation training and testing of severe contrast reactions are related to the concentration, dose, route, and administration of epinephrine.[10–12] Masch and colleagues[44] demonstrated that not having IV access resulted in faster time to medication delivery of epinephrine; however, similar rates of errors of administration still occurred, most commonly administering the intramuscular autoinjector for less than 5 seconds resulting in inadequate dosing. An additional 5 participants autoinjected their thumbs instead of the patient. Asch and colleagues[45] demonstrated fewer errors in epinephrine administration when an autoinjector was used rather than drawing up and administering intramuscular epinephrine. The most common error was the wrong dose of epinephrine followed by attempting to administer the intramuscular concentration (epinephrine 1 mg in 1 mL) intravenously. No errors occurred in the autoinjector group, and the difference between this study and the study by Masch may have been the type of autoinjector used in the simulation scenario: the Auvi-Q (Kaleo, Richmond, VA) versus EpiPen (Mylan, Canonsburg, PA).[44,45] Both experienced and inexperienced caregivers have demonstrated a preference for the Auvi-Q (Kaleo, Richmond, VA) likely because the injector verbalizes instructions, which minimizes potential errors.[46] Having epinephrine autoinjectors stocked in radiology suites may improve patient safety by quicker delivery of the medication as well as reduction in epinephrine administration errors. However, there is a financial consideration because the autoinjectors are approximately 100 times more expensive than the manual device, and only have approximately a 1-year shelf life. Also, the autoinjectors require adequate training to avoid misadministration.[45]

PREVENTION OF HYPERSENSITIVITY REACTIONS
Screening

Identifying which patients will benefit the most from IV contrast administration includes understanding the clinical question to be answered and determining the best imaging test. For most patients, IV contrast is well tolerated, and no special precautions need to be taken. Certain subsets of patients need further consideration and require screening before contrast media administration, particularly those with a history of prior adverse reaction to contrast media.[21] Additional considerations, such as risk of nephrotoxicity, lactic acidosis, nephrogenic systemic fibrosis, or gadolinium deposition, are beyond the scope of this article. Patients with a prior history of severe allergy to the same type of contrast agent have an overall 5- to 6-fold increased risk for a subsequent reaction.[3]

Historically, patients with seafood allergies were thought to have greater risk of reaction to ICM. A systematic review of the literature shows that patients with seafood allergies had similar rates of reactions as patients with allergies to other substances.[47] Iodine cannot be an allergen because it is found throughout our bodies in thyroid hormones and amino acids. Tropomyosins are the major allergen for most patients with seafood allergies.[47] Patients who are allergic to povidone iodine skin preparation react to other allergens in the solution, not the iodine. In addition, this type of reaction is a contact dermatitis rather than a hypersensitivity reaction.[48] Therefore, there is no need to screen patients for seafood allergies or povidone iodine skin preparation allergies, and it is important to clarify when patients report an "iodine allergy" if it is to ICM.

Patients with a history of asthma have a modest increased risk of hypersensitivity reactions; however, well-controlled asthmatics do not appear to be at increased risk for adverse reactions.[49] Patients who have a prior history of reaction to ICM are at no increased risk for GBCAs because they are chemically distinct contrast agents without any known cross-reactivity.[13,50] In general, patients who have unrelated medication or food allergies have a modest 2- to 3-fold increased risk over the general population, but the ACR does not recommend restricting contrast media use and does not consider it alone as an indication for premedication.[21]

Premedication

The greatest risk factor for a hypersensitivity reaction is a prior hypersensitivity reaction to the same type of contrast media. Physiologic reactions, including flushing, metallic taste, nausea, vomiting, and vasovagal reactions, are not hypersensitivity reactions and therefore do not require premedication. Premedication with corticosteroids before contrast administration has been shown to be effective at reducing mild hypersensitivity reactions in average-risk patients to low-osmolality ICM, but no case-controlled studies

have shown efficacy at reducing risk in high-risk patients or for moderate and severe hypersensitivity reactions.[48,51–53] A systematic review of the literature for studies that randomized pretreatment against placebo or no treatment before patient receiving ICM suggests that H_1 antihistamines mainly showed efficacy against cutaneous reactions, while corticosteroids prevent respiratory symptoms; however, no case-controlled study tested the combination of the 2 in high-risk patients.[54] No studies to the authors' knowledge have been published evaluating the efficacy of premedication for oral ICM or GBCAs, and the benefits are extrapolated from the ICM literature.

Although the practice of prophylaxis premedication in high-risk patients is commonly considered the standard of care in the United States, it is not performed in other countries because of the lack of level 1 evidence that it reduces the reaction risk in high-risk patients or the incidence of moderate or severe reactions to LOCM, IOCM, or GBCA.[55] There are also minimal direct risks to premedication, including asymptomatic hyperglycemia and transient leukocytosis.[56–58]

Premedication does not prevent all future reactions, because breakthrough reactions do occur at reported rates between 1.2% and 3.4% for IOCM and or LOCM.[16,59] Breakthrough reactions may partially depend on the indication for the premedication as Mervak and colleagues[59] found a rate of 2.1% for those patients with had a prior contrast reaction compared with 0% for those premedicated for other indications. These ICM breakthrough reactions tend to be of the same severity of as the index reactions, and patients with a mild index reaction are at very low risk of developing a severe breakthrough reaction.[59–61] Breakthrough reactions have also been seen with GBCA, and in 1 study, 56% were of similar severity; however, 33% were more severe than the index reaction.[62] Repeat breakthrough reactions to ICM also occur at a reported rate of 12% and are usually of the same severity.[59] Therefore, it may be more prudent to avoid repeat exposure to contrast media for severe contrast reactions given the higher likelihood of a severe breakthrough reaction rather than rely on corticosteroid premedication.[55] The estimated number of patients needed to treat to prevent 1 severe reaction in patients with a prior reaction is 569 and to prevent 1 lethal reaction is 56,900.[59] In addition, in the in-patient setting, the orally premedicated patients had longer hospital stays and more hospital infections than those not premedicated.[63]

Two common oral premedication regimens and 1 shortened IV premedication regimen are listed in **Box 1**.[51–53,64] Data suggest that a less than 2-hour

---

Box 1
Three possible premedication regimens

- Prednisone 50 mg by mouth 13 hours, 7 hours, and 1 hour plus optional diphenhydramine 50 mg by mouth 1 hour before contrast administration

- Methylprednisolone 32 mg by mouth 12 hours and 2 hours plus optional diphenhydramine 50 mg by mouth 1 hour before contrast administration

- Hydrocortisone 200 mg IV 5 hours and 1 hour plus diphenhydramine 50 mg IV 1 hour before contrast administration

Data from Refs.[51,53,65]

---

oral regimen is not effective compared with placebo.[51] A 5-hour IV premedication regimen was found to be noninferior to a 13-hour oral regimen and could be considered for patients in whom timely diagnosis and treatment are critical, such as the inpatient or emergency room setting.[65]

PREVENTION OF CONTRAST EXTRAVASATION

Warming contrast has been shown to decrease the rate of extravasation for the more viscous iopamidol 370 than iopamidol (Bracco, Milan, Italy) 300.[66] Risk factors for extravasation include older age, female gender, using an existing cannula, using a site other than the antecubital fossa, and using a power injector with a high-injector rate.[28] Using the largest vein available may also reduce the risk of extravasation, such as the larger veins in the antecubital fossa rather than the hands.[67] Other risk mitigating techniques, such as starting a new IV line and avoiding the use of high-injection rate with a power injector, in higher at-risk populations, including elderly women, could also be considered.[28]

SUMMARY

Moderate and severe contrast reactions are rare but can be life threatening. Appropriate contrast reaction management is necessary for the best patient outcome. Radiologists, radiology nurses, and technologists have knowledge gaps on how to manage contrast reactions, which can be closed with appropriate and frequent training that augments traditional didactic lecture with more hands-on or computer-based simulations or online educational modules. Visual aids, treatment algorithm flowcharts, and safety checklists should be posted throughout the radiology suites to help reduce management errors and increase the teams' comfort at

managing these rare events. Errors in epinephrine administration may also be reduced by having epinephrine autoinjectors available in radiology suites, although hands-on and frequent training is advisable, and high cost may hinder adoption. Appropriate screening can be used to reduce the risk for hypersensitivity reactions and extravasations. Corticosteroid prophylaxis is frequently used in the United States to prevent hypersensitivity reactions to ICM and GBCAs in high-risk patients with prior contrast reactions, although breakthrough reactions still occur, usually of similar severity to the index reaction.

DISCLOSURE

The authors have nothing to disclose.

REFERENCES

1. Pasternak JJ, Williamson EE. Clinical pharmacology, uses, and adverse reactions of iodinated contrast agents: a primer for the non-radiologist. Mayo Clin Proc 2012;87(4):390–402.
2. McDonald RJ, Levine D, Weinreb J, et al. Gadolinium retention: a research roadmap from the 2018 NIH/ACR/RSNA workshop on gadolinium chelates. Radiology 2018;289(2):517–34.
3. Beckett KR, Moriarity AK, Langer JM. Safe use of contrast media: what the radiologist needs to know. Radiographics 2015;35(6):1738–50.
4. Wang CL, Cohan RH, Ellis JH, et al. Frequency, outcome, and appropriateness of treatment of nonionic iodinated contrast media reactions. AJR Am J Roentgenol 2008;191(2):409–15.
5. Niell BL, Vartanians VM, Halpern EP. Improving education for the management of contrast reactions: an online didactic model. J Am Coll Radiol 2014;11(2):185–92.e2.
6. Sadler DJ, Parrish F, Coulthard A. Intravenous contrast media reactions: how do radiologists react? Clin Radiol 1994;49(12):879–82.
7. Bartlett MJ, Bynevelt M. Acute contrast reaction management by radiologists: a local audit study. Australas Radiol 2003;47(4):363–7.
8. Lightfoot CB, Abraham RJ, Mammen T, et al. Survey of radiologists' knowledge regarding the management of severe contrast material–induced allergic reactions. Radiology 2009;251(3):691–6.
9. Nandwana SB, Walls DG, Torres WE. Radiology department preparedness for the management of severe acute iodinated contrast reactions: do we need to change our approach? AJR Am J Roentgenol 2015;205(1):90–4.
10. Tubbs RJ, Murphy B, Mainiero MB, et al. High-fidelity medical simulation as an assessment tool for radiology residents' acute contrast reaction management skills. J Am Coll Radiol 2009;6(8):582–7.

11. Wang CL, Davenport MS, Chinnugounder S, et al. Errors of epinephrine administration during severe allergic-like contrast reactions: lessons learned from a bi-institutional study using high-fidelity simulation testing. Abdom Imaging 2014;39(5):1127–33.

12. Gardner JB, Rashid S, Staib L, et al. Benefit of a visual aid in the management of moderate-severity contrast media reactions. Am J Roentgenol 2018;211(4):717–23.

13. Sodagari F, Mozaffary A, Wood CG, et al. Reactions to both nonionic iodinated and gadolinium-based contrast media: incidence and clinical characteristics. Am J Roentgenol 2018;210(4):715–9.

14. Katayama H, Yamaguchi K, Kozuka T, et al. Adverse reactions to ionic and nonionic contrast media. a report from the Japanese Committee on the Safety of Contrast Media. Radiology 1990;175(3):621–8.

15. Abujudeh HH, Kosaraju VK, Kaewlai R. Acute adverse reactions to gadopentetate dimeglumine and gadobenate dimeglumine: experience with 32,659 injections. Am J Roentgenol 2010;194(2):430–4.

16. Jung J-W, Kang H-R, Kim M-H, et al. Immediate hypersensitivity reaction to gadolinium-based MR contrast media. Radiology 2012;264(2):414–22.

17. Aran S, Shaqdan KW, Abujudeh HH. Adverse allergic reactions to linear ionic gadolinium-based contrast agents: experience with 194,400 injections. Clin Radiol 2015;70(5):466–75.

18. Prince MR, Zhang H, Zou Z, et al. Incidence of immediate gadolinium contrast media reactions. AJR Am J Roentgenol 2011;196(2):W138–43.

19. Sánchez-Borges M, Aberer W, Brockow K, et al. Controversies in drug allergy: radiographic contrast media. J Allergy Clin Immunol Pract 2019;7(1):61–5.

20. Macy E. Current epidemiology and management of radiocontrast-associated acute- and delayed-onset hypersensitivity: a review of the literature. Perm J 2018. https://doi.org/10.7812/TPP/17-072.

21. American College of Radiology, Committee on Drugs and Contrast Media. ACR manual on contrast media 2020. Available at: https://www.acr.org/-/media/ACR/Files/Clinical-Resources/Contrast_Media.pdf. Accessed May 15, 2020.

22. Dean KE, Starikov A, Giambrone A, et al. Adverse reactions to intravenous contrast media: an unexpected discrepancy between inpatient and outpatient cohorts. Clin Imaging 2015;39(5):863–5.

23. Loh S, Bagheri S, Katzberg RW, et al. Delayed adverse reaction to contrast-enhanced CT: a prospective single-center study comparison to control group without enhancement. Radiology 2010;255(3):764–71.

24. Wang CL, Cohan RH, Ellis JH, et al. Frequency, management, and outcome of extravasation of nonionic iodinated contrast medium in 69,657 intravenous injections. Radiology 2007;243(1):80–7.

25. Loth TS, Jones DE. Extravasations of radiographic contrast material in the upper extremity. J Hand Surg 1988;13(3):395–8.

26. Ko C-H. Large-volume iodinated contrast medium extravasation: low frequency and good outcome after conservative management in a single-centre cohort of more than 67,000 patients. Eur Radiol 2018;28(12):5376–83.

27. Pond GD, Dorr RT, McAleese KA. Skin ulceration from extravasation of low-osmolality contrast medium: a complication of automation. Am J Roentgenol 1992;158(4):915–6.

28. Heshmatzadeh Behzadi A, Farooq Z, Newhouse JH, et al. MRI and CT contrast media extravasation: a systematic review. Medicine (Baltimore) 2018;97(9):e0055.

29. Bellin M-F, Jakobsen JA, Tomassin I, et al. Contrast medium extravasation injury: guidelines for prevention and management. Eur Radiol 2002;12(11):2807–12.

30. Schild HH, Kuhl CK, Hübner-Steiner U, et al. Adverse events after unenhanced and monomeric and dimeric contrast-enhanced CT: a prospective randomized controlled trial. Radiology 2006;240(1):56–64.

31. Wang CL, Chinnugounder S, Hippe DS, et al. Comparative effectiveness of hands-on versus computer simulation–based training for contrast media reactions and teamwork skills. J Am Coll Radiol 2017;14(1):103–10.e3.

32. Pfeifer K, Staib L, Arango J, et al. High-fidelity contrast reaction simulation training: performance comparison of faculty, fellows, and residents. J Am Coll Radiol 2016;13(1):81–7.

33. LeBedis CA, Rosenkrantz AB, Otero HJ, et al. Contrast reaction training in US radiology residencies: a COAR-DRI study. Clin Imaging 2017;43:140–3.

34. Petscavage JM, Paladin AM, Wang CL, et al. Current status of residency training of allergic-like adverse events to contrast media. Acad Radiol 2012;19(2):252–5.

35. Chinnugounder S, Hippe DS, Maximin S, et al. Perceived barriers to the use of high-fidelity hands-on simulation training for contrast reaction management: why programs are not using it. Curr Probl Diagn Radiol 2015;44(6):474–8.

36. Swensson J, McMahan L, Rase B, et al. Curricula for teaching MRI safety, and MRI and CT contrast safety to residents: how effective are live lectures and online modules? J Am Coll Radiol 2015;12(10):1093–6.

37. Wang CL, Schopp JG, Petscavage JM, et al. Prospective randomized comparison of standard didactic lecture versus high-fidelity simulation for radiology resident contrast reaction management training. AJR Am J Roentgenol 2011;196(6):1288–95.

38. Tofil NM, White ML, Grant M, et al. Severe contrast reaction emergencies. Acad Radiol 2010;17(7):934–40.

39. Coupal TM, Buckley AR, Bhalla S, et al. Management of acute contrast reactions—understanding radiologists' preparedness and the efficacy of simulation-based training in Canada. Can Assoc Radiol J 2018;69(4):349–55.

40. Ali S, Alexander A, Lambrix M, et al. High-fidelity simulation training for the diagnosis and management of adverse contrast media reactions. Am J Roentgenol 2019;212(1):2–8.

41. Petscavage JM, Wang CL, Schopp JG, et al. Cost analysis and feasibility of high-fidelity simulation based radiology contrast reaction curriculum. Acad Radiol 2011;18(1):107–12.

42. Trout AT, Cohan RH, Ellis JH, et al. Teaching management of contrast reactions: does it work and how often do we need to refresh? Acad Radiol 2012;19(4):498–504.

43. Parsian S, O'Malley RB, Hippe DS, et al. A checklist manifesto: effectiveness of checklist use in hands-on simulation examining competency in contrast reaction management in a randomized controlled study. Am J Roentgenol 2018;211(1): W1–12.

44. Masch WR, Ellis JH, Wang CL, et al. Effect of available intravenous access on accuracy and timeliness of epinephrine administration. Abdom Radiol (NY) 2016;41(6):1133–41.

45. Asch D, Pfeifer KE, Arango J, et al. JOURNAL CLUB: benefit of epinephrine autoinjector for treatment of contrast reactions: comparison of errors, administration times, and provider preferences. AJR Am J Roentgenol 2017;209(2):W363–9.

46. Camargo CA, Guana A, Wang S, et al. Auvi-Q versus EpiPen: preferences of adults, caregivers, and children. J Allergy Clin Immunol Pract 2013; 1(3):266–72.e1-3.

47. Schabelman E, Witting M. The relationship of radiocontrast, iodine, and seafood allergies: a medical myth exposed. J Emerg Med 2010;39(5):701–7.

48. Schopp JG, Iyer RS, Wang CL, et al. Allergic reactions to iodinated contrast media: premedication considerations for patients at risk. Emerg Radiol 2013;20(4):299–306.

49. Bettmann MA, Heeren T, Greenfield A, et al. Adverse events with radiographic contrast agents: results of the SCVIR Contrast Agent Registry. Radiology 1997;203(3):611–20.

50. Saleh L, Juneman E, Movahed MR. The use of gadolinium in patients with contrast allergy or renal failure requiring coronary angiography, coronary intervention, or vascular procedure. Catheter Cardiovasc Interv 2011;78(5):747–54.

51. Lasser EC, Berry CC, Talner LB, et al. Pretreatment with corticosteroids to alleviate reactions to intravenous contrast material. N Engl J Med 1987; 317(14):845–9.

52. Lasser EC, Berry CC, Mishkin MM, et al. Pretreatment with corticosteroids to prevent adverse reactions to nonionic contrast media. AJR Am J Roentgenol 1994;162(3):523–6.

53. Greenberger PA, Patterson R. The prevention of immediate generalized reactions to radiocontrast media in high-risk patients. J Allergy Clin Immunol 1991;87(4):867–72.

54. Tramèr MR, von Elm E, Loubeyre P, et al. Pharmacological prevention of serious anaphylactic reactions due to iodinated contrast media: systematic review. BMJ 2006;333(7570):675.

55. Davenport MS, Cohan RH. The evidence for and against corticosteroid prophylaxis in at-risk patients. Radiol Clin North Am 2017;55(2):413–21.

56. Buchman AL. Side effects of corticosteroid therapy. J Clin Gastroenterol 2001;33(4):289–94.

57. Davenport MS, Cohan RH, Caoili EM, et al. Hyperglycemic consequences of corticosteroid premedication in an outpatient population. Am J Roentgenol 2010;194(6):W483–8.

58. Davenport MS, Cohan RH, Khalatbari S, et al. Hyperglycemia in hospitalized patients receiving corticosteroid premedication before the administration of radiologic contrast medium. Acad Radiol 2011; 18(3):384–90.

59. Mervak BM, Davenport MS, Ellis JH, et al. Rates of breakthrough reactions in inpatients at high risk receiving premedication before contrast-enhanced CT. AJR Am J Roentgenol 2015;205(1):77–84.

60. Freed KS, Leder RA, Alexander C, et al. Breakthrough adverse reactions to low-osmolar contrast media after steroid premedication. Am J Roentgenol 2001;176(6):1389–92.

61. Davenport MS, Cohan RH, Caoili EM, et al. Repeat contrast medium reactions in premedicated patients: frequency and severity. Radiology 2009; 253(2):372–9.

62. Bhatti ZS, Mervak BM, Dillman JR, et al. Breakthrough reactions to gadobenate dimeglumine. Invest Radiol 2018;53(9):551–4.

63. Davenport MS, Mervak BM, Ellis JH, et al. Indirect cost and harm attributable to oral 13-hour inpatient corticosteroid prophylaxis before contrast-enhanced CT. Radiology 2016;279(2):492–501.

64. Greenberger PA, Patterson R, Radin RC. Two pretreatment regimens for high-risk patients receiving radiographic contrast media. J Allergy Clin Immunol 1984;74(4 Pt 1):540–3.

65. Mervak BM, Cohan RH, Ellis JH, et al. Intravenous corticosteroid premedication administered 5 hours before CT compared with a traditional 13-hour oral regimen. Radiology 2017;285(2):425–33.

66. Davenport MS, Wang CL, Bashir MR, et al. Rate of contrast material extravasations and allergic-like reactions: effect of extrinsic warming of low-osmolality iodinated CT contrast material to 37°C. Radiology 2012;262(2):475–84.

67. Hardie AD, Kereshi B. Incidence of intravenous contrast extravasation: increased risk for patients with deep brachial catheter placement from the emergency department. Emerg Radiol 2014;21(3): 235–8.

Protocol Optimization for Renal Mass Detection and Characterization

Jason S. Chu, MD, Zhen J. Wang, MD*

KEYWORDS

• Renal mass • Renal cell carcinoma • Imaging protocol • Computed tomography • MR imaging

KEY POINTS

- Computed tomography (CT) protocols for renal mass evaluation should be tailored to the clinical indications with careful considerations of balancing diagnostic accuracy and radiation dose.
- MR imaging serves as a problem-solving tool in renal mass evaluation, and MR imaging protocols should take advantage of its multiparametric capability to provide additional information for renal mass characterization.
- Optimized CT and MR imaging protocols enable analysis of imaging features that help narrow the differential diagnoses and guide management in patients with renal masses.

INTRODUCTION

Renal masses increasingly are found incidentally during work-up for nonrenal indications, largely due to the frequent use of medical imaging. These include renal cysts, benign renal tumors, and renal cell carcinomas (RCCs) that have variable biological aggressiveness. Imaging is essential in renal mass characterization in order to guide appropriate treatment selections, because the management paradigm of localized renal tumors has evolved in recent years to include active surveillance and thermal ablation in addition to partial and radical nephrectomy.[1] Furthermore, imaging plays a key role in the presurgical planning of renal tumors and in surveillance after surgery or systemic therapy for advanced RCCs.

Computed tomography (CT) and MR imaging with intravenous (IV) contrast are the mainstays of renal mass evaluation. This review focuses on the CT and MR imaging protocol selection and optimization for renal mass evaluation. Contrast-enhanced ultrasound with microbubble agents is a useful alternative for characterizing renal masses, especially for patients in whom iodinated CT contrast or gadolinium-based MR imaging

contrast is contraindicated. Contrast-enhanced ultrasound is discussed in detail in a separate chapter.

COMPUTED TOMOGRAPHY

CT is the most commonly used modality for the detection and characterization of renal masses as well as presurgical planning and post-therapy surveillance. Renal masses usually are discovered incidentally on either a non–contrast-enhanced or a single-phase postcontrast CT obtained for unrelated indications. Some masses can be confidently characterized on these images without requiring a subsequent dedicated multiphase renal protocol CT or MR image. For example, renal masses that are homogeneous and have Hounsfield units (HU) measuring fluid density (between −10 HU and 20 HU) on non–contrast-enhanced CT are benign simple cysts.[2] Those that are homogeneous with HU greater than 70 are hemorrhagic or proteinaceous cysts (**Fig. 1**) 99% of the time.[3] For these masses, no further imaging is indicated. Similarly, on a single-phase postcontrast CT, renal masses that are homogeneous and measure fluid density are simple cysts. Recent data also suggest

Department of Radiology and Biomedical Imaging, University of California San Francisco, 505 Parnassus Avenue, Box 0628, San Francisco, CA 94143, USA
* Corresponding author.
E-mail address: zhen.wang@ucsf.edu

Radiol Clin N Am 58 (2020) 851–873
https://doi.org/10.1016/j.rcl.2020.05.003

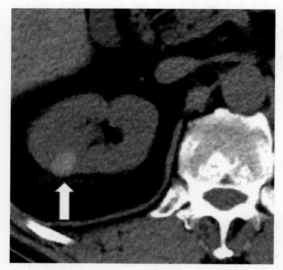

Fig. 1. Precontrast CT in a 62-year-old man shows a homogeneous hyperdense renal lesion (*arrow*) measuring 82 HU in attenuation, consistent with a benign hyperdense cyst, not requiring further characterization because it is homogeneous and greater than 70 HU.

that well-defined homogeneous renal mass with attenuation 30 HU or less on the portal venous phase CT can be considered benign cysts and require no additional imaging.[2,4] When the initial CT is unable to provide a definitive diagnosis, subsequent multiphase renal protocol CT after IV contrast injection commonly is obtained for further characterization of a renal mass.

Multiphase Renal Protocol Computed Tomography

When further work-up for a renal mass is deemed necessary, additional imaging can be obtained using a multiphase renal protocol CT. Enhancement patterns across different phases after IV contrast injection can be used to distinguish renal cysts from solid tumors and may aid in subtyping of renal tumors.

Although the specifics of a renal protocol CT vary by institutions, the following phases in their various combinations commonly are used: precontrast phase, corticomedullary phase, nephrographic phase, and excretory phase (**Fig. 2**A–D). The combination of these phases may be modified depending on the clinical indications, such as for initial lesion characterization, surgical or ablation planning, or post-treatment follow-up. The field of view, whether restricted to the kidneys themselves or expanded to include from the diaphragm to the iliac crest, also depends on the clinical questions.

Precontrast Phase

Precontrast CT provides better detection of small amounts of intralesional fat compared with postcontrast CT (**Fig. 3**).[5] In order to optimally visualize the small foci of fat, thin sections (eg, 1.25 mm) may be required. Similarly, precontrast CT also improves visualization of calcification (**Fig. 4**) compared with postcontrast CT or MR imaging. Angiomyolipomas (AMLs) can be diagnosed confidently once intralesional macroscopic fat has been identified in the absence of other worrisome findings, such as intralesional calcification. On the other hand, the presence of intralesional calcification, regardless of the presence of fat, should prompt suspicion for malignancy, such as RCC.[6–10]

Corticomedullary Phase

Corticomedullary phase typically is acquired 40 seconds to 70 seconds after IV contrast injection (see **Fig. 2**B). During this phase, there is intense enhancement of the renal cortex, allowing differentiation between the cortex and the medulla. This phase is useful in confirming anatomic variants, such as column of Bertin, which can mimic a tumor but which has the same corticomedullary differentiation as normal kidney parenchyma (**Fig. 5**). The renal vasculature also enhances intensely in this phase, which can provide additional information for surgical planning if needed (**Fig. 6**) or identify vascular anomalies, such as pseudoaneurysm and arteriovenous fistula.[9]

Nephrographic Phase

Nephrographic phase is the most sensitive for detecting renal lesions.[11] Obtained at 100 seconds to 120 seconds after IV contrast injection, the timing for this contrast-enhancement phase is later than the typical portal venous phase, allowing for uniform enhancement of the renal parenchyma and in general providing the highest tumor to background distinction compared with the other phases (**Fig. 7**). It has been reported that up to 66% more small renal masses are detected in the nephrographic phase compared with the corticomedullary phase.[11] Nephrographic phase also may improve the assessment of enhancement in poorly vascular tumors. For example, papillary RCCs typically demonstrate low-level progressive enhancement, peaking at the nephrographic phase (**Fig. 8**); therefore, tumor contrast enhancement is more conspicuous on the nephrographic phase compared with the earlier corticomedullary phase.[12] Measurement of HU change after

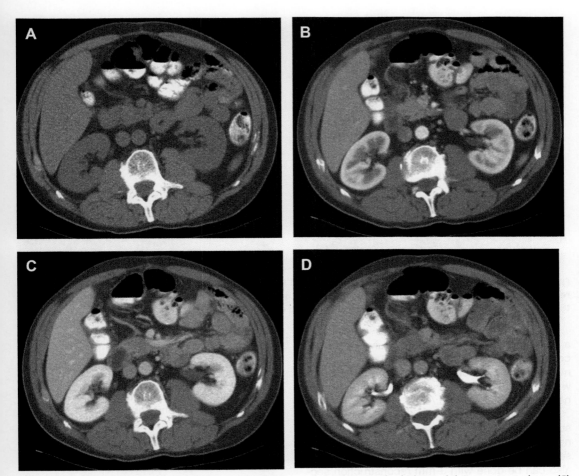

Fig. 2. CT in a 46-year-old man illustrates various enhancement phases in the kidneys. (*A*) Precontrast phase. (*B*) Corticomedullary phase (obtained 40–70 second delay after contrast injection, showing differential enhancement of the renal cortex and medulla). (*C*) Nephrographic phase (100–120 seconds after contrast injection, with uniform enhancement of the entire renal parenchyma). (*D*) Excretory phase (7–10 minutes after contrast injection, with hyperattenuating contrast material in the collecting system).

contrast administration using the earlier corticomedullary phase in a papillary RCC may result in erroneous categorization of the lesion as a nonenhancing cyst (see **Fig. 8**). In the setting of advanced RCCs, tumor extension into the renal vain or inferior vena cava may be best assessed on the nephrographic phase as well.

Excretory Phase

Excretory phase is obtained at 7 minutes to 10 minutes after IV contrast injection. Contrast material is excreted into the renal collection system, ureters, and bladder in this phase, allowing better visualization of these structures. This phase is helpful for identifying RCC involvement of the collecting system as well as diagnosing primary malignancy arising from the collecting system, such as urothelial carcinoma involving the kidney (**Fig. 9**).

Society of Abdominal Radiology Suggested Protocols

The Society of Abdominal Radiology (SAR) Disease-Focused Panel (DFP) on RCC is a multi-institutional working group aimed at addressing the unmet needs in the clinical care, research, and education in RCCs. The group has suggested standardized CT protocols for renal mass evaluation based on different clinical indications, as described later.[13] The suggested imaging protocols are based on expert consensus, with the goal of balancing diagnostic efficacy and radiation exposure (**Table 1**).

IV contrast generally is needed for the characterization, staging, surveillance, and post-treatment follow-up of renal tumors.[14,15] Suggested IV contrast type by the SAR DFP is low-osmolar or iso-osmolar contrast material, at

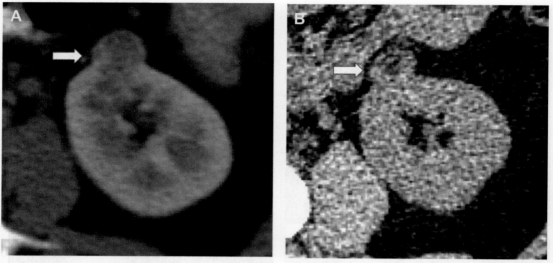

Fig. 3. CT in a 57-year-old woman with a renal AML. (*A*) Postcontrast image shows an exophytic left enhancing renal mass (*arrow*) that is suspicious for an RCC. (*B*) Precontrast image shows a small focus of fat density within the mass (*arrow*), measuring −32 HU, which enables the diagnosis of an AML.

a dose of 35 g to 52.5 g iodine equivalent (ie, for contrast material that contains 350 mg of iodine/mL, the corresponding dose is 100–150 mL), or weight-based dosing. The injection rate is suggested at 2 mL/s to 5 mL/s.

CT images are acquired in the axial plane, with suggested 3-mm reconstruction section thickness. Multiplanar reformats in the coronal and sagittal planes of each postcontrast scan series also can be done with 3-mm reconstruction section thickness without overlap.

Suggested Protocol for Evaluation of Indeterminate Renal Masses

For indeterminate renal masses, the field of view can be restricted to the kidneys only, with precontrast and nephrographic (obtained at 100-second to 120-second delay) phases considered essential for this indication. These 2 phases allow the differentiation between solid and cystic renal masses.

Corticomedullary and excretory phases may be acquired optionally. The excretory phase may be

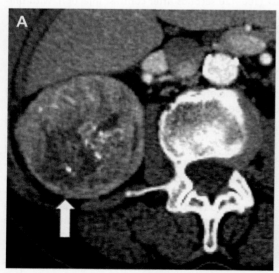
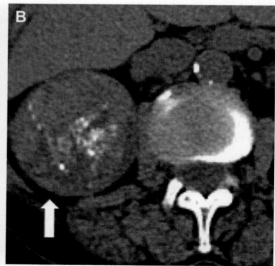

Fig. 4. CT in a 68-year-old woman with a clear cell RCC. (*A*) Postcontrast CT image shows a right renal mass with multiple foci of hyperdensity (*arrow*), which may be either calcification or enhancement. (*B*) Precontrast image shows the hyperdense foci to be calcifications (*arrow*).

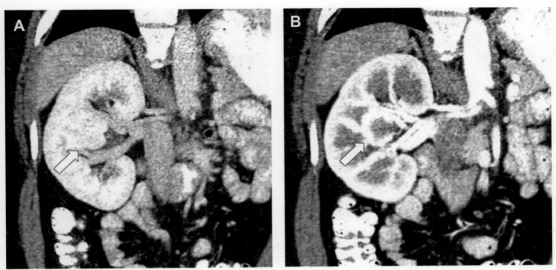

Fig. 5. CT in a 37-year-old woman with hypertrophied column of Bertin. (*A*) Nephrographic phase demonstrates masslike structure (*arrow*) in the right midkidney. (*B*) Corticomedullary phase reveals the masslike structure with similar corticomedullary differentiation as the rest of the renal parenchyma (*arrow*), consistent with a hypertrophied column of Bertin.

helpful for distinguishing urothelial cancers from RCCs and parapelvic or peripelvic cysts from hydronephrosis and for diagnosing calyceal diverticula. The corticomedullary and excretory phases together with the precontrast-phase and nephrographic-phase images may be helpful to subtype renal masses.[13,16] For example, prior studies have shown that clear cell–type RCCs demonstrate peak enhancement during the corticomedullary phase.[17–20] In contrast, papillary RCCs demonstrate greater enhancement at later phases.[17–21] By applying enhancement thresholds, 1 study has shown that 4-phase CT

attenuation profiles enabled differentiation of clear cell RCCs from other solid renal cortical masses, notably from papillary RCCs and lipid-poor AMLs.[12] Such information can be helpful in guiding patient management. For example, a tumor with enhancement features that suggest a papillary RCC can be confirmed with percutaneous biopsy. Given the indolent nature of papillary RCCs in general, these may be appropriate for active surveillance rather than surgical resection, especially in patients who are poor surgical candidates.[22,23] Although multiphase CT for tumor subtyping is promising, there are no prospective studies to

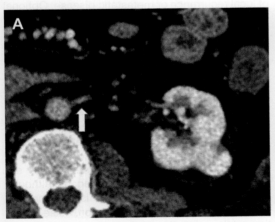
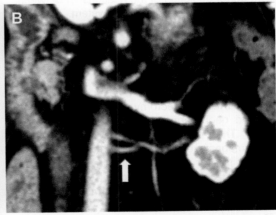

Fig. 6. Presurgical planning CT in a 65-year-old man with a left renal tumor. Axial (*A*) and coronal reformatted (*B*) images acquired in the arterial/corticomedullary phase provide excellent vascular delineation and enable identification of an accessory left renal artery (*arrows*).

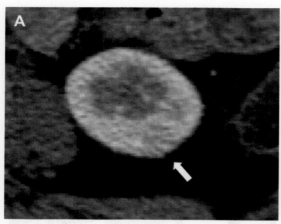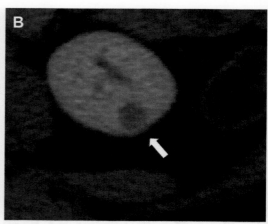

Fig. 7. CT in a 75-year-old woman with a left renal lesion demonstrating higher lesion conspicuity in the nephrographic phase compared with the corticomedullary phase. (*A*) A cortically based renal lesion (*arrow*) was poorly seen on the corticomedullary-phase CT. (*B*) The lesion (*arrow*) was much more conspicuous on the nephrographic-phase CT.

date that have validated the reported enhancement threshold.

Suggested Protocol for Pre–Partial Nephrectomy or Preablation Planning of Renal Masses that Have Been Previously Completely Characterized

For pre–partial nephrectomy or preablation planning of renal masses that have been previously completely characterized, the primary goal is to delineate the tumor and vascular anatomy. Arterial phase (approximately 30-second delay) with field of view focused on the kidneys is recommended to better depict arteries and their relationship to the renal tumor. Nephrographic and excretory phases also are included, with the field of view expanded from diaphragm to iliac crest. The excretory phase allows better depiction of the relationship between the mass and the renal collecting system.

Suggested Protocol for Active Surveillance, Postablation Surveillance, Post–Partial Nephrectomy Surveillance

For active surveillance, postablation surveillance, or post–partial nephrectomy surveillance, precontrast and nephrographic phases should be obtained. The precontrast and nephrographic phase images are used to evaluate for changes of tumor size or enhancement characteristics in cases of active surveillance or detecting enhancing tumor in post-treatment settings (**Fig. 10**).

The precontrast images are acquired with the field of view restricted to the kidneys only, and these may be omitted if the primary goal of surveillance is to assess tumor size changes. The nephrographic phase is acquired with the field of view from diaphragm to iliac crests. Optional acquisition includes the excretory phase at 7-minute to 10-minute delay, from the diaphragm to iliac crests. Inclusion of this phase may be helpful after ablation or partial nephrectomy when collecting system injury is suspected.

Suggested Protocol for Post–Radical Nephrectomy Surveillance or Systemic Therapy Surveillance

For surveillance after radical nephrectomy or systemic therapy, it is suggested to acquire images in the portal venous phase at 60-second to 90-second delay, with the field of view from the diaphragm to iliac crests to optimize the detection of local recurrence or metastatic disease. Optional additional acquisition includes the late arterial phase from diaphragm to iliac crests. This phase can be included in patients with high risks of metastatic disease to improve the detection of hypervascular liver and pancreatic metastases (**Fig. 11**).

Dose Reduction

The major disadvantage of multiphase CT is the increased radiation exposure to patients due to the dose-multiplier effect of extra phases.[24] Reducing radiation dose is desirable while still providing diagnostic quality images. Although filtered back projection (FBP) is the primary method for CT image reconstruction, noise reduction while using this technique entails primarily increasing exposure.[25] The newer iterative reconstruction methods can produce images at lower

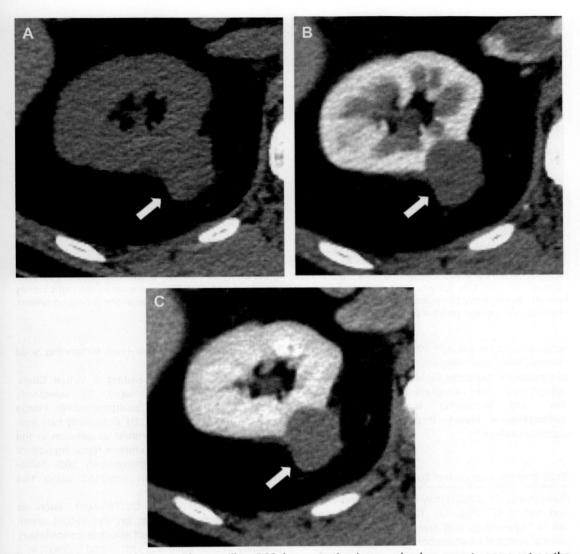

Fig. 8. CT in a 69-year-old man with a papillary RCC demonstrating improved enhancement assessment on the nephrographic phase compared with the corticomedullary phase. Papillary RCCs typically have low-level progressive enhancement that peaks in the nephrographic phase. (*A*) Precontrast-phase, (*B*) corticomedullary-phase, and (*C*) nephrographic-phase images show a right renal mass (*arrows* in *A*, *B*, and *C*) with CT attenuation measurements of 22 HU, 37 HU, and 55 HU, respectively. The changes in CT attenuation in the renal mass after contrast administration were 15 HU using the corticomedullary phase and 33 HU using the nephrographic phase. Using the generally accepted enhancement threshold of 20 HU, the renal mass would be diagnosed as a solid tumor using the nephrographic-phase images but considered indeterminate using the corticomedullary-phase images.

noise level compared with FBP at the same radiation dose through more sophisticated computation on the acquired projection data. Similar diagnostic quality images compared with conventional reconstruction methods, therefore, can be achieved at reduced radiation dose using iterative reconstruction.[26–31] For abdominal imaging, although typically considered a more challenging area for dose optimization due to inherently low

soft tissue contrast attributable to multiple organs of similar attenuation, several iterative reconstruction methods have been shown to reduce image noise while using lower radiation dose, thus improving lesion conspicuity and diagnostic quality compared with standard FBP reconstruction method at reduced radiation risk.[14,15,27,32,33] In the context of renal masses, a study has shown no differences in CT attenuation values when using

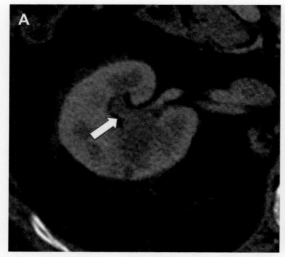
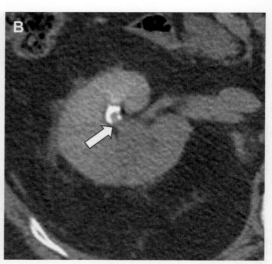

Fig. 9. CT in a 64-year-old man with a renal mass illustrating the utility of excretory phase in delineating involvement of the collecting system. (*A*) Corticomedullary-phase image shows an infiltrative mass in the right kidney (*arrow*). (*B*) Excretory phase-image shows a filling defect (*arrow*) consistent with tumor in the collecting system. The mass was proved to be a central transitional cell carcinoma.

iterative reconstruction.[34] Pitfalls in using iterative construction are related to over-smoothing, which has the potential for alteration of tissue imaging texture, loss of low-contrast spatial resolution, and simulating homogeneity in a heterogeneous lesion, thus influencing lesion characterization.[35–37]

Dual-Energy Computed Tomography

Dual-energy CT (DECT) may further expand on the potential of CT (**Fig. 12**). Through simultaneous use of high-energy and low energy sets of x-ray beams, spectral identification and isolation of material on the basis of the material's energy-related attenuation characteristics allow selective display or removal of materials during image reconstruction.[38,39] The lower-energy beam component also improves the image contrast-to-noise ratio compared with conventional CT. For renal mass imaging, the specific benefits of this technique currently include improved assessment of lesion enhancement and radiation dose reduction.

Uptake of iodinated CT contrast can be visualized using the iodine map, which has been shown to have an advantage over traditional HU-based attenuation measurement in determining lesion enhancement (see **Fig. 12**C).[40–45] Additionally, the ability to produce a virtual monochromatic image can achieve substantial beam-hardening correction, therefore reducing or eliminating renal cyst pseudoenhancement.[38,45] These advantages can aid in distinguishing between nonenhancing

hyperdense cysts and low-level enhancing solid tumors.[40–47]

The capability of generating a virtual unenhanced image (water image), by selectively removing iodine during postprocessing image reconstruction (see **Fig. 12**B), potentially can supplant conventional precontrast acquisition in the renal mass CT protocol, therefore reducing patient radiation exposure.[38] Approximately 50% radiation reduction has been reported using this method.[38,47]

Several limitations in DECT exist, such as persistent iodine contrast on the virtual unenhanced image due to failed spectral cancellation, difficulty in distinguishing iodine and calcium in a lesion, and residual beam-hardening artifact on virtual monochromatic images, resulting in substantial image degradation, especially in extremely large patients.[38,48] Because this technology still is undergoing investigation, standardized algorithmic integration into practice has yet to be established.[39]

MR IMAGING

MR imaging often is utilized as a problem-solving tool for assessing indeterminate renal masses seen on CT or as the initial dedicated study for the work-up of renal masses seen on ultrasound. Small renal masses may be better characterized using MR imaging than CT because of its high specificity for small cysts[49] and because MR imaging is not limited by pseudoenhancement that occurs on CT. MR imaging also is more sensitive

Table 1
Suggested computed tomography protocols from the Society of Abdominal Radiology Disease-focused panel on renal cell carcinoma

Indications		Contrast Phases	Field of View	Timing	Comment
Indeterminate renal mass	Recommended scan series	Precontrast	Kidneys only		
		Nephrographic	Kidneys only	100–120 s delay	
	Optional additional scan series	Corticomedullary	Kidneys only	40–70 s delay	May be helpful in subtyping RCC
		Excretory	Diaphragm to iliac crests	7–10 min delay	May be helpful to differentiate urothelial cancer from RCC and parapelvic or peripelvic cysts from hydronephrosis and to diagnose calyceal diverticula
Pre-partial nephrectomy or preablation planning for renal masses that have been previously completely characterized	Recommended scan series	Arterial	Kidneys only	30 s delay	Better depict the arteries and their relationship to the renal mass
		Nephrographic	Diaphragm to iliac crests	100–120 s delay	Better depict the relationship between the collecting system and the mass.
		Excretory	Diaphragm to iliac crests	7–10 min delay	
Active surveillance; postablation surveillance; post–partial nephrectomy surveillance	Recommended scan series	Precontrast	Kidneys only		May be omitted for active surveillance if the primary goal is to determine renal mass size change
	Optional additional scan series	Nephrographic	Diaphragm to iliac crests	100–120 s delay	May be helpful after ablation or partial nephrectomy when collecting system injury is suspected
		Excretory	Diaphragm to iliac crests	7–10 min delay	

(continued on next page)

Table 1
(continued)

Indications	Contrast Phases	Field of View	Timing	Comment
Post-radical nephrectomy surveillance; systemic therapy surveillance	Recommended scan series	Portal venous	60–90 s delay	Can be included in patients at high risk of metastatic disease to improve detection of liver and pancreatic metastases
	Optional additional scan series	Late arterial	40–50 s delay	

Acquisition: axial, 3-mm reconstruction section thickness with or without 50% overlap.

Recommended additional reformats: coronal and sagittal of each postcontrast scan series; 3-mm reconstruction section thickness without overlap.

IV contrast material type, volume, and injection rate: type, low-osmolar or iso-osmolar contrast material; volume, 35-g to 52.5-g iodine equivalent (ie, for contrast material that contains 350 mg of iodine/mL, the corresponding dose is 100–150 mL); and weight-based dosing injection rate, 2–5 mL/s.

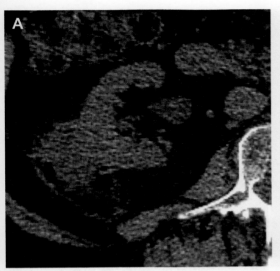
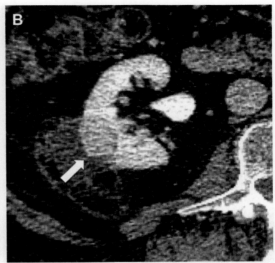

Fig. 10. Surveillance CT in a 76-year-old woman with prior renal tumor ablation. (*A*) Precontrast-phase and (*B*) nephrographic-phase images show enhancing nodule (*arrow*) in the ablated cavity, consistent with recurrent tumor.

to contrast enhancement in renal masses with indeterminate enhancement at CT.[21,50] A drawback of MR imaging compared with CT is the limited ability of MR imaging for detection of calcifications. A typical renal mass MR imaging protocol includes various MR imaging sequences, described later, which provide different soft tissue contrast that aids in the characterization of the mass.

T2-weighted MR Imaging

T2-weighted images usually are acquired using a 2-dimensional (2-D) single-shot fast spin-echo (SSFSE) sequence in the axial and/or coronal plane. Alternatively, 2-D T2-weighted fast spin-echo (FSE) sequence may be used. Routine utilization of fat-suppression for the T2-weighted images allows elimination of competing high signal

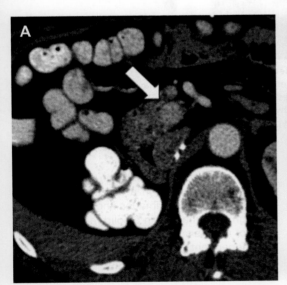
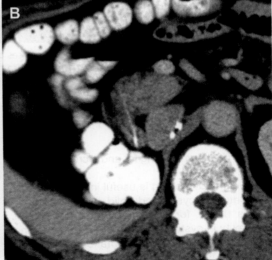

Fig. 11. Surveillance CT in a 55-year-old man after radical nephrectomy for RCC demonstrating the utility of late arterial-phase images for detecting hypervascular metastases. The hypervascular pancreatic metastasis (*arrow*) was conspicuously seen on the (*A*) late arterial phase but was not visible on the (*B*) portal venous phase.

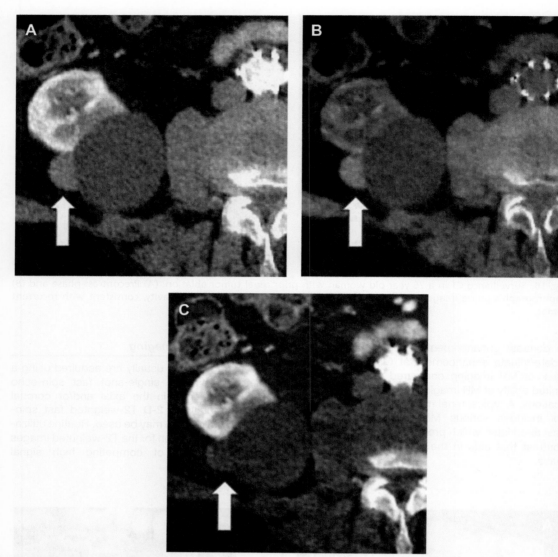

Fig. 12. DECT in a 72-year-old man with renal masses demonstrating the utility of DECT in assessing enhancement. (*A*) Conventional CT image shows a hyperdense renal mass (*arrow*), which may represent either a hyperdense cyst or an enhancing mass on single-phase images. Water (*B*) and iodine (*C*) images derived from DECT acquisition show the renal mass (*arrows* in *B* and *C*) is hyperdense on the water image and is of fluid density on the iodine image, thus enabling the diagnosis of a hyperdense cyst without the need for acquiring separate unenhanced images.

intensity from surrounding fat and increases lesion conspicuity.[51,52]

T2-weighted imaging is useful in the differentiation between cystic and solid renal masses. It also is ideal for assessing the degree of complexity in cystic lesions, including discerning margin irregularity, internal septations, and irregular mural thickening.[53] The presence of predominant cystic components in a renal mass suggests indolent nature. For example, cystic RCCs have better prognosis compared with

solid RCCs, with lower risks of metastasis.[54–57] Necrotic components in a solid mass also can be detected on these images and appear as central high T2 signal within a solid mass. The presence of necrosis in a renal tumor also serves as an independent marker of poor prognosis.[58] T2 signal in a renal tumor provides additional value in tumor subtyping. For example, heterogeneous high T2 signal is seen more commonly in clear cell RCCs[59] (**Fig. 13A**). In contrast, low T2 signal is seen more commonly in papillary

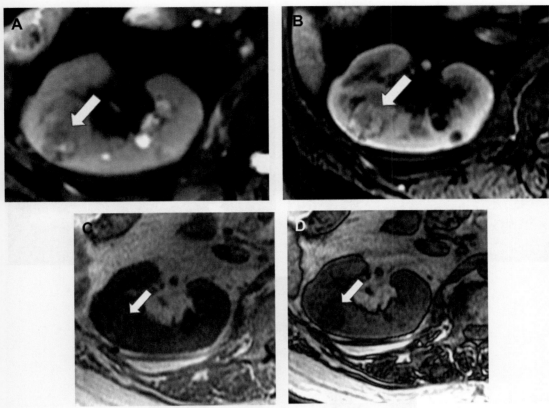

Fig. 13. MR imaging in a 77-year-old man with a clear cell RCC. (*A*) T2-weighted SSFSE with fat saturation image shows a right renal mass (*arrow*) with heterogenous T2 signal. (*B*) T1-weighted 3-D FSPGR postcontrast image shows the mass (*arrow*) to be avidly enhancing. In-phase (*C*) and opposed-phase (*D*) T1 dual-echo images show a loss of signal in the mass (*arrows* in *C* and *D*) on the opposed-phase image compared to the in-phase image, consistent with the presence of intravoxel fat. The combination of these features is highly suggestive of a clear cell RCC, which was proved at surgery.

RCC (**Fig. 14A**), lipid-poor AMLs, or renal leiomyomas.[53,59,60]

Dual-Echo In-phase and Opposed-Phase/Dixon MR Imaging

Dual-echo in-phase and opposed-phase images can be acquired using a 2-D T1-weighted gradient-echo sequence, obtained in the axial plane with 5-mm to 6-mm slice thickness. Alternatively, in-phase and opposed-phase images can be obtained using 3-dimensional (3-D) Dixon technique with thinner (3–4 mm) slice thickness. Multiecho Dixon technique allows reconstruction of images with contribution solely from fat or water protons, achieving improved fat suppression compared with conventional methods. Using a 3-D acquisition, thinner image slices can be obtained and assist in the detection of a small amount of fat within some renal AMLs. It has been reported that 5% of lipid-rich AMLs

detected on 3-D 2-point Dixon sequence were not identified using standard 2-D dual-echo T1 sequence.[17,61] The 3-point Dixon technique, which improves on the 2-point technique by detecting and eliminating phase error due to magnetic field inhomogeneity, has been reported to produce images with more homogeneous fat suppression, better anatomic detail, less susceptibility artifact, and at least equivalent lesion detection compared with conventional T2-weighted fast-recovery FSE imaging.[38] Due to the excellent separation of fat and water signals and improved image quality, this technique also has been applied to gadolinium-enhanced abdominal MR imaging with excellent results.[62]

Dual-echo in-phase and opposed-phase images are helpful in delineating macroscopic fat in a renal mass, with foci of macroscopic fat demonstrating characteristic dark rims on opposed-phase images. A prior study has shown that a

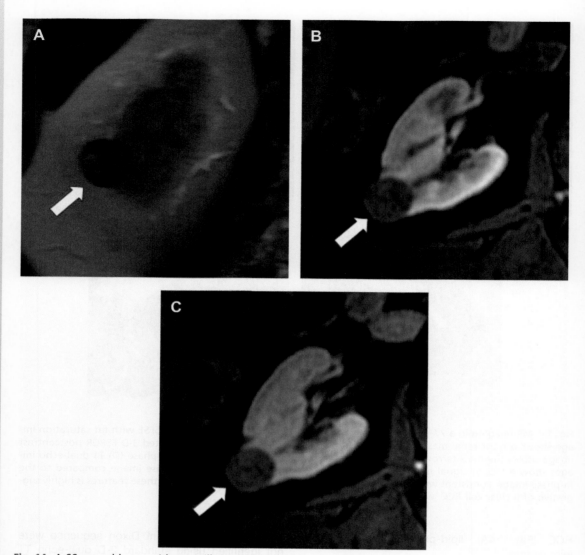

Fig. 14. A 66-year-old man with a papillary RCC. (*A*) Coronal T2-weighted SSFSE image shows a right renal mass (*arrow*) with low T2 signal. (*B*) T1-weighted 3-D FSPGR postcontrast image acquired during the corticomedullary phase demonstrates relative hypoenhancement of the mass compared with the rest of renal parenchyma (*arrow*). (*C*) T1-weighted 3-D FSPGR postcontrast image acquired during the nephrographic phase demonstrates progressive low-level enhancement of the mass (*arrow*). The combination of these features is suggestive of a papillary RCC, which was confirmed at surgery.

small amount of macroscopic fat is more easily recognized as small dark rings on in-phase and opposed-phase images, and this facilitates the diagnosis of renal AMLs[63] (**Fig. 15**). Microscopic fat, on the other hand, manifests as diffuse or ill-defined loss of signal intensity on opposed-phase images. This imaging feature can be seen in both renal AMLs and RCCs.[53,60,64,65] In AMLs, the intermixed adipocytes and other soft tissue elements within each voxel account for the signal reduction on opposed-phase images, whereas in

RCCs this is attributable to intracellular fat.[18] It has been reported that up to 59% of clear cell RCCs have notable signal decrease on the opposed-phase images (**Fig. 16**); therefore, this feature cannot be used to distinguish renal AMLs from RCCs.[16,66]

In-phase and opposed-phase images also aid in the detection of hemosiderin deposition in a renal mass, seen as a signal loss on the in-phase images due to susceptibility effect–related magnetic field distortion, leading to increased T2* dephasing

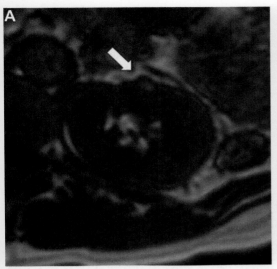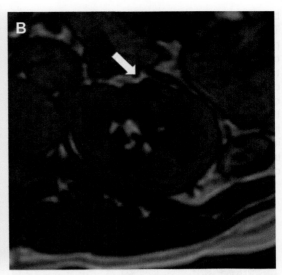

Fig. 15. MR imaging in a 50-year-old woman with a small renal AML. (*A*) In-phase and (*B*) opposed-phase T1-weighted dual-echo images show a small left renal mass (*arrows*) with a characteristic India-ink artifact on the opposed-phase image, highlighting the presence of macroscopic fat in the mass and enabling a confident diagnosis of an AML.

because these images are acquired at a later echo time. Hemosiderin is associated more commonly with papillary RCCs.[17,67]

T1-weighted Precontrast and Dynamic Postcontrast MR Imaging

3-D T1-weighted spoiled gradient-echo (SPGR) with fat saturation is acquired prior to and dynamically following contrast administration, in the axial plane, with 3-mm to 4-mm slice thickness. A variation of this protocol acquires images in the coronal and sagittal planes.[53] Fat-suppressed 3-D

gradient-echo sequences offer comparable or better image quality than 2-D gradient-echo and may be able to detect more focal lesions owing to the advantage of reduced section width with no slice gap, while maintaining or improving image quality.[68,69] The precontrast sequence can reveal hemorrhagic or proteinaceous content within lesions as intrinsic T1 hyperintensity.

After contrast administration, acquisitions should be timed during the corticomedullary (approximately 30 seconds), nephrographic (90–100 seconds), and delayed (180–210 seconds) phases. The dynamic postcontrast images should

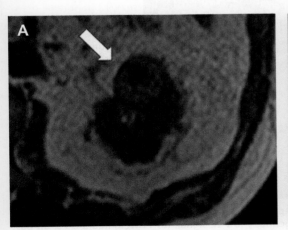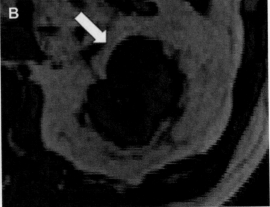

Fig. 16. MR imaging in an 83-year-old man with a clear cell RCC. (*A*) In-phase and (*B*) opposed-phase images show a left renal mass (*arrows*) with diffuse signal loss on the opposed-phase image relative to the in-phase image, consistent with the presence of intravoxel fat.

be obtained in the same plane as the precontrast T1-weighted SPGR, followed by another set of postcontrast images in an orthogonal plane. Additional delayed postcontrast images can be obtained at 5-minute to 7-minute delay in the axial or coronal plane and allow improved visualization of the collecting system. Subtraction imaging of the dynamic series can be obtained and is useful in assessing enhancement in renal masses with intrinsic T1 hyperintensity. One study has shown improved detection of enhancement on the postcontrast subtraction MR images for histologically

proved papillary RCCs that did not meet enhancement criteria on CT.[21] The major challenge in producing accurate subtraction images is ensuring adequate image coregistration, which may be compromised as a result of respiratory motion artifact or inconsistent respiratory effort.[70] Methods of reducing respiratory motion artifact include breath holding, using respiratory gating, phase reordering, and navigator echo.[71]

The dynamic postcontrast images provide information on enhancement pattern in a renal mass and can aid in tumor subtyping. For example,

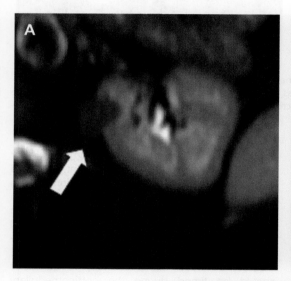
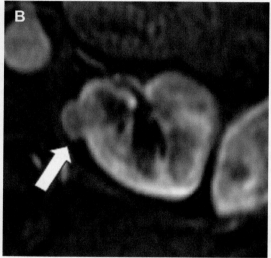
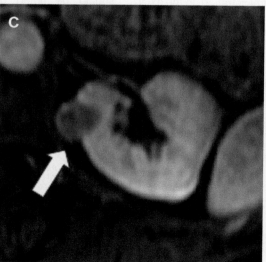

Fig. 17. MR imaging in an 86-year-old man with a lipid-poor renal AML. (A) T2-weighted SSFSE with fat saturation image shows a left renal mass (arrow) with homogenously low T2 signal. (B) T1-weighted 3-D FSPGR postcontrast image in the corticomedullary phase shows the mass (arrow) to be avidly enhancing. (C) T1-weighted 3-D FSPGR postcontrast image in the nephrographic phase shows contrast washout in the mass (arrow). These features are suggestive of a lipid-poor AML, which was confirmed at biopsy.

Table 2
Suggested MR imaging protocols from the Society of Abdominal Radiology Disease-focused panel on renal cell carcinoma

Indication		Sequence	Plane	Slice Thickness/Gap	Comment
Indeterminate renal mass; active surveillance; postablation surveillance; postnephrectomy surveillance	Recommended sequences	2-D T2-weighted SSFSE	Axial and/or coronal	Axial: 4-5 mm/no gap coronal: 5-6 mm/no gap	Alternative: 2-D axial T2-weighted FSE, 4–5 mm/no gap
		2-D T1-weighted gradient-echo in/opposed phase	Axial	5–6 mm/0.5–1 mm	Alternative: 3-D Dixon technique for in/out phase, 3–4 mm/no gap
		3-D T1-weighted SPGR with fat saturation precontrast	Axial and/or coronal	3–4 mm/no gap	
		[a]3-D dynamic T1-weighted SPGR with fat saturation postcontrast	Axial or coronal (same as precontrast)	3–4 mm/no gap	Dynamic timing: 30 s, 90–100 s, 180–210 s Note: precontrast and dynamic postcontrast imaging can be obtained in the axial or coronal plane. After the dynamic series is acquired, obtain the other plane at 240 s. Obtain routine subtraction imaging with the dynamic series.
	Optional additional sequences	3-D T1-weighted SPGR with fat saturation delayed postcontrast	Axial or coronal	3–4 mm/no gap	5–7 min delayed postcontrast scan: perform in the axial plane if the dynamic images are coronal; perform in the coronal plane if the dynamic images are axial; additional sagittal acquisition through the kidneys can also be obtained

(continued on next page)

Table 2
(continued)

Indication	Sequence	Plane	Slice Thickness/Gap	Comment
	DWI	Axial	5–6 mm/no gap	Suggested b values: 0–50 s/mm², 400–500 s/mm², and 800–1000 s/mm² May be helpful for nodal and metastatic disease evaluation

IV contrast material type, volume, and injection rate: type, extracellular gadolinium-based contrast material; volume, 0.1 mL/kg body weight; and injection rate: 1 mL/s to 2 mL/s followed by 10-mL to 20-mL saline flush.

[a] Obtain the precontrast and dynamic postcontrast images in the same plane and with identical acquisition parameters, and acquire preferably at end expiration to facilitate subtraction imaging. Maintain constant receiver gain for all dynamic acquisitions before and after contrast material (ie, set up entire dynamic series with a single prescan before the precontrast acquisition). Fat saturation can be performed with frequency-selective fat saturation strategies or using water-only reconstructed images from Dixon-based acquisitions. The latter provides in-phase/opposed-phase/fat-only reconstructions in the same breath hold.

papillary RCCs typically are noted for their low level of enhancement, which becomes more apparent in later phases of MR imaging.[21] In comparison, clear cell RCCs classically demonstrate hypervascularity after IV contrast administration.[72] Unlike CT, MR imaging allows multiple postcontrast acquisitions with no concern for ionizing radiation.

Diffusion-Weighted Imaging

Diffusion-weighted imaging (DWI) can be useful for improving lesion detection when gadolinium-based contrast is contraindicated, although DWI is less accurate than gadolinium contrast-enhanced MR imaging.[73–75] The renal parenchyma can appear bright on DWI at low to intermediate b values; therefore, at least 1 set of DWIs acquired with b value of 800 s/mm^2 to 1000 s/mm^2 is recommended to enhance conspicuity of renal neoplasms.[18] DWI can be acquired in the axial plane, with 5-mm to 6-mm slice thickness. Although the choice and number of b values have not been standardized, in general, low (0–50 s/mm^2), intermediate (400–500 s/mm^2), and high (800–1000 s/mm^2) b values should be considered.

The precise role of DWI in renal mass characterization has not been clearly established. The use of apparent diffusion coefficient (ADC) calculated from DWI may be helpful for tumor subtyping. For example, significantly lower ADC values have been reported in papillary RCCs, urothelial carcinomas, and lymphomas compared with normal renal parenchyma.[18,76–78]

DWI also has been explored for tumor grading. For example, high nuclear-grade clear cell RCCs have been reported to have significantly lower ADC values than low-grade tumors.[79,80] Diffusional kurtosis imaging, an extension of the DWI model that takes into account deviation of water molecules in biological tissue from gaussian behavior, also has shown promise in distinguishing low-grade RCCs and high-grade RCCs preoperatively.[81–83]

Multiparametric MR Imaging for Improved Renal Mass Characterization

Apart from renal AMLs with macroscopic fat, MR imaging cannot yet reliably differentiate between benign renal tumors and RCCs. The availability of different soft tissue contrast from multiparametric MR imaging, however, can suggest tumor subtypes. For example, clear cell RCCs classically show intermediate to high signal intensity on T2-weighted images and hypervascularity after contrast administration.[72] Some clear cell RCCs also have microscopic/intravoxel fat that is evident

on dual-echo T1-weighted images. Although these features are nonspecific individually, the combination of tumor hypervascularity, intermediate to high T2 signal, and intravoxel lipid is highly suggestive of clear cell RCCs[17] (Fig. 13). In comparison, papillary RCCs usually have lower signal intensity on T2 weighted images and low-level enhancement. Hemosiderin, visualized as signal loss on in-phase images compared with opposed-phase images, is associated more commonly with papillary RCCs.84 The combination of these features is highly suggestive of a papillary RCC[17,84] (Fig. 14). Because papillary RCCs tend to be a less aggressive subtype, the presence of these imaging features may warrant a biopsy for confirmation and may influence the management to active surveillance rather than resection in appropriately selected patients. Lipid-poor AMLs also commonly are hypointense on T2-weighted sequences, similar to papillary RCCs. Unlike the low-level enhancement seen in papillary RCCs, however, lipid-poor AMLs usually have a high level of enhancement with a higher arterial-to-delayed enhancement ratio[60,85] (Fig. 17). The presence of low T2 signal and high level of enhancement may warrant a biopsy for a definitive diagnosis of a lipid-poor renal AML.

Society of Abdominal Radiology Disease-Focused Panel Suggested Renal MR Imaging Protocol

The SAR DFP on RCC has put forth a suggested MR imaging protocol for renal mass evaluation.[86] Because ionizing radiation exposure is not a consideration with MR imaging, the suggested protocol encompasses various MR imaging sequences and is applicable for various clinical indications. Extracellular gadolinium-based contrast material is suggested, with volume of 0.1 mL/kg body weight and injection rate of 1 mL/s to 2 mL/s followed by 10-mL to 20-mL saline flush.

For the purpose of assessing indeterminate renal mass, active surveillance, or surveillance postprocedurally, the suggested MR imaging protocol includes T2-weighted sequence, T1 dual-echo in-phase and opposed-phase sequence, and T1-weighted sequence before and after contrast administration with similar contrast phases, as discussed in the CT protocol. Optional sequences include additional T1-weighted postcontrast acquisition during the delayed phase and DWI (Table 2).

SUMMARY

CT and MR imaging are central to renal mass detection, characterization, treatment planning, and post-treatment surveillance. Suggested CT protocols are tailored to different clinical indications, balancing diagnostic accuracy and radiation exposure. MR imaging protocols are optimized to take advantage of the improved soft tissue contrast for renal tumor diagnosis and staging. Optimized imaging protocols enable analysis of imaging features that help narrow the differential diagnoses and guide management in patients with renal masses.

DISCLOSURE

J. Chu: nothing to disclose. Z.J. Wang: consultant, GE Healthcare; and shareholder, Nextrast.

REFERENCES

1. Campbell S, Uzzo RG, Allaf ME. Renal cancer: renal mass & localized renal cancer guideline - American Urological Association. American Urological Association. 2017. Available at: https://www.auanet.org/guidelines/renal-cancer-renal-mass-and-localized-renal-cancer-guideline. Accessed November 8, 2019.

2. Silverman SG, Pedrosa I, Ellis JH, et al. Bosniak classification of cystic renal masses, version 2019: an update proposal and needs assessment. Radiology 2019;292(2):475–88.

3. Jonisch AI, Rubinowitz AN, Mutalik PG, et al. Can high-attenuation renal cysts be differentiated from renal cell carcinoma at unenhanced CT? Radiology 2007;243(2):445–50.

4. Agochukwu N, Huber S, Spektor M, et al. Differentiating renal neoplasms from simple cysts on contrast-enhanced CT on the basis of attenuation and homogeneity. Am J Roentgenol 2017;208(4):801–4.

5. Davenport MS, Neville AM, Ellis JH, et al. Diagnosis of renal angiomyolipoma with hounsfield unit thresholds: effect of size of region of interest and nephrographic phase imaging. Radiology 2011;260(1):158–65.

6. Lesavre A, Correas J-M, Merran S, et al. CT of papillary renal cell carcinomas with cholesterol necrosis mimicking angiomyolipomas. Am J Roentgenol 2003;181(1):143–5.

7. Richmond L, Atri M, Sherman C, et al. Renal cell carcinoma containing macroscopic fat on CT mimics an angiomyolipoma due to bone metaplasia without macroscopic calcification. Br J Radiol 2010;83(992):e179–81.

8. Prando A. Intratumoral fat in a renal cell carcinoma. AJR Am J Roentgenol 1991;156(4):871.

9. Hélénon O, Merran S, Paraf F, et al. Unusual fat-containing tumors of the kidney: a diagnostic dilemma. Radiographics 1997;17(1):129–44.

10. Lai BMH, Ka SYJ, Kan WK, et al. Case 237: renal cell carcinoma with osseous metaplasia. Radiology 2016;282(1):293–8.

11. Yuh BI, Cohan RH. Different phases of renal enhancement: role in detecting and characterizing renal masses during helical CT. Am J Roentgenol 1999;173(3):747–55.

12. Lee-Felker SA, Felker ER, Tan N, et al. Qualitative and quantitative MDCT features for differentiating clear cell renal cell carcinoma from other solid renal cortical masses. AJR Am J Roentgenol 2014;203(5):W516–24.

13. Wang ZJ, Davenport MS, Silverman SG, et al. CT renal mass protocols v1.0. Society of Abdominal Radiology Disease Focused Panel on Renal Cell Carcinoma 2017. Available at: https://cdn.ymaws.com/www.abdominalradiology.org/resource/resmgr/education_dfp/RCC/RCC.CTprotocolsfinal-7-15-17.pdf.

14. Purysko AS, Nikolaidis P, Dogra VS, et al. ACR appropriateness criteria® post-treatment follow-up and active surveillance of clinically localized renal cell cancer. J Am Coll Radiol 2019;16(11S):S399–416.

15. Heilbrun ME, Casalino DD, Beland MD, et al. ACR appropriateness criteria® indeterminate renal mass. Available at: https://acsearch.acr.org/docs/69367/Narrative/. Accessed October 13, 2019.

16. Wang ZJ, Westphalen AC, Zagoria RJ. CT and MRI of small renal masses. Br J Radiol 2018;91(1087):20180131.

17. Campbell N, Rosenkrantz AB, Pedrosa I. MRI phenotype in renal cancer: is it clinically relevant? Top Magn Reson Imaging 2014;23(2):95–115.

18. Allen BC, Tirman P, Jennings Clingan M, et al. Characterizing solid renal neoplasms with MRI in adults. Abdom Imaging 2014;39(2):358–87.

19. Kang SK, Huang WC, Pandharipande PV, et al. Solid renal masses: what the numbers tell us. Am J Roentgenol 2014;202(6):1196–206.

20. Young JR, Margolis D, Sauk S, et al. Clear cell renal cell carcinoma: discrimination from other renal cell carcinoma subtypes and oncocytoma at multiphasic multidetector CT. Radiology 2013;267(2):444–53.

21. Egbert ND, Caoili EM, Cohan RH, et al. Differentiation of papillary renal cell carcinoma subtypes on CT and MRI. Am J Roentgenol 2013;201(2):347–55.

22. Chawla SN, Crispen PL, Hanlon AL, et al. The natural history of observed enhancing renal masses: meta-analysis and review of the world literature. J Urol 2006;175(2):425–31.

23. Rosales JC, Haramis G, Moreno J, et al. Active surveillance for renal cortical neoplasms. J Urol 2010;183(5):1698–702.

24. Guite KM, Hinshaw JL, Ranallo FN, et al. Ionizing radiation in abdominal CT: unindicated multiphase scans are an important source of medically

unnecessary exposure. J Am Coll Radiol 2011;8(11): 756–61.

25. Mayo-Smith WW, Hara AK, Mahesh M, et al. How I do it: managing radiation dose in CT. Radiology 2014;273(3):657–72.

26. Choudhary S, Rajesh A, Mayer NJ, et al. Renal onco-cytoma: CT features cannot reliably distinguish on-cocytoma from other renal neoplasms. Clin Radiol 2009;64(5):517–22.

27. Yamada Y, Jinzaki M, Tanami Y, et al. Model-based iterative reconstruction technique for ultralow-dose computed tomography of the lung: a pilot study. Invest Radiol 2012;47(8):482–9.

28. Pontana F, Pagniez J, Flohr T, et al. Chest computed tomography using iterative reconstruction vs filtered back projection (part 1): evaluation of image noise reduction in 32 patients. Eur Radiol 2011;21(3): 627–35.

29. Pontana F, Pagniez J, Duhamel A, et al. Reduced-dose low-voltage chest CT angiography with Sinogram-affirmed iterative reconstruction versus standard-dose filtered back projection. Radiology 2013;267(2):609–18.

30. Hur BY, Lee JM, Joo I, et al. Liver computed tomog-raphy with low tube voltage and model-based itera-tive reconstruction algorithm for hepatic vessel evaluation in living liver donor candidates. J Comput Assist Tomogr 2014;38(3):367–75.

31. Yu MH, Lee JM, Yoon J-H, et al. Low tube voltage in-termediate tube current liver MDCT: sinogram-affirmed iterative reconstruction algorithm for detection of hypervascular hepatocellular carci-noma. Am J Roentgenol 2013;201(1):23–32.

32. Gervaise A, Naulet P, Beuret F, et al. Low-dose CT with automatic tube current modulation, adaptive statistical iterative reconstruction, and low tube voltage for the diagnosis of renal colic: impact of body mass index. AJR Am J Roentgenol 2014; 202(3):553–60.

33. Padole A, Ali Khawaja RD, Kalra MK, et al. CT radi-ation dose and iterative reconstruction techniques. Am J Roentgenol 2015;204(4):W384–92.

34. Shampain KL, Davenport MS, Cohan RH, et al. Ef-fect of model-based iterative reconstruction on CT number measurements within small (10–29 mm) low-attenuation renal masses. Am J Roentgenol 2015;205(1):85–9.

35. Greffier J, Macri F, Larbi A, et al. Dose reduction with iterative reconstruction: optimization of CT protocols in clinical practice. Diagn Interv Imaging 2015;96(5): 477–86.

36. Ehman EC, Yu L, Manduca A, et al. Methods for clin-ical evaluation of noise reduction techniques in ab-dominopelvic CT. Radiographics 2014;34(4):849–62.

37. Krishna S, Murray CA, McInnes MD, et al. CT imag-ing of solid renal masses: pitfalls and solutions. Clin Radiol 2017;72(9):708–21.

38. Mileto A, Nelson RC, Paulson EK, et al. Dual-energy MDCT for imaging the renal mass. Am J Roentgenol 2015;204(6):W640–7.

39. Silva AC, Morse BG, Hara AK, et al. Dual-energy (spectral) CT: applications in abdominal imaging. Radiographics 2011;31(4):1031–46.

40. Mileto A, Marin D, Ramirez-Giraldo JC, et al. Accu-racy of contrast-enhanced dual-energy MDCT for the assessment of iodine uptake in renal lesions. Am J Roentgenol 2014;202(5):W466–74.

41. Ascenti G, Mileto A, Krauss B, et al. Distinguishing enhancing from nonenhancing renal masses with dual-source dual-energy CT: iodine quantification versus standard enhancement measurements. Eur Radiol 2013;23(8):2288–95.

42. Kaza RK, Caoili EM, Cohan RH, et al. Distinguishing enhancing from nonenhancing renal lesions with fast kilovoltage-switching dual-energy CT. Am J Roent-genol 2011;197(6):1375–81.

43. Marin D, Davis D, Roy Choudhury K, et al. Charac-terization of small focal renal lesions: diagnostic accuracy with single-phase contrast-enhanced dual-energy CT with material attenuation analysis compared with conventional attenuation measure-ments. Radiology 2017;284(3):737–47.

44. Mileto A, Allen BC, Pietryga JA, et al. Characteriza-tion of incidental renal mass with dual-energy CT: diagnostic accuracy of effective atomic number maps for discriminating nonenhancing cysts from enhancing masses. AJR Am J Roentgenol 2017; 209(4):W221–30.

45. Mileto A, Nelson RC, Samei E, et al. Impact of dual-energy multi–detector row CT with virtual monochromatic imaging on renal cyst pseudoenhancement: in vitro and in vivo study. Radiology 2014;272(3):767–76.

46. Cha D, Kim CK, Park JJ, et al. Evaluation of hyper-dense renal lesions incidentally detected on single-phase post-contrast CT using dual-energy CT. Br J Radiol 2016;89(1062):20150860.

47. Liu X I, Zhou J j, Zeng MS, et al. Homogeneous high attenuation renal cysts and solid masses–differentia-tion with single phase dual energy computed to-mography. Clin Radiol 2013;68(4):e198–205.

48. Mileto A, Sofue K, Marin D. Imaging the renal lesion with dual-energy multidetector CT and multi-energy applications in clinical practice: what can it truly do for you? Eur Radiol 2016;26(10):3677–90.

49. Herts BR, Silverman SG, Hindman NM, et al. Man-agement of the incidental renal mass on CT: a white paper of the ACR incidental findings committee. J Am Coll Radiol 2018;15(2):264–73.

50. Dilauro M, Quon M, McInnes MDF, et al. Comparison of contrast-enhanced multiphase renal protocol CT versus MRI for diagnosis of papillary renal cell carci-noma. Am J Roentgenol 2016;206(2):319–25.

51. Low RN, Ma J, Panchal N. Fast spin-echo triple-echo Dixon: initial clinical experience with a novel

pulse sequence for fat-suppressed T2-weighted abdominal MR imaging. J Magn Reson Imaging 2009;30(3):569–77.

52. Lu DS, Saini S, Hahn PF, et al. T2-weighted MR imaging of the upper part of the abdomen: should fat suppression be used routinely? AJR Am J Roentgenol 1994;162(5):1095–100.

53. Pedrosa I, Sun MR, Spencer M, et al. MR imaging of renal masses: correlation with findings at surgery and pathologic analysis. Radiographics 2008; 28(4):985–1003.

54. Smith AD, Remer EM, Cox KL, et al. Bosniak category IIF and III cystic renal lesions: outcomes and associations. Radiology 2012;262(1):152–60.

55. Jhaveri K, Gupta P, Elmi A, et al. Cystic renal cell carcinomas: do they grow, metastasize, or recur? AJR Am J Roentgenol 2013;201(2):W292–6.

56. Hindman NM, Bosniak MA, Rosenkrantz AB, et al. Multilocular cystic renal cell carcinoma: comparison of imaging and pathologic findings. Am J Roentgenol 2012;198(1):W20–6.

57. Suzigan S, López-Beltrán A, Montironi R, et al. Multilocular cystic renal cell carcinoma: a report of 45 cases of a kidney tumor of low malignant potential. Am J Clin Pathol 2006;125(2):217–22.

58. Pedrosa I, Chou MT, Ngo L, et al. MR classification of renal masses with pathologic correlation. Eur Radiol 2008;18(2):365–75.

59. Oliva MR, Glickman JN, Zou KH, et al. Renal cell carcinoma: t1 and t2 signal intensity characteristics of papillary and clear cell types correlated with pathology. AJR Am J Roentgenol 2009;192(6): 1524–30.

60. Hindman N, Ngo L, Genega EM, et al. Angiomyolipoma with minimal fat: can it be differentiated from clear cell renal cell carcinoma by using standard MR techniques? Radiology 2012;265(2): 468–77.

61. Rosenkrantz AB, Raj S, Babb JS, et al. Comparison of 3D two-point Dixon and standard 2D dual-echo breath-hold sequences for detection and quantification of fat content in renal angiomyolipoma. Eur J Radiol 2012;81(1):47–51.

62. Low RN, Panchal N, Vu AT, et al. Three-dimensional fast spoiled gradient-echo dual echo (3D-FSPGR-DE) with water reconstruction: preliminary experience with a novel pulse sequence for gadolinium-enhanced abdominal MR imaging. J Magn Reson Imaging 2008;28(4):946–56.

63. Israel GM, Hindman N, Hecht E, et al. The use of opposed-phase chemical shift MRI in the diagnosis of renal angiomyolipomas. Am J Roentgenol 2005; 184(6):1868–72.

64. Karlo CA, Donati OF, Burger IA, et al. MR imaging of renal cortical tumours: qualitative and quantitative chemical shift imaging parameters. Eur Radiol 2013;23(6):1738–44.

65. Yoshimitsu K, Honda H, Kuroiwa T, et al. MR detection of cytoplasmic fat in clear cell renal cell carcinoma utilizing chemical shift gradient-echo imaging. J Magn Reson Imaging 1999;9(4):579–85.

66. Outwater EK, Bhatia M, Siegelman ES, et al. Lipid in renal clear cell carcinoma: detection on opposed-phase gradient-echo MR images. Radiology 1997; 205(1):103–7.

67. Granter SR, Perez-Atayde AR, Renshaw AA. Cytologic analysis of papillary renal cell carcinoma. Cancer 1998;84(5):303–8.

68. Rofsky NM, Lee VS, Laub G, et al. Abdominal MR imaging with a volumetric interpolated breath-hold examination. Radiology 1999;212(3):876–84.

69. Kim MJ, Mitchell DG, Ito K, et al. Hepatic MR imaging: comparison of 2D and 3D gradient echo techniques. Abdom Imaging 2001;26(3):269–76.

70. Zhang J, Pedrosa I, Rofsky NM. MR techniques for renal imaging. Radiol Clin North Am 2003;41(5): 877–907.

71. Morelli JN, Runge VM, Ai F, et al. An image-based approach to understanding the physics of MR artifacts. Radiographics 2011;31(3):849–66.

72. Sun MRM, Ngo L, Genega EM, et al. Renal cell carcinoma: dynamic contrast-enhanced MR imaging for differentiation of tumor subtypes—correlation with pathologic findings. Radiology 2009;250(3): 793–802.

73. Sandrasegaran K, Sundaram CP, Ramaswamy R, et al. Usefulness of diffusion-weighted imaging in the evaluation of renal masses. AJR Am J Roentgenol 2010;194(2):438–45.

74. Kim S, Jain M, Harris AB, et al. T1 hyperintense renal lesions: characterization with diffusion-weighted MR imaging versus contrast-enhanced MR imaging. Radiology 2009;251(3):796–807.

75. Taouli B, Thakur RK, Mannelli L, et al. Renal lesions: characterization with diffusion-weighted imaging versus contrast-enhanced MR imaging. Radiology 2009;251(2):398–407.

76. Wang H, Cheng L, Zhang X, et al. Renal cell carcinoma: diffusion-weighted MR imaging for subtype differentiation at 3.0 T. Radiology 2010;257(1): 135–43.

77. Yoshida S, Masuda H, Ishii C, et al. Usefulness of diffusion-weighted MRI in diagnosis of upper urinary tract cancer. AJR Am J Roentgenol 2011;196(1): 110–6.

78. Nguyen DD, Rakita D. Renal lymphoma: MR appearance with diffusion-weighted imaging. J Comput Assist Tomogr 2013;37(5):840–2.

79. Aslan A, İnan İ, Aktan A, et al. The utility of ADC measurement techniques for differentiation of low- and high-grade clear cell RCC. Pol J Radiol 2018; 83:e446–51.

80. Yoshida R, Yoshizako T, Hisatoshi A, et al. The additional utility of apparent diffusion coefficient

values of clear-cell renal cell carcinoma for predicting metastasis during clinical staging. Acta Radiol Open 2017;6(1). https://doi.org/10.1177/2058460116687174.

81. Wang K, Cheng J, Wang Y, et al. Renal cell carcinoma: preoperative evaluate the grade of histological malignancy using volumetric histogram analysis derived from magnetic resonance diffusion kurtosis imaging. Quant Imaging Med Surg 2019; 9(4):671–80.

82. Jensen JH, Helpern JA. MRI quantification of non-Gaussian water diffusion by kurtosis analysis. NMR Biomed 2010;23(7):698–710.

83. Jensen JH, Helpern JA, Ramani A, et al. Diffusional kurtosis imaging: the quantification of non-gaussian water diffusion by means of magnetic resonance imaging. Magn Reson Med 2005;53(6):1432–40.

84. Murray CA, Quon M, McInnes MDF, et al. Evaluation of T1-weighted MRI to detect intratumoral hemorrhage within papillary renal cell carcinoma as a feature differentiating from angiomyolipoma without visible fat. Am J Roentgenol 2016;207(3):585–91.

85. Sasiwimonphan K, Takahashi N, Leibovich BC, et al. Small (<4 cm) renal mass: differentiation of angiomyolipoma without visible fat from renal cell carcinoma utilizing MR imaging. Radiology 2012;263(1): 160–8.

86. Wang ZJ, Davenport MS, Silverman SG, et al. MRI renal mass protocols v1.0. Society of Abdominal Radiology Disease Focused Panel on Renal Cell Carcinoma 2017. Available at: https://cdn.ymaws.com/www.abdominalradiology.org/resource/resmgr/education_dfp/RCC/RCC.MRIprotocolfinal-7-15-17.pdf.

Image Interpretation
Practical Triage of Benign from Malignant Renal Masses

Evan Allgood, MD[a],*, Steven S. Raman, MD[b]

KEYWORDS

- Kidney • Small enhancing renal mass • Clear cell renal cell carcinoma
- Papillary renal cell carcinoma • Chromophobe renal cell carcinoma • Oncocytoma
- Fat-poor angiomyolipoma

KEY POINTS

- Renal lesions not characterized as Bosniak I/II cysts or angiomyolipoma are indeterminate and require additional imaging characterization.
- Multiphase contrast-enhanced imaging has emerged as a means of characterizing indeterminate renal masses, with clear cell renal cell carcinoma (RCC), papillary RCC, chromophobe RCC, fat-poor angiomyolipoma, and oncocytoma as primary differential considerations.
- Relative corticomedullary enhancement greater than that of adjacent renal cortex of an indeterminate renal mass is a strong predictor for clear cell RCC.
- Multiphase contrast-enhanced imaging allows for quantitative analysis of renal lesions with many emerging applications, such as radiocytogenetics.

INTRODUCTION

Incidentally discovered renal masses that don't require immediate treatment and are not definitively characteristic of angiomyolipoma (AML) or Bosniak I/II cysts at initial imaging are indeterminate and require further imaging characterization.[1] For indeterminate renal masses, size is the leading determinant of renal mass triage. The larger an indeterminate renal mass, the greater the likelihood of high-grade/malignant disease.[2] Smaller indeterminate masses, conversely, are more likely benign.[2] Despite these observations, small (pT1a or <4 cm in size) indeterminate renal masses comprise 38% of surgically resected renal masses with 20% to 30% found benign on pathologic analysis.[3] Furthermore, given slow growth and low rate of progression/metastasis of small renal cell carcinoma (RCC) lesions, Jewett and colleagues[4] advocate for active surveillance with serial imaging for small RCC. Although these small indeterminate renal masses are traditionally presumed malignant with partial nephrectomy as preferred treatment,[5] accurate image characterization of these lesions will optimize triage to biopsy or ablative/surgical treatment and allow for better selection for active surveillance and to optimize follow-up based on risk of malignancy/benignity. This review focuses on current and evolving methods to triage indeterminate renal masses at multiphase imaging based on assessment of their enhancement characteristics.

NORMAL ANATOMY AND IMAGING TECHNIQUE

Current Society of Abdominal Radiology (SAR) computed tomographic (CT) protocol guidelines

[a] Department of Radiology, University of Southern California, 1500 San Pablo Street 2nd Floor, Los Angeles, CA 90033, USA; [b] Department of Radiology, University of California - Los Angeles, 757 Westwood Plaza Suite 1621, Los Angeles, CA 90095, USA
* Corresponding author.
E-mail address: Evan.Allgood@med.usc.edu

Radiol Clin N Am 58 (2020) 875–884
https://doi.org/10.1016/j.rcl.2020.06.002
0033-8389/20/© 2020 Elsevier Inc. All rights reserved.

advocate for a minimum of unenhanced and nephrographic (120 sec) phases to assess for renal mass enhancement (**Fig. 1**; **Table 1**).[6] Unenhanced imaging provides a baseline to assess for lesion enhancement on subsequent phases and is also sufficient to assess for lesion homogeneity, macroscopic fat, and calcification.[7] Uniform enhancement of the renal cortex and medulla during the nephrographic phase optimizes detection of heterogeneously enhancing lesions.

Corticomedullary and excretory postcontrast CT phases are optional per the SAR, but can be very helpful in delineating renal vascular and collecting system anatomy before any intervention that may be pursued.[6] These additional phases also provide additional postcontrast time points to assess enhancement characteristics of renal masses.

Radiation exposure represents a significant risk for those undergoing CT surveillance, particularly given the prevalence of this modality in the medical community. Radiation dose of CT must be minimized, particularly in younger patients, because the equivalent of 8 lifetime CT scans theoretically increases lifetime cancer risk from 1/1000 to 1/82.[8] As more is understood about differentiation of small indeterminate masses, directed measures must be taken to minimize radiation dose.

Dynamic contrast-enhanced MRI is a robust alternative technique for indeterminate renal mass characterization with similar lesion enhancement characteristics demonstrated as compared with CT (see **Fig. 1**, **Table 1**).[9] In addition to assessment of enhancement characteristics, MRI has the added benefit of T2-weighted, opposed phase, and diffusion-weighted imaging (DWI). Although generally tolerated well, MRI has unique limitations, primarily related to patient factors, such as motion, body habitus, claustrophobia, metallic implanted devices, and foreign bodies. In addition, MRI acquisition times are generally significantly longer than for CT, and the examinations are more costly.

Contrast-enhanced ultrasound (CEUS) evaluation of indeterminate renal masses has been promising with less scan time than MRI, minimal risk of contrast morbidity, and no radiation exposure.[10] Unlike CT and MRI, CEUS contrast boluses can be given multiple times during imaging acquisition, although this modality can be significantly limited in patients with large body habitus. CEUS image acquisition can also be difficult to reproduce, with a high level of interoperator variability.

Effective and safe active imaging surveillance of indeterminate renal masses requires judicious use of CT to minimize radiation dose. Periodic use of MRI and CEUS can allow for longer intervals between CT scans during the surveillance period with resultant decrease in patient radiation exposure.

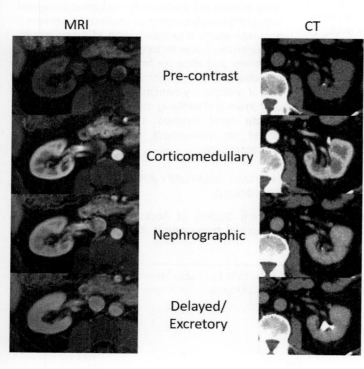

MRI   CT

Pre-contrast

Corticomedullary

Nephrographic

Delayed/
Excretory

Fig. 1. Precontrast, corticomedullary, nephrographic, and delayed/excretory phases on both CT and MRI.

Table 1
Imaging protocols

CT[6]

Contrast: Low or isoosmolar, 35–52.5 g iodine (approximately 100–150 mL of 350 mg iodine/mL), rate: 2–5 mL/s

Phase	Anatomic Coverage	Acquisition	Reconstructions	Additional reformats
Precontrast	Kidneys only	Axial	3-mm slices, with or without 50% overlap	
Corticomedullary	Kidneys only	Axial, 40- to 70-s delay	3-mm slices, with or without 50% overlap	Coronal/sagittal, 3-mm slices without overlap
Nephrographic	Kidneys only	Axial, 100- to 120-s delay	3-mm slices, with or without 50% overlap	Coronal/sagittal, 3-mm slices without overlap
Excretory	Diaphragm to iliac crests	Axial, 7- to 10-min delay	3-mm slices, with or without 50% overlap	Coronal/sagittal, 3-mm slices without overlap

MRI[9]

Contrast: Extracellular gadolinium-based, 0.1 mL/kg, rate: 1–2 mL/s followed by 10–20 mL saline

Sequence	Planes/Thickness/Gap	Details/Alternatives
2D T2 SSFSE	Axial/4–5 mm/no gap Coronal/5–6 mm/no gap	2D T2 FSE/4- to 5-mm slice thickness/no gap
2D T1 GRE in/out of phase	Axial/5–6 mm/0.5–1 mm	3D Dixon/3 to 4-mm slice thickness/no gap
3D T1 SPGR fat saturation, precontrast	Axial/3–4 mm/no gap Coronal/3–4 mm/no gap	
3D T1 dynamic SPGR fat saturation, postcontrast	Axial/3–4 mm/no gap Coronal/3–4 mm/no gap	Postcontrast timing: 30, 90–100, 180–210 s, 5–7 min Obtain subtraction images as well
Diffusion-weighted imaging	Axial/5–6 mm/no gap	B values: 0–50, 400–500, 800–1000 s/mm^2

Abbreviations: GRE, gradient echo; SSFSE, single-shot fast spin echo; SPGR, spoiled gradient recalled.

IMAGING FINDINGS/PATHOLOGY

Incidentally discovered renal masses with macroscopic fat and absence of calcification on any precontrast or postcontrast phase enables confident diagnosis of AML, especially if the lesion is exophytic and of soft contour conforming to the surrounding renal parenchyma and perirenal tissues.[1] Bosniak I/II cysts are characterized on unenhanced imaging based on homogeneity, CT attenuation values, or magnetic resonance (MR) T1 and T2 characteristics. Bosniak I/II cysts should also demonstrate absence of enhancement on all modalities. In lesions that enhance in the nephrographic phase and that lack macroscopic fat, the 5 primary differential considerations are clear cell, papillary or chromophobe RCC, oncocytoma, and fat-poor (FP) AML.

Under the current paradigm, these 5 subtypes of enhancing renal mass cannot be reliably differentiated based on enhancement characteristics derived only from unenhanced and nephrographic phases. If an enhancing small renal mass is detected, resection or ablation of the lesion with preservation of as many nephrons as possible represent the most definitive treatment options. Tissue diagnosis of the lesion is derived from the surgical specimen or a biopsy performed in conjunction with ablation. Accurate imaging-based subtyping of enhancing indeterminate renal masses will enable appropriate triage to biopsy, ablative or surgical treatment and will improve active surveillance.

Given the broad differential diagnosis of small enhancing renal masses, which includes both malignant and benign entities, additional postcontrast phases are used to more specifically characterize indeterminate renal masses. Corticomedullary and excretory phases provide additional time points at which to assess lesion enhancement. Birnbaum and colleagues[11] recognized the need for both corticomedullary and nephrographic phases to best assess for indeterminate renal mass enhancement, particularly for lesions that demonstrate peak enhancement later than the corticomedullary phase. In a small pilot study in 2000, Jinzaki and colleagues[12] initially demonstrated differences between the most common renal mass subtypes based on their absolute peak enhancement and deenhancement in the corticomedullary and nephrographic phases, although these differences were not found to be statistically significant.

Generally, clear cell renal cell carcinomas (ccRCC) are round, oval, or lobular lesions that enhance heterogeneously and have a peak absolute HU greater than 160 on corticomedullary phase with unenhanced HU between 25 and 40, nephrographic HU at about 120, and excretory phase HU of approximately 100. Oncocytomas, the most common benign mimic of ccRCC, tend to be round or oval lesions that enhance more homogenously with peak corticomedullary HU 140 to 160 with deenhancement in the nephrographic phase near 120 HU and excretory phase HU values of about 100. Chromophobe RCC tend to be larger and more heterogenous compared with oncocytoma with peak enhancement in the nephrographic phase and excretory phase HU of 60 to 80. Patients with FP AML tend to be younger than patients with RCC. FP AML

lesions tend to be ovoid- or mushroom-shaped space-occupying lesions that are typically 45 to 55 HU on unenhanced scans, with homogenous peak absolute enhancement of about 140 HU in the corticomedullary phase with deenhancement in the nephrographic and excretory phases at 100 to 120 and 80 to 100 HU, respectively. Finally, papillary RCCs tend to measure 40 to 50 HU on unenhanced scans and have absolute peak attenuation of 80 HU in the nephrographic phase with mild deenhancement to about 60 HU in the excretory phase.[13] Unfortunately, there is overlap between several of the above characteristics that make indeterminate renal mass characterization difficult under the current paradigm (Fig. 2).

MRI can add more information, with T2 signal (tends to be low in FP AML and papillary RCC with higher signal noted in ccRCC; Figs. 3 and 4), opposed phase imaging (signal drop of 20% may be seen in 20%–40% of FP AML and ccRCC because of microscopic fat, whereas signal gain may be seen in papillary RCC because of hemosiderin), and DWI (papillary RCC has increased restriction and low ADC compared with ccRCC; Fig. 5) demonstrating additional utility in the characterization of indeterminate renal masses alongside qualitative and quantitative absolute and relative lesion enhancement.[14]

More recent CT and MR studies in the past 10 years with much larger cohorts have confirmed that the absolute peak enhancement of ccRCC is significantly greater than all other lesions in the corticomedullary phase with rapid deenhancement in the nephrographic and excretory phases,

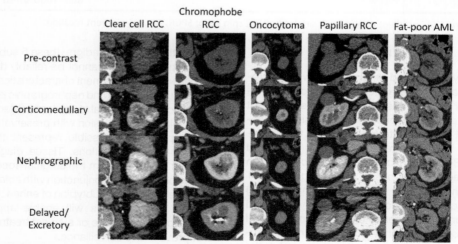

Fig. 2. Differential considerations for indeterminate renal masses shown at precontrast, corticomedullary, nephrographic, and excretory/delayed phases. Although there are some characteristics that allow for differentiation between these lesions, there is significant overlap in the subjective appearances of oncocytoma, FP AML, clear cell, papillary, and chromophobe RCC.

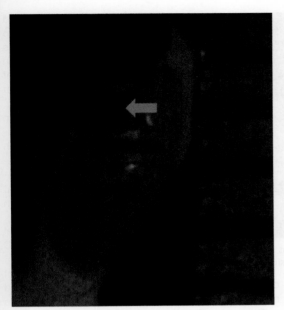

Fig. 3. A T2-weighted image shows characteristic hypointensity of a papillary RCC (*arrow*).

enabling quantitative and qualitative discriminative signatures and quantitative subtyping of enhancing indeterminate renal masses.[13–15] Lee-Felker and colleagues[13] also reported that the peak relative enhancement of ccRCC (enhancement above the renal cortical background) was

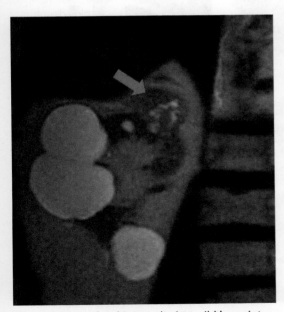

Fig. 4. A T2-weighted image depicts mild hyperintensity and heterogeneity within a ccRCC (*arrow*). Additional homogeneous T2 hyperintense simple cysts are also seen within the right kidney.

significantly higher in comparison to the other common lesions. Similar absolute and relative enhancement features of ccRCC have also been demonstrated on contrast ultrasound (CEUS).[10] Refinement of methods and increasing sample sizes over the years have demonstrated more reliable and accurate differentiation of enhancing indeterminate renal masses at imaging. This review summarizes many of these methods.

Mean Enhancement

Bird and colleagues[16] demonstrated a statistically significant difference in mean enhancement between oncocytoma and all types of RCC. This study used the entire lesion as a region of interest (ROI), including areas of hypoenhancing scar and necrosis. Because RCC has a much higher propensity for necrosis than oncocytoma, using the entire lesion likely underestimated the peak enhancement of these lesions and may have precluded differentiation between the subtypes of RCC in this study.

Absolute Enhancement

Absolute enhancement is based on the peak Hounsfield unit attenuation (HU) of small ROIs placed on the most enhancing portions of the lesion in the corticomedullary phase and in the same location across other phases (unenhanced, nephrographic, and excretory). Overall, there is statistically significant increased absolute enhancement of ccRCC compared with papillary RCC, chromophobe RCC, FP AML, and oncocytoma in the corticomedullary phase with narrow confidence intervals[13,15] (see **Fig. 2**).

Peak enhancement in the nephrographic phase has been shown to be suboptimal for lesion characterization because the mean peak HU for almost all lesions except papillary RCC tends to cluster in a narrow range between 70 and 90 HU. Papillary RCC tends to have peak absolute enhancement during the nephrographic phase near 70 to 80 HU, which is significantly less than the peak enhancement of ccRCC during the corticomedullary phase. Chromophobe RCC lesions can show peak enhancement in either the corticomedullary or the nephrographic phase[15] (Fig. 6). Absolute nephrographic phase enhancement of high Fuhrman grade ccRCC lesions was statistically significantly decreased compared with low-grade lesions.[17] These results were further corroborated by Coy and colleagues,[18] more specifically showing that nephrographic phase enhancement less than 52.1 HU is a statistically significant predictor of high-grade ccRCC lesions.

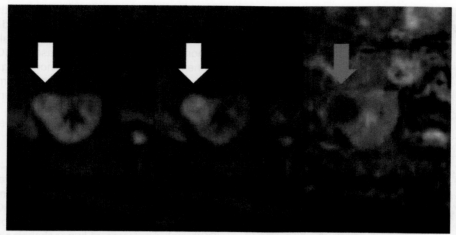

Fig. 5. A papillary RCC depicts increasing signal on DWI as the b value increases from 400 to 800 (*white arrows*) compatible with restriction of diffusion with diminished signal on ADC (*red arrow*).

Absolute enhancement at the excretory phase is derived from HU values taken from ROIs, including the same portion of the indeterminate renal mass on both unenhanced and excretory phases. The difference between these 2 values results in the absolute excretory phase enhancement of the mass.

There was statistically significant increased absolute enhancement of ccRCC compared with

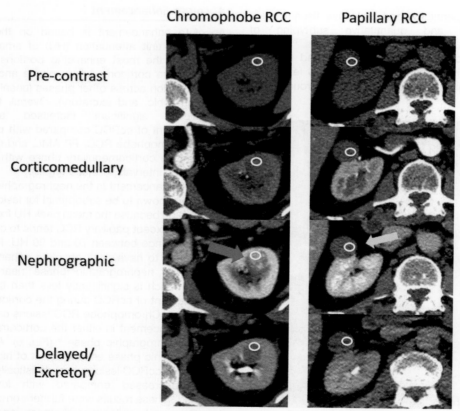

Fig. 6. Precontrast and postcontrast phases of chromophobe and papillary RCC depicting subtle absolute peak enhancement in the nephrographic phase (*red and yellow arrows*, respectively). ROIs placed on these lesions demonstrate precontrast, corticomedullary, nephrographic, and excretory phase HU of 13, 39, 144, and 50 for the chromophobe lesion and 29, 35, 42, and 25 for the papillary lesion, respectively.

papillary RCC, chromophobe RCC, and oncocytoma at the excretory phase with nonoverlapping confidence intervals.[15] Absolute excretory phase enhancement of high Fuhrman grade ccRCC lesions was statistically significantly decreased compared with low-grade ccRCC lesions on excretory phase.[17]

Although most research focused on absolute enhancement characteristics of indeterminate renal masses have been derived from CT, both Sun and colleagues[14] and Young and colleagues[19] have shown similar results on dynamic contrast-enhanced multiphasic MRI, with ccRCC showing the greatest magnitude of peak absolute enhancement and deenhancement, followed by FP AML, oncocytoma, and chromophobe with papillary RCC demonstrating the least absolute enhancement.

The magnitude of absolute enhancement has also been correlated with radiocytogenetics. The gain of chromosome 12 in ccRCC is associated with higher tumor grade and worse prognosis. Absolute enhancement of ccRCC with gain of chromosome 12 has been shown to be significantly higher on nephrographic and excretory phases compared with ccRCC with no gain of chromosome 12.[20]

Relative Enhancement

Relative enhancement is a novel variant quantitative concept that has been used to successfully differentiate subtypes of indeterminate renal masses. Relative enhancement is calculated as peak absolute enhancement of the mass subtracted from the peak enhancement of background uninvolved renal cortex with a comparably sized ROI on each phase, thus controlling for patients who may have intrinsic renal dysfunction or variable enhancement owing to diminished cardiac output or renal artery stenosis. The formula is as follows, with all values taken from the same postcontrast phase: [(Mass ROI − Uninvolved cortex ROI)/Uninvolved cortex ROI] × 100%.[13] Relative corticomedullary attenuation greater than 0% supports a positive predictive value of 90% in favor of ccRCC[13] (Fig. 7). Lesions greater than 45 HU on unenhanced phases that have less than 10% relative corticomedullary attenuation can be differentiated from ccRCC with 97% negative predictive value.[13]

Analysis of relative enhancement characteristics has been applied to differentiate between type 1 and type 2 papillary RCC, with significantly greater relative attenuation of type 2 papillary RCC compared with type 1 on excretory phase.[21]

Similar to absolute enhancement, most studies on relative enhancement have focused on CT. In their 2007 study, Sun and colleagues[14] initially showed that ccRCC had the greatest relative enhancement compared with chromophobe and papillary RCC. Young and colleagues[19] reproduced their multidetector CT results on MRI and showed that ccRCC is the only lesion to routinely enhance above background cortex compared with both chromophobe RCC and papillary RCC. Oncocytoma and FP AML showed a similar relationship, but with narrower confidence intervals. A similar relationship between lesion enhancement and that of adjacent cortex has been demonstrated on CEUS as well.[10]

In correlating markers of aggressive ccRCC, such as those lacking phosphatase and tension homolog (PTEN) expression, relative corticomedullary CT enhancement was found to be

Clear cell RCC

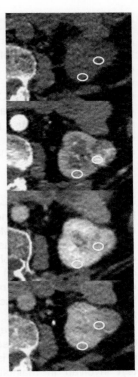

Pre-contrast

Corticomedullary

Nephrographic

Delayed/
Excretory

Fig. 7. Precontrast and postcontrast CTs depict relative enhancement assessment of a ccRCC with ROIs placed over the area with peak corticomedullary enhancement as well as an area of uninvolved cortex on all phases. The relative enhancement of this lesion, as calculated with the formula described in the text, is 77% in the corticomedullary phase, −24% in the nephrographic phase, and −29% in the excretory phase.

significantly less in PTEN-negative ccRCC compared with PTEN expressing RCC. PTEN is implicated in tumor cell growth, metabolism, and tumorigenesis, and lack of its expression is associated with worse survival, poor response to anti-VEGF and anti-EGF therapies, higher Fuhrman grade, and higher likelihood of lymph node metastasis.[22]

Cytogenetic correlations with CT-based relative enhancement have also been significant. Relative nephrographic phase enhancement was significantly lower in ccRCC with loss of Y chromosome compared with those without loss of Y. ccRCC lesions with loss of Y chromosome have been associated with higher T stage, higher Fuhrman grade, and greater risk of metastatic disease.[23] ccRCC with gain of chromosome 20 had significantly less relative nephrographic and excretory enhancement compared with lesions without gain of 20. Gain of chromosome 20 is associated with a higher rate of tumor recurrence.[24]

Absolute Deenhancement

Absolute deenhancement is derived from subtracting the peak ROI of a lesion in the nephrographic phase from peak ROI in the corticomedullary phase. This parameter is significantly increased in ccRCC compared with oncocytoma. Lee-Felker and colleagues[13] also showed a 90% positive predictive value favoring ccRCC in lesions that demonstrate less than 50 HU of absolute deenhancement.

Relative Washout

Relative washout is another quantitative tool and is calculated as follows: [(Mass attenuation, corticomedullary phase – Mass attenuation, nephrographic, OR excretory phase)/(Mass attenuation, corticomedullary phase)] × 100%. This equation can be used to calculate relative washout for either the nephrographic or excretory phase, as shown above.

Levels of carbonic anhydrase-IX (CA-IX) in ccRCC have been assessed using relative nephrographic washout. CA-IX is a transmembrane protein involved in maintaining cellular pH. Low levels are associated with poor prognosis, and high levels are associated with good response to interleukin-2 immunotherapy. ccRCC lesions with high levels of CA-IX showed significantly higher relative nephrographic washout and a trend toward significantly higher relative excretory washout compared with lesions with low levels of CA-IX.[25]

SUMMARY

Quantitative parameters derived from multiphase imaging of small indeterminate masses have proven useful for differentiation of ccRCC from chromophobe/papillary RCC, FP AML, and oncocytoma. More investigation is needed to more reliably differentiate between chromophobe/papillary RCC, FP AML, and oncocytoma by multiphase imaging, although early results show promise. Accurate differentiation of these lesions by multiphase imaging at initial characterization will allow for better triage of patients for renal mass biopsy, ablation, and resection and also will strengthen the role of multiphase imaging in active surveillance.

Diagnostic Features Useful for Characterization

Clear cell renal cell carcinoma

- Heterogeneous, even at small size
- Peak enhancement in corticomedullary phase
- Relative enhancement in corticomedullary phase greater than 0
- Mild T2 hyperintensity
- Can have signal drop out on out-of-phase imaging, owing to microscopic fat

Papillary renal cell carcinoma

- More likely to be homogeneous than clear cell renal cell carcinoma at small size
- Peak enhancement in nephrographic phase
- Relative enhancement less than 0 in all phases
- Restricted diffusion
- T2 hypointense

Chromophobe renal cell carcinoma

- Peak enhancement in corticomedullary or nephrographic phase
- Relative enhancement less than 0 in all phases

Oncocytoma

- Mimic of clear cell renal cell carcinoma
- Peak enhancement in corticomedullary phase
- Relative enhancement less than 0 in all phases

Fat-poor angiomyolipoma

- Peak enhancement in corticomedullary phase
- Relative enhancement less than 0 in all phases
- Tends to be >45 HU on unenhanced CT
- T2 hypointense

Summary Points

- Clear cell RCC is the only lesion with relative enhancement reliably greater than 0

- FP AML tends to be >45 HU on unenhanced CT

- Despite the findings above, RCC cannot and should not be excluded in lesions that do not fulfill diagnostic criteria of lipid rich AML or Bosniak I/II cysts

- T2 hypointensity is most strongly associated with FP AML and papillary RCC

What the Referring Physician Needs to Know

- RCC cannot be excluded based on imaging alone, but if an indeterminate renal mass also has characteristics of a benign lesion, this should be clearly stated as an additional differential consideration.

REFERENCES

1. Herts BR, Silverman SG, Hindman NM, et al. Management of the incidental renal mass on CT: a White Paper of the ACR Incidental Findings Committee. J Am Coll Radiol 2018;15(2):264–73.

2. Frank I, Blute ML, Cheville JC, et al. Solid renal tumors: an analysis of pathological features related to tumor size. J Urol 2003;170(6):2217–20.

3. Gill IS, Aron M, Gervais DA, et al. Small renal mass. N Engl J Med 2010;362(7):624–34.

4. Jewett MAS, Mattar K, Basiuk J, et al. Active surveillance of small renal masses: progression patterns of early stage kidney cancer. Eur Urol 2011;60(1):39–44.

5. Motzer RJ, Jonasch E, Agarwal N. NCCN guidelines. Kidney Cancer 2018;59.

6. Wang ZJ, Davenport MS, Silverman SG, et al. CT renal mass protocols v1.0. Society of Abdominal Radiology. 2017. Available at: https://www.abdominalradiology.org/resource/resmgr/education_dfp/RCC/%20RCC.CTprotocolsfinal-7-15-17.pdf. Accessed October 2019.

7. O'Connor SD, Silverman SG, Cochon LR, et al. Renal cancer at unenhanced CT: imaging features, detection rates, and outcomes. Abdom Radiol (NY) 2018;43(7):1756–63.

8. Costello JE, Cecava ND, Tucker JE, et al. CT radiation dose: current controversies and dose reduction strategies. Am J Roentgenol 2013;201(6):1283–90.

9. Wang ZJ, Davenport MS, Silverman SG, et al. MRI renal mass protocol v1.0. Society of Abdominal Radiology. 2017. Available at: https://www.abdominalradiology.org/resource/resmgr/education_dfp/RCC/%20RCC.MRIprotocolfinal-7-15-17.pdf. Accessed October 2019.

10. King KG, Gulati M, Malhi H, et al. Quantitative assessment of solid renal masses by contrast-enhanced ultrasound with time–intensity curves: how we do it. Abdom Imaging 2015;40(7):2461–71.

11. Birnbaum BA, Jacobs JE, Ramchandani P. Multiphasic renal CT: comparison of renal mass enhancement during the corticomedullary and nephrographic phases. Radiology 1996;200(3):753–8.

12. Jinzaki M, Tanimoto A, Mukai M, et al. Double-phase helical CT of small renal parenchymal neoplasms: correlation with pathologic findings and tumor angiogenesis. J Comput Assist Tomogr 2000;24(6):835–42.

13. Lee-Felker SA, Felker ER, Tan N, et al. Qualitative and quantitative MDCT features for differentiating clear cell renal cell carcinoma from other solid renal cortical masses. Am J Roentgenol 2014;203(5):W516–24.

14. Sun MRM, Ngo L, Genega EM, et al. Renal cell carcinoma: dynamic contrast-enhanced MR imaging for differentiation of tumor subtypes—correlation with pathologic findings. Radiology 2009;250(3):793–802.

15. Young JR, Margolis D, Sauk S, et al. Clear cell renal cell carcinoma: discrimination from other renal cell carcinoma subtypes and oncocytoma at multiphasic multidetector CT. Radiology 2013;267(2):444–53.

16. Bird VG, Kanagarajah P, Morillo G, et al. Differentiation of oncocytoma and renal cell carcinoma in small renal masses (<4 cm): the role of 4-phase computerized tomography. World J Urol 2011;29(6):787–92.

17. Coy H, Young JR, Douek ML, et al. Association of qualitative and quantitative imaging features on multiphasic multidetector CT with tumor grade in clear cell renal cell carcinoma. Abdom Radiol (NY) 2019;44(1):180–9.

18. Coy H, Young JR, Pantuck AJ, et al. Association of tumor grade, enhancement on multiphasic CT and microvessel density in patients with clear cell renal cell carcinoma. Abdom Radiol (NY) 2019. https://doi.org/10.1007/s00261-019-02271-1.

19. Young JR, Coy H, Kim HJ, et al. Performance of relative enhancement on multiphasic MRI for the differentiation of clear cell renal cell carcinoma (RCC) from papillary and chromophobe RCC subtypes and oncocytoma. Am J Roentgenol 2017;208(4):812–9.

20. Young JR, Coy H, Douek M, et al. Clear cell renal cell carcinoma: identifying the gain of chromosome 12

on multiphasic MDCT. Abdom Radiol (NY) 2017; 42(1):236–41.

21. Young JR, Coy H, Douek M, et al. Type 1 papillary renal cell carcinoma: differentiation from type 2 papillary RCC on multiphasic MDCT. Abdom Radiol (NY) 2017;42(7):1911–8.

22. Young JR, Coy H, Kim HJ, et al. Clear cell renal cell carcinoma: identifying PTEN expression on multiphasic MDCT. Abdom Radiol (NY) 2018;43(12): 3410–7.

23. Young JR, Coy H, Douek M, et al. Clear cell renal cell carcinoma: identifying the loss of the Y chromosome

on multiphasic MDCT. Am J Roentgenol 2017; 209(2):333–8.

24. Young JR, Young JA, Margolis DJA, et al. Clear cell renal cell carcinoma: identifying the gain of chromosome 20 on multiphasic MDCT. Abdom Radiol (NY) 2016;41(11):2175–81.

25. Young JR, Coy H, Kim HJ, et al. Utility of multiphasic multidetector computed tomography in discriminating between clear cell renal cell carcinomas with high and low carbonic anhydrase-IX expression. Abdom Radiol (NY) 2018;43(10): 2734–42.

Mimics and Pitfalls in Renal Imaging

Erick M. Remer, MD

KEYWORDS

- Technical pitfall • Phase of contrast enhancement • Region of interest • Renal pseudotumor
- Fat-containing renal mass

KEY POINTS

- Not all focal renal abnormalities are malignant tumors; benign neoplasms and posttraumatic, infectious, vascular, and treatment changes can mimic malignancy.
- Attention to technical details when interpreting renal images is paramount; radiologists must consider factors such as the imaging protocol, imaging plane, phase of enhancement, and region-of-interest placement.
- Identification of fat within a renal mass and characterization of the type of fat can narrow the differential diagnosis.

INTRODUCTION

In general terms, much of what we do when characterizing renal lesions involves a binary determination: an abnormality either enhances and is thus more likely to be a tumor or does not enhance and is thus more likely to be a benign lesion. However, there are many instances in which these simplistic rules do not apply. In such cases, clues to making the correct diagnosis may be historical (such as the presence of pyuria and fever or a history of renal trauma or surgery) or may relate to specific imaging features of a focal abnormality (such as shape or the presence of intralesional fat). Further, several technical pitfalls may be encountered when interpreting renal images. These pitfalls may be related to contrast delivery, phase of enhancement, or collecting system opacification after contrast administration; imaging plane orientation with respect to a renal abnormality; use of proper window and level settings during image interpretation; and placement of regions of interest (ROIs) to measure attenuation or signal intensity. In addition, several focal renal lesions can mimic tumors. These pseudotumors may be congenital, may have a vascular origin, may result from prior infection or trauma, or may be related to therapy for renal cell carcinoma (RCC) such as partial nephrectomy or tumor ablation. Finally, the detection of either microscopic or macroscopic fat within renal masses affects the differential diagnosis, and so appropriate methods must be used to detect fat and interpret the resulting images. This article reviews these potential pitfalls in renal imaging.

TECHNICAL PITFALLS

Technical pitfalls in renal imaging may be patient related, image acquisition related, or interpretation related (**Table 1**). When patients move or fail to hold their breath during image acquisition, attenuation measurements may be spuriously increased or decreased, and image degradation and blurring may occur. These misregistration artifacts usually seem as shading or streaking in the reconstructed image.[1]

Sometimes, renal abnormalities may be less well depicted or difficult to identify based on their position in the kidney with respect to the imaging plane. For example, a renal mass in the upper or lower pole may be easily scrolled past when

Imaging Institute and Glickman Urological and Kidney Institute, Cleveland Clinic, 9500 Euclid Avenue, A21, Cleveland, OH 44195, USA
E-mail address: remere1@ccf.org

Radiol Clin N Am 58 (2020) 885–896
https://doi.org/10.1016/j.rcl.2020.05.001
0033-8389/20/© 2020 Elsevier Inc. All rights reserved.

radiologic.theclinics.com

Table 1
Technical pitfalls

Element	Description
Motion	Spurious increased or decreased attenuation
Window level settings	Altered lesion detectability
Imaging plane with respect to lesion location	Decreased lesion visibility in some planes vs in others
Phase of contrast	Diminished detectability in corticomedullary phase
Pseudoenhancement	Spurious increased attenuation in contrast-enhanced phase vs in unenhanced phase

viewed on the PACS workstation but may be more obvious to the reader when visualized in the coronal or sagittal plane (**Fig. 1**). Multiplanar reformatted images can improve the reader's confidence in the identification of small masses that more clearly deform the renal contour when viewed in one plane than in another.[2] A study that assessed missed imaging findings by radiology residents found that 5.5% of missed findings on abdomen and pelvic computed tomographic (CT) images were cases of pyelonephritis and that residents believed that the use of coronal images would help to provide a thorough evaluation of the renal cortices.[3]

The phase of contrast during which imaging occurs can also greatly affect the detectability of renal masses. One study found that nephrographic phase images, when compared with medullary phase images, can show 1.3 times more masses in the renal cortex[4] and 4 to 5 times more masses

in the medulla[3,5] (**Fig. 2**). Although the phases of renal enhancement may vary based on the rate of delivery of contrast material, generally speaking, the corticomedullary phase occurs approximately 30 to 40 seconds after the beginning of contrast administration and the nephrographic phase begins at 80 to 120 seconds.[6] Because the speed of CT scanners has increased, the kidneys are now often visualized during the corticomedullary phase on single-phase, routine abdominal protocol CT scans. Small hyperenhancing clear cell RCCs (ccRCCs) can be particularly difficult to detect during this phase, as these lesions may be isoattenuating to normal parenchyma in the corticomedullary phase and may only be discernible based on subtle interruption of normal corticomedullary enhancement or heterogeneous tumor enhancement (**Fig. 3**).

Another technical pitfall encountered in renal imaging is the phenomenon of pseudoenhancement, which involves mischaracterizing a renal cyst as an enhancing neoplasm because of a false attenuation change between unenhanced and enhanced images. Pseudoenhancement is thought to be the result of multidetector, spiral CT image reconstruction algorithms that adjust for beamhardening effects.[7] Several factors may affect the degree of pseudoenhancement, including lesion size or location, degree of renal parenchymal enhancement, number of CT detector rows, peak tube voltage, and reconstruction kernel.[8] This phenomenon tends to occur most notably with small (<1 cm) and intraparenchymal lesions (**Fig. 4**). If pseudoenhancement is suspected, ultrasound imaging or MR imaging can be used to determine whether the mass is truly cystic or solid.

REGION-OF-INTEREST PLACEMENT AND INTERPRETATION

The placement and interpretation of ROI attenuation measurements for the evaluation of renal masses can also be problematic. The most

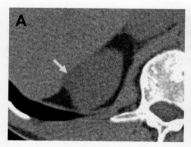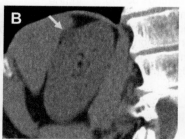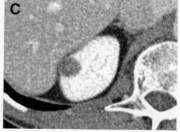

Fig. 1. (*A*) Axial unenhanced CT of right kidney shows barely discernible upper pole pRCC (*arrow*) that is more obvious (*arrow*) on coronal unenhanced multiplanar reformatted (MPR) (*B*) and axial-enhanced images (*C*).

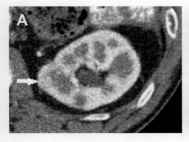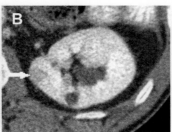

Fig. 2. (A) Corticomedullary phase and (B) nephrographic phase axial contrast-enhanced CT images of the left kidney show improved detectability of 1.2-cm ccRCC (arrows) when there is greater enhancement difference between the tumor and renal cortex in the nephrographic phase.

fundamental pitfall is using visual inspection alone to assess the attenuation of a renal lesion. One's eye can be tricked by homogeneous low-attenuation solid lesions mimicking cysts, so routine ROI use and proper placement is essential. Radiologists should ensure that the ROIs are placed well within the boundaries of the renal mass to avoid volume averaging with normal renal parenchyma. In addition, if the image slice thickness is less than one-half of the lesion diameter, normal parenchyma cephalad or caudad to the lesion can be volume averaged into the ROI, artificially altering it.

ROIs are placed on renal abnormalities to determine a lesion's attenuation, to assess for attenuation change between unenhanced and enhanced images (enhancement), or to detect fat within a lesion. Heterogeneity of renal lesions and the impact on ROI measurements can affect interpretation, leading to erroneous conclusions in several ways. On unenhanced CT, if a focal lesion measures less than 20 HU, has no wall thickening, is homogeneous, has no or minimal calcifications, and has no or few septa, it can be considered benign.[9,10] Discernment of heterogeneity is important to detect the uncommon RCC that measures less than 20 HU (Fig. 5).[11] In one series, RCC was found in approximately 0.5% of more than 15,000 patients, and 37% of these lesions were missed on initial interpretation, especially when the lesions were smaller than 3 cm.[12]

Typical papillary RCCs (pRCCs) are hyperattenuating to renal parenchyma on unenhanced scans, enhance only modestly, and tend to be homogeneous.[13–15] Rarely those with lower unenhanced attenuation values can mimic renal cysts on unenhanced CT scans. One study[16] found that of 114 pRCCs, 3 were homogeneous and measured less than 20 HU on unenhanced scans (Fig. 6). In another series, 24 of 104 RCCs (both ccRCCs and pRCCs) measured less than 20 HU when an ROI encompassing most of the lesion was used. However, of these 24 lesions, 21 were heterogeneous, and small ROIs could be used to detect regions within these lesions measuring more than 20 HU in the 3 that were homogeneous.[17]

If a lesion demonstrates high attenuation on an unenhanced CT image, assessment for homogeneity is again of paramount importance. The attenuation of hemorrhagic cysts and RCC can overlap on unenhanced CT images. However, if a lesion is both homogeneous and measures 70 HU or greater, it is almost certainly benign,[18] representing a hemorrhagic cyst (Fig. 7).

Detection of enhancement in pRCCs can be difficult, as these lesions tend to enhance only modestly.[12–14] In one series, a substantial number of pRCCs showed no CT enhancement (17% [7/41]) or equivocal enhancement (9.8% [4/41]) (Fig. 8).[13] Another series found that 25% of malignant lesions characterized as Bosniak III cysts

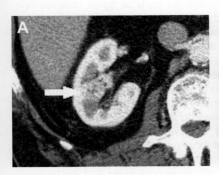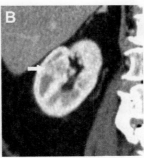

Fig. 3. (A) Axial and (B) coronal corticomedullary phase contrast-enhanced CT images of the right kidney show a ccRCC (arrows) that is difficult to detect because its attenuation is similar to that of the surrounding medullary renal parenchyma. One clue to the correct diagnosis is the heterogeneity of enhancement.

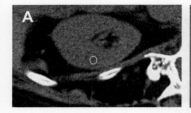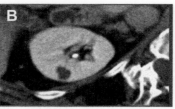

Fig. 4. Pseudoenhancement can occur when small intracortical cysts are mischaracterized as enhancing tumors. (A) Unenhanced and (B) enhanced images of the right kidney show an ROI (*circle*) used to measure the attenuation of a renal cyst before (A) and (B) after contrast administration. The unenhanced attenuation was 9 HU and the postcontrast attenuation was 30 HU, erroneously suggesting a mildly enhancing tumor.

were pRCCs.[19] This may, in part, be explained by the pathologic features of cystic change or necrosis in pRCC.[10,20] For such marginally enhancing tumors, the use of small ROIs rather than medium or large ROIs to detect enhancement has been shown to provide superior performance.[8] More particularly, researchers found that in lesions lacking enhancement that could be identified by visual observation alone, small ROIs performed statistically significantly better than whole-lesion ROIs in distinguishing any RCC from a cyst (area under the receiver operating characteristic curve [AUC]: small ROI, 0.792; whole-lesion ROI, 0.602) and in distinguishing between pRCC and a cyst (AUC: small ROI, 0.883; whole lesion ROI, 0.642) (Fig. 9).[8]

Because of challenges with the interpretation of CT for minimally enhancing renal masses, MR imaging can be used to problem solve by aiding in delineating tumor types and specifically identifying enhancing tissue.[21] In addition, machine learning has also been investigated as a method to differentiate between renal neoplasms and cysts; the

detection of high entropy on CT texture analysis has been found to be comparable to the assessment of expert readers and superior to the assessment of novice readers in distinguishing between low-attenuation RCCs and cysts, with a sensitivity of 84% and a specificity of 80%.[22]

On contrast-enhanced CT images, a homogeneous lesion with attenuation less than 20 HU is almost certainly a cyst.[23] Emerging data from small series suggest that the attenuation threshold for benign lesions could potentially be increased to 30 or 40 HU,[24–26] with the caveat that a pRCC may rarely be missed using this new threshold.[16]

PSEUDOTUMORS

Several masslike renal abnormalities detected on imaging are not RCCs. When first approaching a renal abnormality, it is therefore good practice for the radiologist to question whether the finding could be developmental, posttraumatic, infectious or postinfectious, vascular, or postprocedural in origin (Box 1).

Congenital anatomic variants include a prominent column of Bertin, which occurs as a result of incomplete resorption of junctional parenchyma during organogenesis. This variant seems as a tongue of tissue extending into the renal sinus in contiguity with renal parenchyma. Enhancement that is similar to the surrounding parenchyma (for CT, MR imaging, or contrast-enhanced ultrasound) or uptake on cortical agent radioisotope imaging and characteristic morphology are clues to the diagnosis of this anatomic variant. In the corticomedullary phase of enhancement, a normal corticomedullary pattern also helps to distinguish potential anatomic variants from real lesions. For instance, a dromedary hump is a focal protrusion of parenchyma in the lateral midleft renal parenchyma adjacent to the spleen that should, otherwise, follow the imaging characteristics of the remainder of renal parenchyma.

Inflammatory masses such as focal pyelonephritis (Fig. 10), immunoglobulin G-4 (IgG4) renal

Fig. 5. Unenhanced axial CT image demonstrating poorly defined ccRCC. Although some portions measure less than 20 HU, there are areas of heterogeneous higher attenuation (*arrows*).

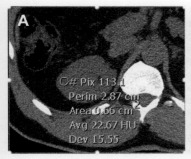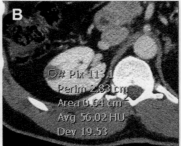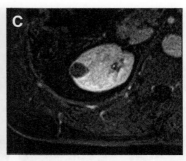

Fig. 6. Images of homogeneous low-attenuation pRCC. (*A*) ROI on unenhanced axial CT image shows a lesion attenuation of 22 HU. (*B*) Contrast-enhanced axial CT image shows a mass with an enhancement of 56 HU. (*C*) Same tumor on MR imaging with faint visual enhancement is confirmed on subtracted postcontrast axial T1-weighted fat-suppressed image.

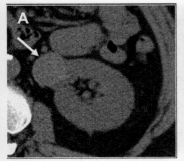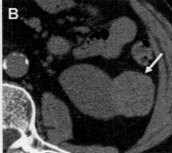

Fig. 7. Unenhanced axial CT images from a 57-year-old woman with 2 left renal masses. (*A*) Hyperdense cyst is homogeneous and measures 72 HU (*arrow*). (*B*) pRCC is mildly heterogeneous, has angular margins, and measures 58 HU (*arrow*).

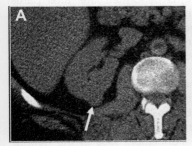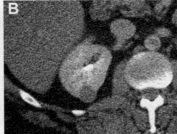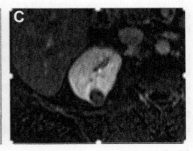

Fig. 8. Images of pRCC. (*A*) Axial unenhanced CT image shows a renal mass that measures 31 HU (*arrow*). (*B*) Nephrographic phase–enhanced axial CT image shows a mass with an attenuation of 42 HU. (*C*) Subtracted contrast-enhanced T1-weighted axial MR image of the same tumor shows minimal detectable enhancement.

disease, and abscess may have the appearance of a focal neoplasm. Combing the medical record for pertinent clinical clues can keep the radiologist from wandering down the wrong diagnostic path. For instance, focal compensatory hypertrophy or renal cortical preservation in the setting of extensive renal scarring after infection or infarction can have a masslike appearance (**Fig. 11**). After an acute inflammatory event, imaging clues to the

correct diagnosis include multifocal areas of scarring, preserved corticomedullary differentiation, and stability over time.

Similarly, vascular malformations such as aneurysms or arteriovenous fistulas may appear masslike on unenhanced images or during certain phases of contrast administration. Confirmation of a vascular cause of the finding can be made with arterial phase imaging or Doppler ultrasound.

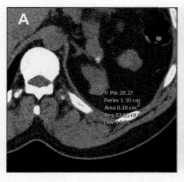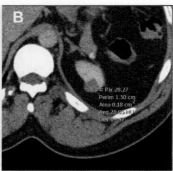

Fig. 9. Use of small ROIs to detect enhancement. (*A*) Hyperdense pRCC on unenhanced axial CT image with a small ROI demonstrates an attenuation of 53 HU. (*B*) Nephrographic phase CT image ROI measures an attenuation of 75 HU, confirming enhancement (>20 HU difference). ROIs encompassing two-thirds of the mass measured attenuation values of 55 HU and 64 HU and were, thus, unable to detect enhancement.

Findings on imaging after partial nephrectomy or renal tumor ablation can mimic findings of a residual or recurrent tumor. The resection approach used for renal tumors depends on tumor size and tumor location within the kidney with respect to the collecting system and vascular structures; these factors affect the amount of parenchyma that must be resected. Preserved renal function after resection is strongly correlated with preserved parenchymal mass and renal reconstruction, so preservation of normal renal parenchyma is imperative.[27,28] The renal remnant will have different appearances based on the amount of parenchyma that was resected and the method of renorrhaphy to achieve hemostasis closure of the renal capsule. Often, the renal capsule is reapproximated over bolsters of oxidized cellulose or other hemostatic agents, which can appear masslike, especially in the immediate postoperative period.[29]

Typically, imaging should not be performed in the immediate postoperative period unless a complication (such as hematoma with or without pseudoaneurysm, urinoma, or abscess) is suspected. Oxidized cellulose can mimic an abscess at the resection site, as it may have the appearance of a water attenuation collection with gas bubbles interspersed within it even if uninfected (Fig. 12).[30] A renal parenchymal defect, perinephric fat infiltration, and fluid collections (75%) are other common findings after renal mass resection.[31] Some postoperative patients will have round or ovoid mildly enhancing residual tissue at the resection site; this is usually referred to as a pseudotumor[32] or granuloma (Fig. 13).[33] Generally, this tissue involutes over time. Although the American Urologic Association guidelines recommend follow-up for T1 renal tumors (up to 7 cm localized to the kidney),[34] early recurrence is rare and postoperative imaging findings can be confusing. Based on these factors, the investigators of one study suggested that imaging might be best deferred until 1 year after surgery.[35]

When imaging is performed later after partial nephrectomy, normal changes may be difficult to distinguish from tumor recurrence. The investigators of one small series suggested that the degree of enhancement, morphology of imaging findings, and temporal change can be used to distinguish tumor recurrence from scarring after partial nephrectomy.[36] In this study, recurrent tumors (presumably ccRCC) had greater enhancement than scarring (median 119 HU vs 48 HU) and showed enhancement loss in the nephrographic and excretory phases as opposed to increased enhancement for scarring. Also, the true recurrent tumors appeared as spiculated masses rather than as thin spidery projections and increased rather than decreased in size over time (Fig. 14).

Imaging findings after ablation will also vary over time. Shortly after either radiofrequency ablation or cryoablation, the treatment zone should be larger than the original tumor, because a margin of normal parenchyma is intentionally ablated. The ablation zone does not typically enhance and should decrease in size over time.[37] However, early residual enhancement in the first few days

---

Box 1
Types of pseudotumors

Congenital (column of Bertin, dromedary hump)

Masslike compensatory hypertrophy (multifocal scarring)

Inflammatory (pyelonephritis, abscess, IgG4 disease)

Vascular abnormality—aneurysm/pseudoaneurysm

Partial nephrectomy pseudotumor/granuloma

Oxidized cellulose pseudoabscess

Early postablation enhancement

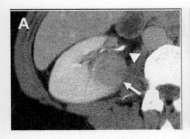
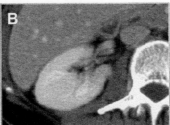

Fig. 10. (*A*) Axial contrast-enhanced CT image in a patient with flank pain shows a focal rounded masslike abnormality (*arrow*) with mild stranding in perirenal fat (*arrowhead*). The mass was initially interpreted as a neoplasm until information about pyuria and fever became available. (*B*) A follow-up–enhanced CT image obtained 4 months later shows resolution of focal infectious nephritis.

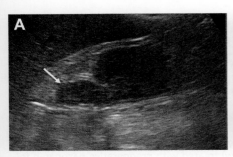
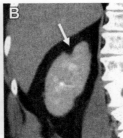

Fig. 11. A 73-year-old man with urinary obstruction. (*A*) Sagittal ultrasound image of the right kidney shows bulbous protrusion from the upper pole of the kidney (*arrow*). (*B*) Coronal contrast-enhanced CT MPR image shows that the region represents normal parenchyma adjacent to a parenchymal scar (*arrow*).

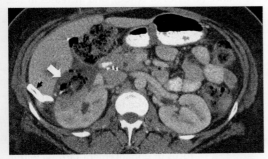

Fig. 12. Oxidized cellulose placed at renal tumor resection site (*white arrow*) is visualized as a low-attenuation collection with interspersed gas foci, mimicking an abscess on the enhanced CT image. A surgical drain (*black arrow*) can also be seen.

after ablation can be detected at the site of the tumor in 60% to 80% of ablation zones (**Fig. 15**).[38–40] This early enhancement, which may be homogeneous or curvilinear, occurs more commonly in cases of ccRCC and typically resolves within a month. Therefore, many centers have abandoned the use of early imaging to assess for ablation completeness, waiting until 3 months after the procedure to begin imaging follow-up.

When disease progression (recurrence) after tumor ablation does occur, it is most common at the periphery of the ablation site, has variable morphology depending on the ablation method and device, and is characterized by new nodular enhancement or internal enhancement.[31] Comparing postablation images with preablation images is extremely beneficial, as information on the exact site and morphology of the original tumor is crucial for proper interpretation of postablation images (**Fig. 16**).

FAT-CONTAINING RENAL MASSES

Some renal masses contain fat, which can aid in making a correct diagnosis based on imaging findings. However, the amount of fat, its location with respect to the cellular makeup of the lesion, and the method of detection all contribute to the complexity of deciphering and categorizing renal masses that contain fat.

The prototypical fat-containing renal mass is the angiomyolipoma (AML), a benign neoplasm that contains components of vascular tissue, smooth muscle, and adipocytes or fat cells. Most of the AMLs thus have macroscopic fat[41] (sometimes referred to as bulk fat), indicating an adequate number of adipocytes to be detected by imaging. Detection of macroscopic fat can be accomplished by finding an ROI on unenhanced CT that measures less than −10 HU.[42] For tiny foci of fat, thin-section CT reconstruction can improve sensitivity.

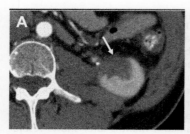
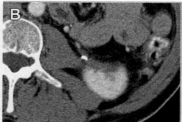
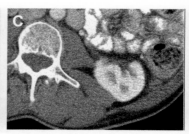

Fig. 13. Images of pseudotumor after partial nephrectomy. (*A*) CT image obtained 2 months after surgery shows mildly enhancing soft tissue at the resection site (*arrow*) that diminishes by 6 months (*B*) and resolves thereafter (7 years) (*C*).

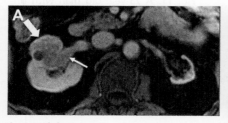
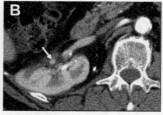
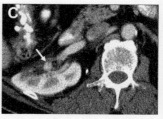

Fig. 14. (*A*) Contrast-enhanced T1-weighted MR image from a 67-year-old man with atrophic left kidney and right renal tumor (*large arrow*) with renal vein invasion (*small arrow*) treated with preoperative pazopanib followed by partial nephrectomy. (*B*) One-year follow-up CT image shows a 5-mm enhancing nodule (*arrow*) at the resection site, not identified by the interpreting radiologist. (*C*) Two-year follow-up CT image shows increase in size of nodule (*arrow*) to 1.2 cm. The patient underwent cryoablation for recurrence. Recurrent disease most commonly demonstrates rounded, convex margins, may hyperenhance (in cases of ccRCC), and increases in size over time.

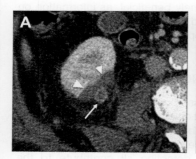
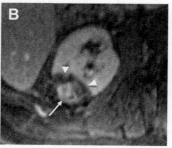

Fig. 15. Early postablation enhancement in 2 patients. (*A*) CT image obtained 1 day after ablation shows small rounded focus of enhancement (*arrow*) within ablation zone (*arrowheads*). (*B*) MR image obtained 1 day after ablation shows large rounded focus of enhancement (*arrow*) within ablation zone (*arrowheads*).

Macroscopic fat on MR imaging can be identified using several methods. Signal intensity loss after the application of chemical selective fat suppression or fat and water separation Dixon techniques can confirm the presence of macroscopic fat. Alternatively, curvilinear or linear chemical shift artifact (of the second kind) causes an India-ink artifact at the boundary of a macroscopic fat-containing lesion on T1-weighted gradient-recalled echo images. Central high signal intensity should be maintained, matching the signal intensity of other macroscopic fat (such as retroperitoneal or subcutaneous fat) and thus confirming the presence of macroscopic fat (Fig. 17).[35] Research has shown that MR imaging may be more sensitive to fat than unenhanced CT in small AMLs.[43]

Not all renal masses with macroscopic fat are AMLs. Rarely, macroscopic fat can be seen in RCCs, most often with coexistent calcifications.[35] When a renal mass engulfs retroperitoneal fat, leading to intralesional macroscopic fat, RCC should be suspected.

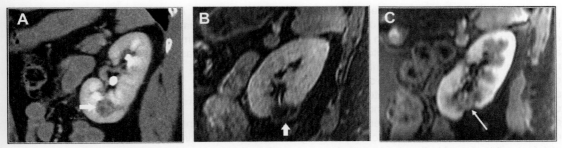

Fig. 16. Recurrence after cryoablation. (*A*) Preprocedural sagittal reformatted CT image shows small lower pole tumor (*arrow*). (*B*) Six-month fat-saturated T1-weighted sagittal MR image after cryoablation shows a normal finding of thin rim enhancement at the ablation zone boundary (*arrow*) without other enhancement. (*C*) Two-year sagittal MR image shows rounded, enhancing nodule (*arrow*) at the deep margin of the ablation zone extending into the central sinus indicating tumor recurrence.

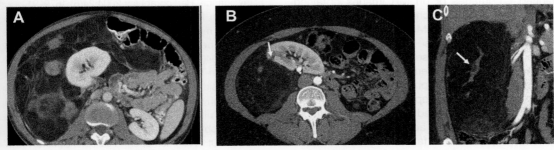

Fig. 17. Liposarcoma versus large AML. (*A*) CT image of dedifferentiated retroperitoneal liposarcoma with abundant fat and soft tissue nodules. (*B*) Large AML also appears as predominantly fat attenuation but also demonstrates a tiny renal parenchymal notch (*arrow*) and (*C*) has large central vessels (*arrow*).

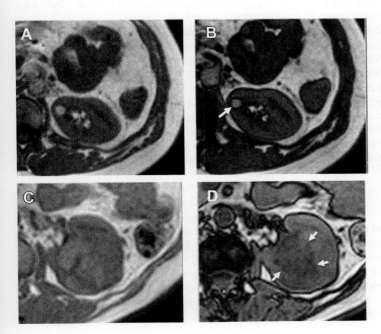

Fig. 18. Microscopic versus macroscopic fat on in-phase and opposed-phase T1-weighted gradient-recalled echo MR imaging. (*A*) In-phase and (*B*) opposed-phase images of AML show maintained central hyperintensity (as is also seen with retroperitoneal fat) with India ink artifact at the boundary of the AML and renal parenchyma on opposed-phase image (*arrow*). (*C*) In-phase and (*D*) opposed-phase images in ccRCC show diffuse signal intensity loss on opposed-phase image (*arrows*), indicating microscopic (intracellular) fat not macroscopic (bulk) fat.

As in other areas of the body, when a large mass is first detected, identifying the site of origin can be challenging. For instance, when an AML presents as a large fat-containing retroperitoneal mass, it may be misidentified as a retroperitoneal liposarcoma, as these masses can have a similar appearance. In these cases, an accurate diagnosis is crucial; an AML is benign and may not require therapy, whereas a liposarcoma requires radical resection. Because AMLs arise from the kidney, a defect will be found in the renal parenchyma at the location of origin. AMLs also tend to contain large vessels, whereas sarcomas tend to be hypovascular, and AMLs are often multiple, whereas liposarcomas are a unicentric process (see **Fig. 17**).[44]

Approximately 5% of AMLs contain so few adipocytes that they cannot be discerned on unenhanced CT images or on MR images obtained with fat-suppression techniques; these masses are known as fat-poor AMLs (fpAMLs). The scarcity of fat cells can cause signal intensity loss in a noncurvilinear or diffuse manner on opposed-phase T1-weighted gradient-recalled echo images when compared with in-phase images, indicating the presence of microscopic fat. Microscopic fat, however, can be detected in 2 different settings: from a scarce number of adipocytes (as in fpAML) or from the presence of fat within tumor cells (as can be seen in ccRCC) (**Fig. 18**).[35] This distinction cannot be made with chemical shift imaging alone, and so additional features must be considered to determine the diagnosis. fpAMLs are more common in women and are generally small and hyperattenuating on unenhanced CT images due to a high percentage of smooth muscle component.[36] These masses also tend to be T2 hypointense (T2 signal intensity ratio <0.9) and hyperenhance after contrast administration (arterial-to-delayed enhancement ratio >1.5).[45] These findings are in contradistinction to those seen with pRCC; these masses are T2 hypointense but hypoenhance after contrast administration. The findings are also different from those seen with ccRCCs, which hyperenhance after contrast administration but are T2 hyperintense. Both fpAMLs and pRCCs generally show restricted diffusion.

SUMMARY

Radiologists face several pitfalls when interpreting images of the kidneys. Clinical history is paramount to guiding an appropriate evaluation, and attention to technical details, use of multiplanar imaging, and appropriate use of attenuation measurements can help readers avoid interpretation mistakes. Knowledge of the expected imaging appearance of kidneys after various treatments for RCC and patterns of fat within renal masses and how they impact the differential diagnosis of a focal renal mass will also help to minimize diagnostic errors.

ACKNOWLEDGMENTS

The author thanks Megan Griffiths for her careful review and editing of this article.

DISCLOSURES

None.

REFERENCES

1. Barrett JF, Keat N. Artifacts in CT: recognition and avoidance. Radiographics 2004;24(6):1679–91.
2. Johnson PT, Horton KM, Fishman EK. How not to miss or mischaracterize a renal cell carcinoma: protocols, pearls, and pitfalls. AJR Am J Roentgenol 2010;194(4):W307–15.
3. Wildman-Tobriner B, Allen BC, Maxfield CM. Common resident errors when interpreting computed tomography of the abdomen and pelvis: a review of types, pitfalls, and strategies for improvement. Curr Probl Diagn Radiol 2019;48(1):4–9.
4. Szolar DH, Kammerhuber F, Altziebler S, et al. Multiphasic helical CT of the kidney: increased conspicuity for detection and characterization of small (< 3-cm) renal masses. Radiology 1997;202(1):211–7.
5. Cohan RH, Sherman LS, Korobkin M, et al. Renal masses: assessment of corticomedullary-phase and nephrographic-phase CT scans. Radiology 1995;196(2):445–51.
6. Sheth S, Fishman EK. Multi-detector row CT of the kidneys and urinary tract: techniques and applications in the diagnosis of benign diseases. Radiographics 2004;24(2):e20.
7. Israel GM, Bosniak MA. How I do it: evaluating renal masses. Radiology 2005;236(2):441–50.
8. Rosenkrantz AB, Matza BW, Portnoy E, et al. Impact of size of region-of-interest on differentiation of renal cell carcinoma and renal cysts on multi-phase CT: preliminary findings. Eur J Radiol 2014;83(2):239–44.
9. O'Connor SD, Pickhardt PJ, Kim DH, et al. Incidental finding of renal masses at unenhanced CT: prevalence and analysis of features for guiding management. AJR Am J Roentgenol 2011;197(1):139–45.
10. O'Connor SD, Silverman SG, Ip IK, et al. Simple cyst-appearing renal masses at unenhanced CT: can they be presumed to be benign? Radiology 2013;269(3):793–800.
11. Schieda N, Vakili M, Dilauro M, et al. Solid renal cell carcinoma measuring water attenuation (-10 to 20

HU) on unenhanced CT. AJR Am J Roentgenol 2015;205(6):1215–21.

12. O'Connor SD, Silverman SG, Cochon LR, et al. Renal cancer at unenhanced CT: imaging features, detection rates, and outcomes. Abdom Radiol (NY) 2018;43(7):1756–63.

13. Herts BR, Coll DM, Novick AC, et al. Enhancement characteristics of papillary renal neoplasms revealed on triphasic helical CT of the kidneys. AJR Am J Roentgenol 2002;178(2):367–72.

14. Egbert ND, Caoili EM, Cohan RH, et al. Differentiation of papillary renal cell carcinoma subtypes on CT and MRI. AJR Am J Roentgenol 2013;201(2):347–55.

15. Young JR, Margolis D, Sauk S, et al. Clear cell renal cell carcinoma: discrimination from other renal cell carcinoma subtypes and oncocytoma at multiphasic multidetector CT. Radiology 2013;267(2):444–53.

16. Corwin MT, Loehfelm TW, McGahan JP, et al. Prevalence of Low-Attenuation Homogeneous Papillary Renal Cell Carcinoma Mimicking Renal Cysts on CT. AJR Am J Roentgenol 2018;211(6):1259–63.

17. McGahan JP, Sidhar K, Fananapazir G, et al. Renal cell carcinoma attenuation values on unenhanced CT: importance of multiple, small region-of-interest measurements. Abdom Radiol (NY) 2017;42(9):2325–33.

18. Jonisch AI, Rubinowitz AN, Mutalik PG, et al. Can high-attenuation renal cysts be differentiated from renal cell carcinoma at unenhanced CT? Radiology 2007;243(2):445–50.

19. Smith AD, Remer EM, Cox KL, et al. Bosniak category IIF and III cystic renal lesions: outcomes and associations. Radiology 2012;262(1):152–60.

20. Brinker DA, Amin MB, de Peralta-Venturina M, et al. Extensively necrotic cystic renal cell carcinoma: a clinicopathologic study with comparison to other cystic and necrotic renal cancers. Am J Surg Pathol 2000;24(7):988–95.

21. Kang SK, Huang WC, Panharipande PV, et al. Solid renal masses: What the numbers tell us. AJR Am J Roentgenol 2014;202:1196–206.

22. Kim NY, Lubner MG, Nystrom JT, et al. Utility of CT Texture analysis in differentiating low-attenuation renal cell carcinoma from cysts: A bi-Institutional retrospective study. AJR Am J Roentgenol 2019;213(6):1259–66.

23. Silverman SG, Israel GM, Trinh QD. Incompletely characterized incidental renal masses: emerging data support conservative management. Radiology 2015;275(1):28–42.

24. Agochukwu N, Huber S, Spektor M, et al. Differentiating Renal Neoplasms From Simple Cysts on Contrast-Enhanced CT on the Basis of Attenuation and Homogeneity. AJR Am J Roentgenol 2017;208(4):801–4.

25. Corwin MT, Hansra SS, Loehfelm TW, et al. Prevalence of solid tumors in incidentally detected homogeneous renal masses measuring >20 HU on portal venous phase CT. AJR Am J Roentgenol 2018;211(3):W173–7.

26. Hu E, Ellis JH, Silverman SG, et al. Expanding the definition of a benign renal cyst on contrast-enhanced CT: can incidental homogeneous renal masses measuring 21-39 HU be safely ignored? Acad Radiol 2018;25(2):209–12.

27. Mir MC, Ercole C, Takagi T, et al. Decline in renal function after partial nephrectomy: etiology and prevention. J Urol 2015;193(6):1889–98.

28. Dong W, Zhang Z, Zhao J, et al. Excised parenchymal mass during partial nephrectomy: functional implications. Urology 2017;103:129–35.

29. Pai D, Willatt JM, Korobkin M, et al. CT appearances following laparoscopic partial nephrectomy for renal cell carcinoma using a rolled cellulose bolster. Cancer Imaging 2010;10:161–8.

30. Sarwani NI, Motta-Ramirez GA, Remer EM, et al. Imaging findings after minimally invasive nephron-sparing renal therapies. Clin Radiol 2007;62(4):333–9.

31. Hecht EM, Bennett GL, Brown KW, et al. Laparoscopic and open partial nephrectomy: frequency and long-term follow-up of postoperative collections. Radiology 2010;255(2):476–84.

32. Kshirsagar AV, Choyke PL, Linehan WM, et al. Pseudotumors after renal parenchymal sparing surgery. J Urol 1998;159(4):1148–51.

33. Lee MS, Oh YT, Han WK, et al. CT findings after nephron-sparing surgery of renal tumors. AJR Am J Roentgenol 2007;189(5):W264–71.

34. American Urological Association. Follow-up for clinically localized renal neoplasms guidelines. 2013. Avaialble at: https://www.auanet.org/guidelines/renal-cancer-follow-up-for-clinically-localized-renal-neoplasms-guideline. Accessed November 25, 2019.

35. Tubre RW, Parker WP, Dum T, et al. Findings and impact of early imaging after partial nephrectomy. J Endourol 2017;31(3):320–5.

36. Lang EK, Thomas R, Davis R, et al. Multiphasic helical CT criteria for differentiation of recurrent neoplasm and desmoplastic reaction after laparoscopic resection of renal mass lesions. J Endourol 2004;18(2):167–71.

37. Allen BC, Remer EM. Percutaneous cryoablation of renal tumors: patient selection, technique, and postprocedural imaging. Radiographics 2010;30(4):887–902.

38. Javadi S, Ahrar JU, Ninan E, et al. Characterization of contrast enhancement in the ablation zone immediately after radiofrequency ablation of renal tumors. J Vasc Interv Radiol 2010;21(5):690–5.

39. Porter CA 4th, Woodrum DA, Callstrom MR, et al. MRI after technically successful renal cryoablation:

early contrast enhancement as a common finding. AJR Am J Roentgenol 2010;194(3):790–3.

40. Takaki H, Nakatsuka A, Cornelis F, et al. False-positive tumor enhancement after cryoablation of renal cell carcinoma: a prospective study. AJR Am J Roentgenol 2016;206(2):332–9.

41. Schieda N, Davenport MS, Pedrosa I, et al. Renal and adrenal masses containing fat at MRI: Proposed nomenclature by the Society of Abdominal Radiology Disease-focused Panel on Renal Cell Carcinoma. J Magn Reson Imaging 2019;49(4):917–26.

42. Jinzaki M, Silverman SG, Akita H, et al. Renal angiomyolipoma: a radiological classification and update on recent developments in diagnosis and management. Abdom Imaging 2014;39(3): 588–604.

43. Schieda N, Avruch L, Flood TA. Small (<1 cm) incidental echogenic renal cortical nodules: chemical shift MRI outperforms CT for confirmatory diagnosis of angiomyolipoma (AML). Insights Imaging 2014; 5(3):295–9.

44. Israel GM, Bosniak MA. Pitfalls in renal mass evaluation and how to avoid them. Radiographics 2008; 28(5):1325–38.

45. Sasiwimonphan K, Takahashi N, Leibovich BC, et al. Small (<4 cm) renal mass: differentiation of angiomyolipoma without visible fat from renal cell carcinoma utilizing MR imaging. Radiology 2012;263(1):160–8.

Approach to Renal Cystic Masses and the Role of Radiology

Andrew D. Smith, MD, PhD*, Asser Abou Elkassem, MD

KEYWORDS

- Bosniak classification system • Renal cysts • Cystic renal masses

KEY POINTS

- The first step in evaluation of a renal mass is to determine if it is cystic or solid and apply the Bosniak classification system version 2019.
- The need for additional characterization depends on the initial imaging modality and the imaging features that can be used for Bosniak classification.
- The Bosniak classification should not be applied to cystic appearing infectious, inflammatory, or vascular etiologies; for all other renal cystic masses with imaging that allows for a complete characterization, the Bosniak classification should be applied.

IS IT A RENAL CYST?

The first step in the evaluation of a renal mass is to determine if it is cystic or solid.[1] Completing this task is critical for management, and the imaging modality is important. The Bosniak classification system version 2019 considers a renal lesion with less than 25% enhancing tissue as cystic, but multiple other definitions for defining a renal cyst now apply and are described elsewhere in this article.[1] In general, the use of colloquial terms that lack standard definitions, such as "complicated cyst" or "complex cyst," should be avoided, although these terms are common in clinical practice for indeterminate renal cysts that require further characterization by renal computed tomography (CT) scan or MR imaging or renal ultrasound examination.

One of the most commonly encountered renal lesions on CT scan are those that are considered too small to characterize (TSTC) owing to problems with volume averaging when attempting to assess the attenuation.[1–4] Homogeneous low-attenuating renal lesions that are TSTC are now considered benign cystic masses.[1] By comparison, a heterogenous renal lesion that is TSTC by CT scan is rarely encountered, but is indeterminate and cannot be assumed to represent a renal cyst, because some of these lesions may represent solid renal neoplasms (**Fig. 1**).[1,2]

To characterize a larger renal lesion on CT scan, a region of interest is used to assess the attenuation in Hounsfield units (HU). If the attenuation of 75% or more of a renal lesion on noncontrast or contrast-enhanced CT scanning measures as fluid attenuation (−9 to 20 HU), it can be considered cystic.[1,2,5–7] The cystic component of a renal cyst may not measure fluid in attenuation, and enhancement is key to differentiating a hyperdense renal cyst from a solid renal neoplasm. Renal masses with less than 25% enhancing tissue are considered cystic, with enhancement on CT scans defined as an increase of 20 HU or more between noncontrast and contrast-enhanced images, most commonly from dedicated renal protocol CT acquisition.[1,8] In addition, homogeneous hyperattenuating (≥70 HU) renal

Department of Radiology, University of Alabama at Birmingham, JTN 452, 619 19th Street South, Birmingham, AL 35249-6830, USA
* Corresponding author.
E-mail address: andrewdennissmith@uabmc.edu

Radiol Clin N Am 58 (2020) 897–907
https://doi.org/10.1016/j.rcl.2020.05.007
0033-8389/20/© 2020 Elsevier Inc. All rights reserved.

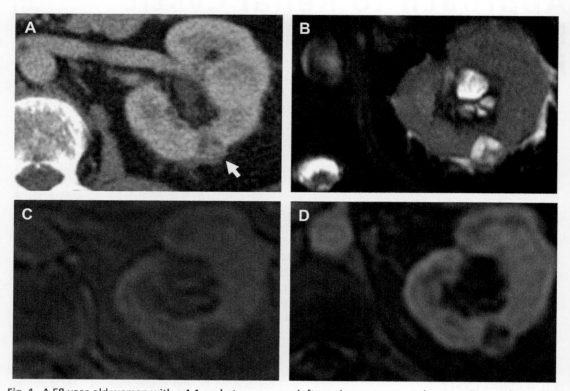

Fig. 1. A 58-year-old woman with a 1.1-cm heterogeneous left renal mass on a portal venous CT scan that is TSTC (*arrow, A*). This lesion was indeterminate owing to heterogeneity and further evaluated by renal MR imaging and found to be hyperintense with septations on T2-weighted imaging (*B*), hypointense on pre-contrast T1-weighted fat-saturated images (*C*), and had enhancing septations on post-contrast T1-weighted fat-saturated images (*D*). The lesion was characterized as a Bosniak type IIF renal cystic mass.

lesions at noncontrast CT scanning and homogenous renal lesions measuring −9 to 30 HU at portal venous phase CT scanning are considered benign cystic masses.[1,3,9–13] By comparison, all heterogeneous masses at noncontrast CT scanning are considered indeterminate and could be cystic or solid in nature.[1,2]

The role and reliability of dual energy CT scanning for characterizing renal masses is under investigation in research studies and not yet incorporated into the Bosniak classification system.[14,15] More validation is needed in this area of research. Given the decreased importance of renal enhancement in the Bosniak classification system version 2019, characterization and Bosniak classification of many well-defined renal cysts on dual energy CT images may be possible, especially if 75% or more of the renal mass measures fluid attenuation (−9 to 20 HU) at 120 kV imaging.

On MR imaging, a renal cyst is defined as a renal mass with less than 25% enhancing tissue, with enhancement defined as an increase of 15% or more in signal intensity between contrast-enhanced and noncontrast images or as definitive visual enhancement on high-quality subtraction images.[1,16] On noncontrast MR imaging, homogeneous masses markedly hyperintense at T2-weighted imaging (similar to cerebrospinal fluid) and homogeneous masses markedly hyperintense at fat-saturated T1-weighted imaging (approximately 2.5 times normal renal parenchymal signal intensity) are considered benign cystic masses (Bosniak type II).[1,17–19] Conversely, homogeneous renal masses with mild to moderate intensity at T1- or T2-weighted imaging or heterogenous masses on noncontrast MR imaging are indeterminate and cannot be classified as cystic without further characterization.[1] Furthermore, heterogeneously hyperintense renal masses at fat-saturated T2-weighted imaging cannot be classified as cysts, because some represent necrotic papillary cancers.[1]

On ultrasound examination, a renal cyst is anechoic or hypoechoic with posterior acoustic enhancement (or increased through-transmission).[1] The posterior acoustic enhancement is a key feature, as some solid masses can be hypoechoic but lack posterior acoustic enhancement. Additional features such as debris, wall thickening, color flow, and number, thickness, and nodularity of septations can also be evaluated and should be used to assist with characterization.[1] On contrast-enhanced ultrasound examination, a renal cyst is defined as a renal lesion with less than 25% enhancing tissue.[1]

DOES THIS RENAL MASS NEED FURTHER CHARACTERIZATION?

The need for additional characterization of a renal mass depends on the initial imaging modality and the imaging features that can be used for Bosniak classification (Table 1).[1] With the exception of homogeneous renal lesions that are TSTC, if a renal lesion is not well-defined or not clearly cystic, further characterization by imaging is needed.[1–4] Most renal lesions are detecting on noncontrast or portal venous CT examinations that are obtained for other purposes, and the Bosniak 2019 classification leads to confident characterization as benign cystic lesion, although for a minority of cases the Bosniak rules cannot be applied completely without additional imaging.[1] A review of renal masses requiring further characterization by additional imaging is presented in Table 2.

Notable changes in the Bosniak classification system are that the presence or absence of contrast enhancement and extent of calcifications are less important, whereas wall and septation thickness and protrusions are now key features.[1] Even a simple cyst may have wall enhancement in version 2019. Given this change, the Bosniak classification system can be applied to the majority of well-defined renal cysts that lack thickened walls and are identified on portal venous CT scans (Fig. 2).

Many renal lesions that are incompletely characterized on CT scans are considered low risk and do not need additional characterization. For example, homogeneous low-attenuating renal lesions that are TSTC on CT images are Bosniak II renal masses and do not require further imaging or workup.[1–4,8] Despite the limitations of noncontrast CT imaging, several types of cystic lesions are considered low risk and do require additional imaging or follow-up. Homogeneous hyperattenuating (≥70 HU) renal masses on noncontrast CT scans are considered Bosniak II renal cystic masses and do not require additional imaging or follow-up.[1,3,9,10] Furthermore, homogeneous fluid attenuating (−9 to 20 HU) renal masses on noncontrast CT scans are considered Bosniak type II renal cystic masses and do not need additional imaging or follow-up.[1–4,8] Importantly, the term "simple cyst" does not apply to noncontrast CT scans and should only apply to contrast-enhanced CT scans, because contrast enhancement is needed

to confirm the absence of wall thickening or septations that are needed to classify a Bosniak type I renal cyst.[1]

Several renal lesions identified on noncontrast CT scans need further characterization with imaging, including any renal lesion with a heterogeneous appearance or any lesion measuring soft tissue in attenuation (>20 to <70 HU).[1,2,8] The rarely encountered heterogenous renal lesion that is TSTC on noncontrast or contrast-enhanced CT scanning (see Fig. 1) should be further characterized by renal MR imaging to determine if the heterogeneous appearance is due to septations in a cystic renal mass or indicative of a solid renal mass, although this distinction can often be made 6 to 12 months after the initial discovery owing to the small size.[1,2,8] The homogeneous soft tissue attenuating (21–69 HU) renal mass on a noncontrast CT scan is typically evaluated by ultrasound imaging to determine if it is a hyperdense cyst or solid renal mass (Fig. 3); however, larger patients may be best evaluated with a renal CT scan or MR imaging owing to suboptimal ultrasound penetration related to attenuation by large amounts of body fat.[1,2,8]

On a contrast-enhanced CT scan, a simple renal cyst does not require additional imaging or workup and is defined as a renal cyst with a well-defined, thin (≤2 mm), smooth wall that may enhance, homogeneous simple fluid (−9 to 20 HU), and no septa or calcifications.[1] In the past, homogenous renal lesions measuring 21 HU or more on portal venous CT scans required additional workup to differentiate solid from cystic components.[1,2,5–8] Recent evidence suggests that well-defined homogeneous masses measuring 40 HU or more on portal venous CT scans are likely benign cysts, but the optimal attenuation threshold is unclear, and the Bosniak classification system now considers renal masses that measure −9 to 30 HU on portal venous CT scans as a benign Bosniak type II renal mass that do not need further characterization or follow-up.[1,11–13]

Conversely, any mass on a portal venous CT scan with an attenuation of greater than 30 HU should be further evaluated, because it could represent a solid renal mass.[1] Again, ultrasound imaging is typically used to differentiate solid from cystic renal masses, although larger patients may be best evaluated by renal CT scans or MR imaging.[1,2,8]

A well-defined cystic renal mass on a portal venous CT scan with 75% or more of the lesion measuring fluid attenuation, does not necessarily need additional characterization if the walls and septations are clearly delineated (see Fig. 2), because the Bosniak classification system can be applied to these renal masses.[1] Heterogeneous

Table 1
Bosniak classification system version 2019 of cystic renal masses

Class	CT Scan[a]	MR Imaging[a]	Ultrasound Examination[c]
I	Well-defined cyst with thin (<2 mm) smooth wall; homogeneous simple fluid (−9 to 20 HU); no septa or calcifications; the wall may enhance	Well-defined cyst, thin (≤2 mm) smooth wall; homogeneous simple fluid (signal intensity similar to CSF); no septa or calcifications; the wall may enhance	Well-defined cyst (anechoic with posterior acoustic enhancement), thin (≤2 mm) smooth wall; no septa or calcifications
II	Well-defined cyst with thin (<2 mm) smooth walls: 1. Cystic masses with thin (<2 mm) and few (1–3) septa; septa and wall may enhance; may have calcification of any type[b] 2. Homogeneous hyperattenuating (>70 HU) masses at noncontrast CT scan 3. Homogeneous nonenhancing masses >20 HU at renal mass protocol CT scan, may have calcification of any type[b] 4. Homogeneous masses −9 to 20 HU at noncontrast CT scan 5. Homogeneous masses 21–30 HU at portal venous phase CT scan 6. Homogeneous low-attenuation masses that are TSTC	Well-defined cyst with thin (≤2 mm) smooth walls: 1. Cystic masses with thin (≤2 mm) and few (1–3) enhancing septa; any nonenhancing septa; may have calcification of any type[b] 2. Homogeneous masses markedly hyperintense at T2-weighted imaging (similar to cerebrospinal fluid) at noncontrast MR imaging 3. Homogeneous masses markedly hyperintense at T1-weighted imaging (approximately 2.5 times normal parenchymal signal intensity) at noncontrast MR imaging	Well-defined cyst with thin (≤2 mm) smooth walls: 1. Cystic masses that are anechoic or hypoechoic and contain thin (≤2 mm) and few (1–3) septa; septa and wall may have color flow; may have well-defined calcification that does not obstruct other imaging features 2. Cystic masses that are hypoechoic or that contain debris; no septations, may have well-defined calcification that does not obstruct other imaging features
IIF	Cystic masses with a smooth minimally thickened (3 mm) enhancing wall, or smooth minimal thickening (3 mm) of ≥1 enhancing septa, or many (>4) smooth thin (<2 mm) enhancing septa	1. Cystic masses with a smooth minimally thickened (3 mm) enhancing wall, or smooth minimal thickening (3 mm) of ≥1 enhancing septa, or many (≥4) smooth thin (≤2 mm) enhancing septa 2. Cystic masses that are heterogeneously hyperintense at unenhanced fat-saturated T1-weighted imaging	Cystic masses with a smooth minimally thickened (3 mm) wall that may have color flow, or smooth minimal thickening (3 mm) of ≥1 septa that may have color flow, or many (≥4) smooth thin (≤2 mm) septa that may have color flow; may have well-defined calcification that does not obstruct other imaging features
III	≥1 enhancing thick (>4 mm width) or enhancing irregular (displaying <3-mm obtusely margined convex protrusion[s]) walls or septa	≥1 enhancing thick (≥4 mm width) or enhancing irregular (displaying ≤3-mm obtusely margined convex protrusion[s]) walls or septa	Not applicable to routine renal ultrasound examination[c]

(continued on next page)

Table 1 (continued)			
Class	CT Scan[a]	MR Imaging[a]	Ultrasound Examination[c]
IV	≥1 enhancing nodule(s) (>4-mm convex protrusion with obtuse margins, or a convex protrusion of any size that has acute margins)	≥1 enhancing nodule(s) (≥4-mm convex protrusion with obtuse margins, or a convex protrusion of any size that has acute margins)	Not applicable to routine renal ultrasound examination[c]

Abbreviation: CSF, cerebrospinal fluid.

  [a] The Bosniak classification is intended for cystic renal masses after infectious, inflammatory, or vascular etiologies and necrotic solid masses are excluded. If a cystic mass has features described in >1 Bosniak class, the highest Bosniak class is assigned. In rare cases, a mass may have an unusual combination of features (undefined, not fitting a specific Bosniak class) that may warrant inclusion into Bosniak type IIF. Other than for the diagnosis of Bosniak type I simple cysts, the role of ultrasound examination with or without contrast material in assigning a Bosniak class is uncertain.

  [b] Renal masses that at CT scan have abundant thick or nodular calcifications; are hyperattenuating, homogeneous, nonenhancing, and >3 cm; or are heterogeneous (including but not limited to many [≥4] nonenhancing septa or ≥3 mm nonenhancing septa or wall) might best be visualized at MR imaging before the assignment of a Bosniak class to determine if there are occult enhancing elements that might affect classification.

  [c] Ultrasound criteria were not specifically discussed in the Bosniak classification system version 2019 table, but are inferred from the text.[1] Cystic renal masses with thickened walls (>4 mm width) or thickened or irregular septations without or with color flow should be further evaluated by renal CT scan or MR imaging. Many radiology practices choose to follow Bosniak type IIF renal cysts by ultrasound examination, but it is unclear if this is sufficient to identify changes in complexity that are associated with a higher malignancy rate.

renal masses that are not clearly cystic, that have ill-defined features on portal venous CT scans, or that are evaluated on another contrast-enhanced phase (eg, arterial phase) need further characterization by renal CT scans or MR imaging.[1,2,8] In cases where the renal mass is not clearly cystic, renal ultrasound examination may be of benefit; however a renal CT scan or MR imaging may be needed if the patient is too large for a high-quality ultrasound examination to be obtained or if the entire lesion is cannot be fully characterized using ultrasound examination, or the if walls are thickened (≥4 mm) on ultrasound imaging.[1,2,8]

In the past, there were few guidelines on how to characterize a renal mass as cystic on noncontrast MR imaging. The Bosniak classification system version 2019 provides new and important information. Homogeneous renal masses that are markedly hyperintense at T2-weighted imaging (similar to cerebrospinal fluid) on noncontrast MR imaging are considered Bosniak II renal cystic masses (Fig. 4). Lesions meeting this criteria are commonly encountered on abdominal and spinal noncontrast MR imaging and no longer need further characterization.[1,19] In addition, homogeneous renal masses that are hyperintense at T1-weighted imaging (approximately 2.5 times normal parenchymal signal intensity) at noncontrast MR imaging are also considered benign Bosniak II renal masses and do not need further characterization.[1,17,18] By comparison, renal masses with low to intermediate signal on T1- or T2-weighted intensity on noncontrast MR imaging are

indeterminate and require further characterization by renal CT scans or MR imaging without and with intravenous contrast.[1,8]

The most widely accepted use of renal ultrasound examination for the characterization of renal masses is to differentiate a solid from a cystic renal mass identified on CT scan or MR imaging.[1,2,8] In addition, cystic renal masses are frequently first identified on a routine renal ultrasound examination, and many radiologists choose to characterize the renal cystic masses using inferences from the Bosniak classification system, as in Table 1. Simple cysts that are anechoic with well-defined smooth borders and posterior acoustic enhancement do not require further characterization.[1] In addition, an anechoic or hypoechoic well-defined cystic renal mass with thin (≤2 mm) smooth walls and few (1–3) septa does not require further characterization. However, if the cystic renal mass cannot be fully characterized on ultrasound examination or has thickened or irregular walls or septations, many (≥4) septations, or nodularity in the septations or walls, then further CT scans or MR imaging characterization is needed.[1]

SHOULD THE BOSNIAK CLASSIFICATION SYSTEM BE APPLIED?

The Bosniak classification system stratifies the risk of malignancy of cystic renal masses and is designed to be applied to definitive cystic renal masses and incompletely characterized lesions that are highly likely to be benign cystic renal

Table 2
Renal masses requiring further characterization before the Bosniak classification system can be applied

Modality	Renal Mass Finding(s)	Recommendation for Further Characterization
CT scan	Heterogeneous and TSTC	Renal MR imaging at 6–12 mo to differentiate solid from cystic and better characterize; renal CT scan may be suitable in some cases
	Heterogeneous on noncontrast CT scan	Renal CT scan or MR imaging to differentiate solid from cystic and better characterize
	Indeterminate potentially cystic lesion on dual energy CT scan	Renal CT scan or MR imaging to better characterize
	Solid appearing (21–69 HU) on noncontrast CT scan	Renal ultrasound or multiphasic renal CT scan or MR imaging in larger patients to differentiate solid vs cystic
	Potentially solid (≥31 HU) on portal venous CT scan	Renal CT scan or MR imaging to better characterize and differentiate enhancement or calcification in a solid renal neoplasm vs hyperdense (hemorrhagic or proteinaceous) renal cyst
	Heterogeneous or not well-defined on contrast-enhanced CT scan	Renal CT scan or MR imaging to better characterize
	Cystic mass with thickened walls (≥4 mm)	Renal CT scan or MR imaging to better characterize and differentiate higher category Bosniak renal cysts
MR imaging	Low to intermediate T1- or T2-weighted signal intensity on noncontrast MR imaging	Renal CT scan or MR imaging to better characterize
	Heterogeneous T1- or T2-weighted signal intensity on noncontrast MR imaging	Renal CT scan or MR imaging to better characterize and differentiate a necrotic papillary malignancy from a renal cystic mass[1]
	Not well-defined owing motion artifact on multiphasic MR imaging	Renal CT scan to reduce motion artifact; may consider renal MR imaging
Ultrasound examination	Not well-defined on ultrasound examination	Renal CT scan or MR imaging to better characterize
	Thickened walls	Renal CT scan or MR imaging to better characterize
	Many septations	Renal CT scan or MR imaging to better characterize
	Nodular areas or protrusions	Renal CT scan or MR imaging to better characterize

A renal CT scan or MR imaging acquisition is assumed to be a multiphasic examination without and with intravenous contrast. An indeterminate renal mass with contraindications to both renal CT scan and MR imaging should be evaluated by contrast-enhanced ultrasound examination.

masses.[1] However, the Bosniak classification should not be applied to cystic-appearing infectious, inflammatory, or vascular etiologies.[1,2,8] A common mistake encountered in the emergency radiology setting is to incorrectly apply the Bosniak classification system to a cystic-appearing renal mass in a patient with a urinary tract infection, with the cystic-appearing renal mass later identified as a renal abscess (Fig. 5). Some aneurysms can also seem to be cystic on grayscale ultrasound

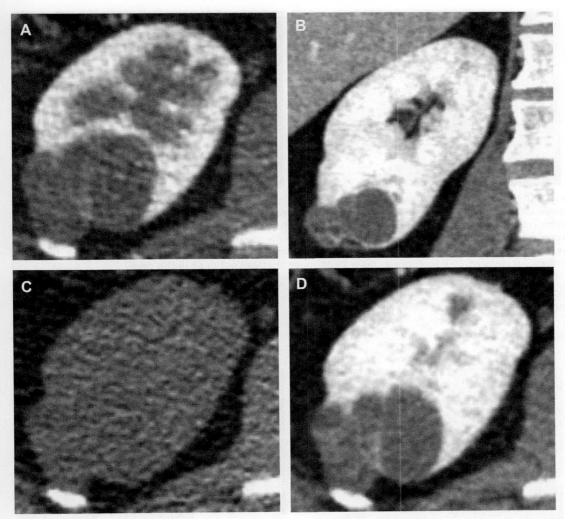

Fig. 2. A 63-year-old man with incidental discovery of a well-defined right renal mass on axial (*A*) and coronal (*B*) portal venous CT images. The hypoattenuating component of the mass measures fluid in attenuation and comprises 75% or more of the mass, indicating that it is cystic. Multiple thin internal septations are seen with probable enhancement. This mass could be classified as a Bosniak type IIF renal cystic mass based on these features, but a subsequent renal CT scan was ordered. Axial noncontrast (*C*) and axial corticomedullary phase (*D*) images from the renal CT scan confirm the presence of multiple thin enhancing septations, and this was correctly classified as a Bosniak type IIF renal cystic mass.

examination or noncontrast CT scans, but can be easily differentiated from a cystic mass on color flow ultrasound imaging (by visualizing the internal vascular flow) or on contrast-enhanced CT scans (with enhancement that matches the aorta). One additional special case is the calyceal diverticulum. Most calyceal diverticuli appear as cystic renal masses and cannot be prospectively identified as non-neoplastic, but the radiologist should look for layering stones as a clue that a calyceal diverticulum may be present (**Fig. 6**). If it is unclear whether calcifications represent layering stones versus wall calcifications, then a CT urogram could be

performed, because a calyceal diverticulum should fill with contrast on the excretory phase, and the Bosniak classification system would not apply.

For all other cystic renal masses, the Bosniak classification should be applied (see **Table 1**). There are now 6 types of Bosniak II renal cysts identifiable by CT scans, 3 by MR imaging, and 2 by ultrasound examination (see **Table 1**).[1] Most of these can be characterized on single phase CT scans or MR imaging. For example, a well-defined cystic mass with thin (<2 mm) smooth walls, few (1–3) septa, and the presence or absence of calcifications can be identified on a portal venous CT

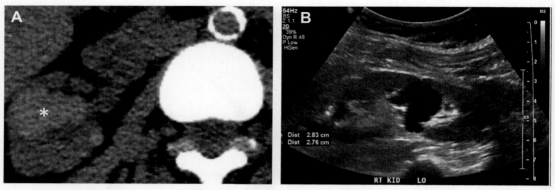

Fig. 3. A 66-year-old man with a 3.2-cm homogeneous right renal mass on noncontrast CT scan (*asterisk*), with a mean attenuation of 42 HU (*A*). A renal ultrasound examination was performed and demonstrated a hypoechoic cystic renal mass with small amounts of internal debris (*B*), most likely representing a hemorrhagic renal cyst and compatible with a Bosniak type II renal cystic mass. Given the size of this renal cystic mass on noncontrast CT scan, renal MR imaging could have been ordered instead of a renal ultrasound examination to look for occult enhancing elements (see footnote in **Table 1**), although that was not done in this case.

scan as a Bosniak type II cystic renal mass that needs no further characterization or follow-up.

The Bosniak classification system cannot be applied to heterogeneous appearing lesions on noncontrast CT scans or MR imaging without further characterization.[1] One notable difference in the Bosniak classification system version 2019 is the lack of a need to differentiate perceivable

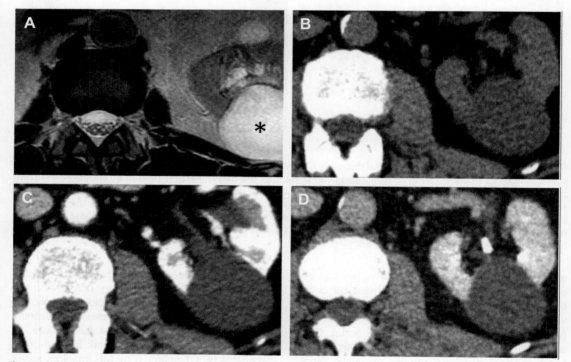

Fig. 4. A 55-year-old man with an incompletely imaged 4.5-cm homogeneous left renal mass (*asterisk*) that is markedly hyperintense at T2-weighted imaging (similar to cerebrospinal fluid) from a noncontrast spinal MR imaging that was obtained in 2018 (*A*), before the latest updates to the Bosniak classification system. A follow-up renal CT scan demonstrated a mildly hyperdense lesion (25 HU) on unenhanced phase (*B*), and no enhancement on corticomedullary phase (*C*) or nephrographic phase (*D*). This was characterized as a Bosniak type II renal cystic mass. According to the Bosniak classification system version 2019, the noncontrast MR imaging findings are sufficient to classify this as a Bosniak type II renal cystic mass, and no further characterization is needed.

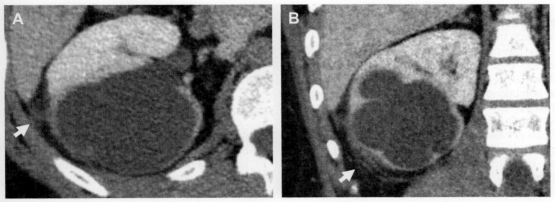

Fig. 5. A 45-year-old woman with abdominal pain, leukocytosis, and lower urinary tract symptoms. On the portal venous CT scan, a cystic-appearing renal mass with thickened walls and multiple thin internal septations is present, along with mild edema (*arrows*) in the surrounding perirenal fat (*A, B*). This lesion was correctly identified as a renal abscess, and the Bosniak classification system was not applied. The abscess subsequently resolved on intravenous antibiotic therapy (*B*).

from measurable enhancement.[1] Thereby, if a complex renal cystic mass is well-defined and clearly meets criteria for a cyst on portal venous CT scans (eg, ≥75% with fluid attenuation), it is often possible to fully characterize these renal cystic masses without the need for a dedicated

renal CT scan or MR imaging (see **Fig. 2**). A renal mass on a CT scan or MR imaging is needed to fully characterize any renal mass with ill-defined features and to confirm enhancement, because a cystic renal mass with thickened (≥4 mm) or irregular walls that do not enhance would not strictly fall

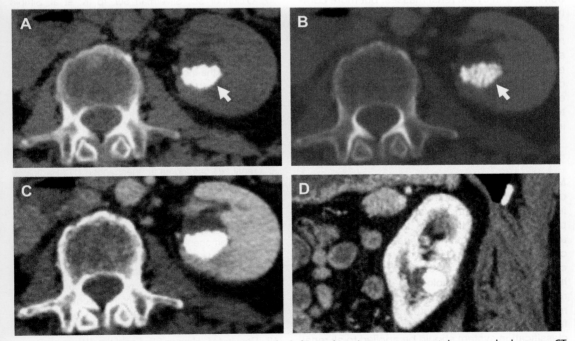

Fig. 6. A 57-year-old man with incidental discovery of a left renal cystic mass on a portal venous dual energy CT scan. The virtual nonenhanced images show multiple layering stones (*arrows*) within the renal cystic mass on soft tissue (*A*) and bone (*B*) windows. The cyst walls are thin, smooth, and enhance on contrast-enhanced axial (*C*) and coronal (*D*) images. This was interpreted as a calyceal diverticulum containing stones. No additional imaging was obtained, and the Bosniak classification system was not applied.

into any particular category and would default into the Bosniak IIF category (see **Table 1** footnote), although this occurrence is likely rare.[1]

The use of noncontrast MR imaging as it applies to the Bosniak classification system has been described elsewhere in this article and is limited to homogenous masses that are markedly hyperintense at T2-weighted imaging or at T1-weighted imaging, both of which are features of Bosniak type II renal cystic masses.[1] Features on contrast-enhanced MR imaging can and should be used to classify renal cystic masses (see **Table 1**).

Although the role of ultrasound examination has not been fully established in the classification of renal cystic masses, some inferences can be extracted and are permissible by the Bosniak classification system (see **Table 1**).[1] The role of contrast-enhanced ultrasound examination is less clear and cystic renal masses are often assigned a higher Bosniak class compared with renal CT imaging, owing to increased conspicuity of septa and previously undetected enhancement.[1] In addition, contrast-enhanced ultrasound examination is typically a focused examination and is not commonly used to survey for additional contralateral or other occult renal lesions or for coexisting retroperitoneal lymphadenopathy (uncommon with cystic renal masses, but more common with solid renal malignancies). For these reasons, the Bosniak classification system does not currently incorporate contrast-enhanced ultrasound examination as an accepted tool for further evaluating cystic renal masses.[1] However, contrast-enhanced ultrasound examination is an excellent choice when there are contraindications to both contrast-enhanced CT scans and MR imaging.

SUMMARY

Most renal masses are first encountered as incidental findings on abdominal CT scans, MR imaging, and ultrasound examination. The main purpose of this article was to provide a simple approach to evaluation of renal masses that are cystic or potentially cystic. Updates to the Bosniak classification system as captured in version 2019 have improved the radiologist's ability to define a renal cystic mass on multiple different imaging modalities and better determine the need for further characterization by imaging. The Bosniak classification system should be applied to all renal cystic masses that have appropriate high-quality images for complete characterization, except for specific clinical scenarios including cystic-appearing abscesses, aneurysms, or cystic masses containing stones that are likely to represent calyceal diverticuli.

DISCLOSURE

Nothing to disclose.

REFERENCES

1. Silverman SG, Pedrosa I, Ellis JH, et al. Bosniak classification of cystic renal masses, version 2019: an update proposal and needs assessment. Radiology 2019;292(2):475–88.
2. Bosniak MA. The current radiological approach to renal cysts. Radiology 1986;158(1):1–10.
3. Bosniak MA. The Bosniak renal cyst classification: 25 years later. Radiology 2012;262(3):781–5.
4. Israel GM, Bosniak MA. An update of the Bosniak renal cyst classification system. Urology 2005; 66(3):484–8.
5. Herts BR, Silverman SG, Hindman NM, et al. Management of the incidental renal mass on CT: a white paper of the ACR Incidental Findings Committee. J Am Coll Radiol 2018;15(2):264–73.
6. O'Connor SD, Pickhardt PJ, Kim DH, et al. Incidental finding of renal masses at unenhanced CT: prevalence and analysis of features for guiding management. AJR Am J Roentgenol 2011;197(1):139–45.
7. O'Connor SD, Silverman SG, Ip IK, et al. Simple cyst-appearing renal masses at unenhanced CT: can they be presumed to be benign? Radiology 2013;269(3):793–800.
8. Silverman SG, Israel GM, Herts BR, et al. Management of the incidental renal mass. Radiology 2008; 249(1):16–31.
9. Pooler BD, Pickhardt PJ, O'Connor SD, et al. Renal cell carcinoma: attenuation values on unenhanced CT. AJR Am J Roentgenol 2012;198(5):1115–20.
10. Jonisch AI, Rubinowitz AN, Mutalik PG, et al. Can high-attenuation renal cysts be differentiated from renal cell carcinoma at unenhanced CT? Radiology 2007;243(2):445–50.
11. Agochukwu N, HuberS, Spektor M, et al. Differentiating renal neoplasms from simple cysts on contrast-enhanced CT on the basis of attenuation and homogeneity. AJR Am J Roentgenol 2017; 208(4):801–4.
12. Hu EM, Ellis JH, Silverman SG, et al. Expanding the definition of a benign renal cyst on contrast-enhanced CT: can incidental homogeneous renal masses measuring 21-39 HU be safely ignored? Acad Radiol 2018;25(2):209–12.
13. Corwin MT, Hansra SS, Loehfelm TW, et al. Prevalence of solid tumors in incidentally detected homogeneous renal masses measuring > 20 HU on portal venous phase CT. AJR Am J Roentgenol 2018; 211(3):W173–7.

14. Mileto A, Sofue K, Marin D. Imaging the renal lesion with dual-energy multidetector CT and multi-energy applications in clinical practice: what can it truly do for you? Eur Radiol 2016;26(10):3677–90.

15. Mileto A, Nelson RC, Paulson EK, et al. Dual-energy MDCT for imaging the renal mass. AJR Am J Roentgenol 2015;204(6):W640–7.

16. Ho VB, Allen SF, Hood MN, et al. Renal masses: quantitative assessment of enhancement with dynamic MR imaging. Radiology 2002;224(3): 695–700.

17. Kim CW, Shanbhogue KP, Schreiber-Zinaman J, et al. Visual assessment of the intensity and pattern of T1 hyperintensity on MRI to differentiate hemorrhagic renal cysts from renal cell carcinoma. AJR Am J Roentgenol 2017;208(2): 337–42.

18. Davarpanah AH, Spektor M, Mathur M, et al. Homogeneous T1 hyperintense renal lesions with smooth borders: is contrast-enhanced MR imaging needed? Radiology 2016;280(1):128–36.

19. Nelson SM, Oettel DJ, Lisanti CJ, et al. Incidental renal lesions on lumbar spine MRI: who needs follow-up? AJR Am J Roentgenol 2019;212(1): 130–4.

Imaging of Renal Infections and Inflammatory Disease

Maria Zulfiqar, MD[a],*, Cristián Varela Ubilla, MD[b], Refky Nicola, MS, DO[c], Christine O. Menias, MD[d]

KEYWORDS

- Renal infection • Pyelonephritis • Urinary tract infection • Imaging

KEY POINTS

- Pyelonephritis commonly occurs as a complication of ascending urinary tract infection manifesting as a unilateral or bilateral striated nephrogram on imaging.
- Complications of pyelonephritis include emphysematous pyelonephritis appearing as gas within the renal parenchyma on imaging and renal abscess signified by a rim-enhancing cystic renal mass.
- Pyonephrosis is one of the few urologic emergencies requiring urgent drainage. A peripherally enhancing, thickened, and dilated renal pelvis is concerning for pyonephrosis.
- Chronic pyelonephritis is a spectrum of long-standing renal infection including xanthogranulomatous pyelonephritis and renal replacement lipomatosis.

INTRODUCTION

Urinary tract infection (UTI) is the most common urologic disease in the United States, accounting for more than 10 million office and 2 to 3 million emergency department visits every year.[1] Typically, in adults the diagnosis of a UTI is established with patient history, physical examination, and urinalysis. Per American College of Radiology appropriateness criteria, diagnostic imaging is reserved for complex patients with either treatment failure or when there is concern for complications such as pyelonephritis or an abscess, especially in the setting of diabetes mellitus, immunosuppression, or stones.[2]

ETIOLOGY
Ascending Infection

The urinary tract is a tubular system that opens at the body's surface as the urethra, which makes it susceptible to colonization by infectious organisms that include both gram-negative and gram-positive bacteria, as well as certain fungi. The most common causative agent is *Escherichia coli*. UTIs are more common in women than men because of the shorter length of the urethra.[3] In most cases, the infection is confined to the urinary bladder. An ascending migration of the pathogens through the ureters into the kidneys can lead to a complicated UTI,[4] which includes a spectrum of acute and chronic renal infectious pathology, discussed as follows.

Descending Infection

In patients with bacteremia, sepsis, or infective endocarditis, the bloodborne pathogens can seed into the kidneys by crossing the tubular epithelium barrier followed by parenchymal colonization and infection.[5]

[a] Mallinckrodt Institute of Radiology, Washington University School of Medicine, 510 South Kingshighway Boulevard, St Louis, MO 63110, USA; [b] Radiology Department, Clinica Davila, Avenida Recoleta 464, Recoleta, Santiago 8431657, Chile; [c] Division of Body Imaging, Department of Radiology, Roswell Park Cancer Institute, Elm and Carlton Street, Buffalo, NY 14203, USA; [d] Mayo Clinic School of Medicine, Mayo Clinic Hospital, 5777 East Mayo Boulevard, Phoenix, AZ 85054, USA
* Corresponding author.
E-mail address: mariazulfiqar@wustl.edu

Radiol Clin N Am 58 (2020) 909–923
https://doi.org/10.1016/j.rcl.2020.05.004
0033-8389/20/© 2020 Elsevier Inc. All rights reserved.

Renal Stones

The presence of renal stones increases the risk of complicated UTI. The obstruction of the urinary tract by renal stones leads to urinary stasis with entrapment and proliferation of bacteria.[6] The major types of renal stones include calcium oxalate (most common), calcium phosphate, struvite, uric acid, cysteine, xanthine, and protein matrix stones.[7] The struvite stones are composed of magnesium ammonium phosphate and calcium carbonate-apatite and can cause chronic upper UTI with urease-producing organisms such as *Proteus* and *Klebsiella*.[8] Overall, renal stones are more common in men with a prevalence of 10.6%, compared with 7.1% among women.[9] However, struvite stones are more common in women, with a frequency of 10% to 15% and can grow rapidly into a large calculus involving and conforming to the shape of the entire renal collecting system that resembles a staghorn or coral (**Fig. 1**). If left untreated, the complication rate can reach up to 75%, including renal failure and life-threatening urosepsis.[10]

PATHOLOGY
Acute Pyelonephritis

Acute pyelonephritis denotes an infection of the renal pelvis, calyces, and parenchyma and presents predominantly in adult women. Almost always, the infection ascends from the urinary bladder or spreads to the kidneys hematogenously. Clinically, the patient presents with fever, dysuria, flank pain, and costovertebral angle tenderness. The diagnosis is confirmed with bacterial growth in the urine culture.[5]

Imaging features

The diagnosis of acute pyelonephritis is clinical, and imaging is generally used to assess for complications. Ultrasound is frequently used as the initial imaging modality, but the most common finding is a normal examination.[11] When present, sonographic features of acute pyelonephritis include loss of corticomedullary differentiation, increased renal size, loss of renal sinus fat due to edema, dilated renal pelvis, and urothelial thickening. The change in renal echogenicity commonly occurs in a linear or wedge-shaped pattern that could be increased due to hemorrhage, or decreased due to edema.[12] The alternating pattern of increased renal echogenicity with normal renal parenchyma is termed as echogenic "striation." Focal pyelonephritis can appear as a masslike area of abnormal echogenicity, especially in patients with diabetes mellitus or immunosuppression.[2] On Doppler interrogation, areas of hypoperfusion are identified that correspond to the changes in echogenicity[11] (**Fig. 2A**).

Computed tomography (CT) is preferred in the evaluation of acute pyelonephritis because of its excellent ability to detect complications such as

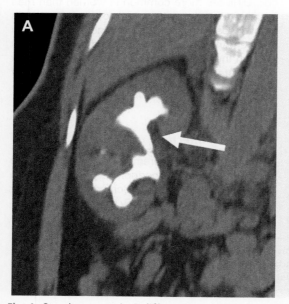
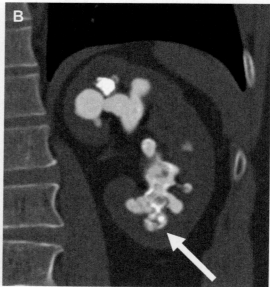

Fig. 1. Struvite stones in 2 different patients. Coronal CT of the abdomen in a 39-year-old woman (*A*) shows a large staghorn calculus conforming to the shape of the renal pelvis and extending into the major calyces (*arrow*) in a configuration resembling a stag's antler. Coronal CT of the abdomen in a 42-year-old woman (*B*) shows smaller stones with an irregular texture within the calyces resembling a more coraliform configuration (*arrow*).

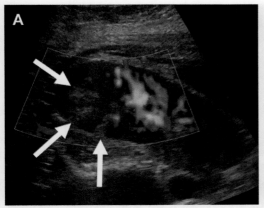
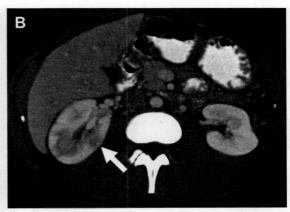

Fig. 2. Acute pyelonephritis. Power Doppler image with grayscale in a 24-year-old woman shows the character-istic echogenic striated appearance of the kidney with distinct echogenic wedge-shaped areas of increased paren-chymal echogenicity and associated hypoperfusion (*A, arrows*). Axial CT image of the abdomen of a 30-year-old woman shows an enlarged edematous right kidney with areas of cortical hypoenhancement consistent with py-elonephritis (*B, arrow*).

gas, hemorrhage, obstruction, or stones.[13] The "striated nephrogram" is the classic appearance that occurs as inflammation selectively increases parenchymal pressure leading to intratubular edema and obstruction, which is then manifested as alternating bands of high and low parenchymal attenuation on CT oriented to the axis of the renal tubules and collecting ducts[14] (**Fig. 2**B). This can be unilateral or bilateral, and the affected kidney is often enlarged and edematous with or without peri-nephric fat stranding. In addition, smooth urothelial thickening and enhancement also may be seen.[15]

Differential diagnosis and pitfalls

The "striated nephrogram" is not specific for acute pyelonephritis (**Table 1**). Any process that in-creases the pressure within the renal parenchyma can lead to this pattern of enhancement.[16] Unilat-eral etiologies include renal vein thrombosis, renal contusion, or ureteric obstruction.[14,17]

Differentiation between focal pyelonephritis and segmental renal infarction can be challenging (**Ta-ble 2**). In such cases, the "cortical rim sign" can be very helpful, which is seen due to preserved outer rim of renal cortex being perfused by perforating collateral vessels in the presence of occlusion of main or smaller renal arteries in the affected kid-ney[18] (**Fig. 3**A). Bilateral striated nephrograms are associated with contrast-associated acute kidney injury, hypotension, renal infarcts, and autosomal recessive polycystic kidney disease (**Fig. 3**B). Another potential pitfall is infiltrating tran-sitional cell carcinoma that invades the renal pa-renchyma, thus causing a delayed cortical nephrogram that can mimic a "striated nephro-gram" appearance (**Fig. 3**C).[19]

Emphysematous Pyelonephritis

Emphysematous pyelonephritis is a life-threatening necrotizing infection of the renal parenchyma with gas-forming organisms. Patients with

---

Table 1
Differential diagnosis for the "striated nephrogram"

Unilateral	Bilateral
• Acute pyelonephritis	• Acute pyelonephritis
• Renal vein thrombosis	• Contrast-associated acute kidney injury
• Renal infarction/contusion	• Hypotension
• Ureteric obstruction	• Renal infarcts
• Transitional cell carcinoma	• Autosomal recessive polycystic kidney disease

---

Table 2
Differentiating imaging features between focal pyelonephritis and segmental renal infarction

Focal Pyelonephritis	Segmental Renal Infarction
• No cortical rim sign	• Cortical rim enhance-ment in 50% cases due to extrarenal arterial capsular supply
• Delayed enhancement	• No enhancement within wedge

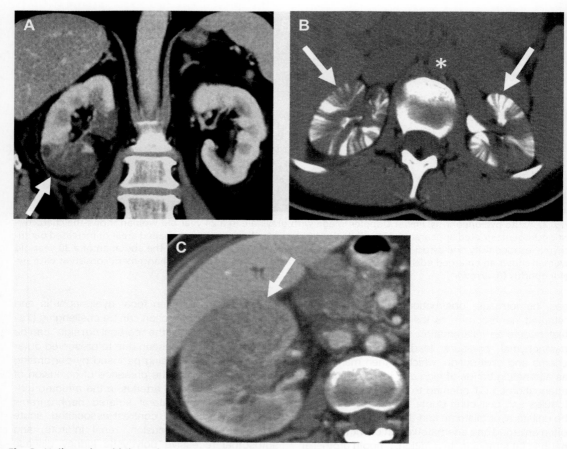

Fig. 3. Unilateral and bilateral striated nephrograms. Coronal contrast-enhanced CT image of the abdomen (*A*) shows a wedge-shaped area of decreased enhancement in the right kidney inferior pole with preserved outer rim of enhancement (*arrow*) representing an infarct. Axial CT image of the abdomen without intravenous contrast (*B*), shows areas of contrast retention in both kidneys alternating bands of nonretention (*arrows*) representing changes of contrast-associated acute kidney injury from recent cardiac catheterization. Note absence of contrast within the aorta (*asterisk*). Axial contrast-enhanced CT image of the abdomen (*C*) shows wedge-shaped area of hypoenhancement (*arrow*) in the right kidney mimicking a striated nephrogram, in this patient with infiltrating transitional cell carcinoma.

emphysematous pyelonephritis are extremely ill with fever and flank pain.[20] When gas is confined to the collecting system, the term emphysematous pyelitis, an important differentiator from parenchymal gas, is implied, which can be managed conservatively with antibiotic treatment.[21] The most common gas-forming organism is *E coli* (68%) followed by *Klebsiella pneumoniae* (10%).[22] Emphysematous pyelonephritis almost exclusively occurs in patients with poorly controlled diabetes mellitus, where the elevated levels of glucose inhibit the normal function of leukocytes, impairing the body's defense against infection.[22,23]

Imaging features
Conventional radiography has a sensitivity of 66% to 70% for detection of gas in the kidneys.[24] The

gas is commonly present in a radial pattern along the renal pyramids[25] (**Fig. 4**A). On gray scale ultrasound, highly echogenic areas within the renal sinuses and parenchyma are identified with associated ring down artifact representing gas, commonly referred to as "dirty shadowing" (**Fig. 4**B).[26] When present in the perinephric space, gas can obscure the visualization of the kidney. On CT, the characteristic finding is intraparenchymal, intracaliceal, or intrapelvic gas, often extending into the subcapsular space or even across the Gerota fascia, indicative of a more advanced stage of renal necrosis (**Fig. 4**C).[25]

Wan and colleagues[27] identified 2 types of emphysematous pyelonephritis depending on presence of fluid and their gas pattern. The mortality rate in the 2 subtypes correlates with degree of

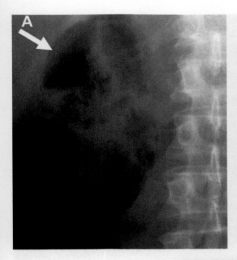

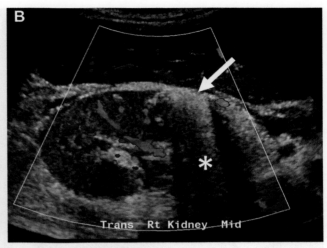

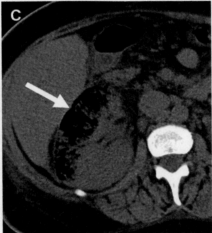

Fig. 4. Emphysematous pyelonephritis. Plain radiograph of the abdomen (*A*) shows mottled appearance of the right renal silhouette from parenchymal gas (*arrow*). Long view of the kidney on ultrasound (*B*) shows a crescentic echogenic region along the renal margin (*arrow*) with "dirty posterior acoustic shadowing" (*asterisk*) representing gas. Axial noncontrast CT image of the abdomen (*C*) shows an enlarged right kidney with intraparenchymal gas (*arrow*).

parenchymal destruction. Type 1 emphysematous pyelonephritis is more fulminant and occurs in approximately 33% of cases. There is destruction of more than one-third of the renal parenchyma, however, without any fluid collection (**Fig. 5**A). Gas may be intraparenchymal, or present with in a crescentic pattern in the subcapsular or perinephric region. The associated mortality rate is as high as 69%. Treatment is nephrectomy (**Fig. 5**B).[28] Type 2 emphysematous pyelonephritis is associated with destruction of less than one-third of the renal parenchyma, with gas associated with renal or perirenal abscesses (**Fig. 5**C). The gas is typically confined to the abscess or may be seen within the renal pelvis and has a lower mortality at 18%.[27] Treatment is percutaneous drainage or in severe cases, nephrectomy.

Renal Abscess

Renal abscess is defined as necrosis of the renal parenchyma that commonly develops as a complication of focal pyelonephritis. These are usually solitary and unilateral. The complications include rupture of the abscess into surrounding spaces leading to perinephric, subdiaphragmatic, or pelvic spread.[29] A renal abscess should be suspected if appropriate treatment for pyelonephritis does not demonstrate any significant clinical improvement. Approximately 15% to 20% of patients with a renal abscess will have negative urine cultures.[2]

Imaging features

On grayscale ultrasound, an abscess presents as a hypoechoic well-circumscribed mass with poor

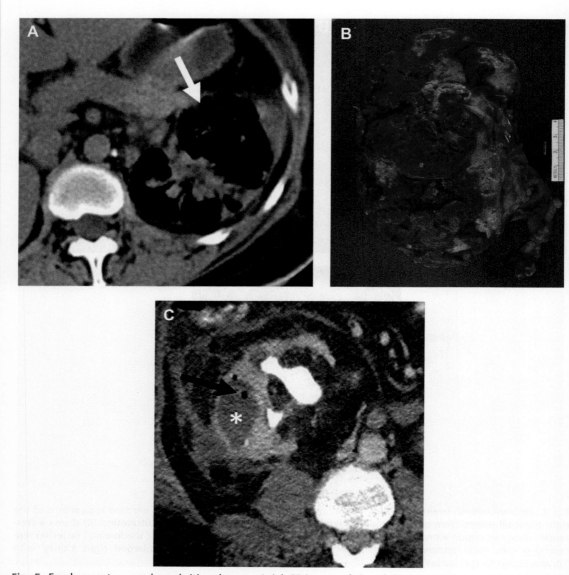

Fig. 5. Emphysematous pyelonephritis subtypes. Axial CT image of the abdomen (*A*) shows extensive paren-chymal gas in the left kidney (*arrow*) representing type 1 emphysematous pyelonephritis that was treated with nephrectomy with gross pathology specimen demonstrating global necrosis (*B*). Axial CT image of the abdomen in another patient (*C*) shows a rim-enhancing fluid collection in the right renal parenchyma (*asterisk*) with internal foci of gas (*arrow*) representing an abscess consistent with type 2 emphysematous pyelonephritis that was treated with percutaneous drainage and antibiotics.

through transmission, but without internal vascular flow on Doppler (**Fig. 6**A). Low-level internal echoes representing hemorrhage or debris are often identified. Gas within the abscess will cause dirty shadowing. Internal complexity is indicated by the presence of septations.[12] On CT, an abscess presents as a cystic mass with thick periph-eral enhancement called the "rim sign," with perinephric fat stranding indicating an inflamma-tory process[29,30] (**Fig. 6**B).

In patients with elevated serum creatinine, iodine contrast allergy, or need for serial imaging, magnetic resonance imaging (MR imaging) may be used to evaluate for renal abscesses. An addi-tional important consideration is evaluation in chil-dren and patients who are pregnant in whom radiation may want to be used sparingly. On MR imaging, a T1 hypointense and T2 hyperintense heterogeneous cystic lesion with thick rim enhancement, perinephric fat stranding, and

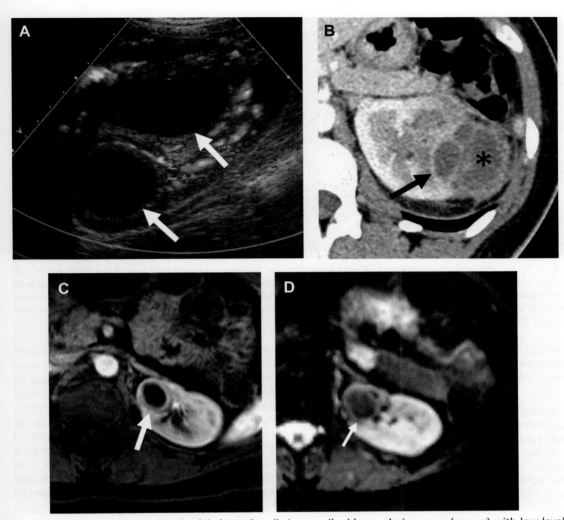

Fig. 6. Renal abscess. Power Doppler (*A*) shows 2 well-circumscribed hypoechoic masses (*arrows*) with low-level internal echoes representing debris consistent with abscesses. (*B*) Axial CT image of the abdomen with intravenous contrast demonstrates a cystic mass in the left kidney (*asterisk*) with thick rim enhancement (*arrow*) and perinephric fat stranding representing an abscess. Post contrast axial T1 (*C*) and apparent diffusion coefficient MR imaging sequences (*D*) in another patient show a left renal abscess demonstrating thick rim enhancement and central diffusion restriction (*arrow*).

central diffusion restriction is consistent with a renal abscess (**Fig. 6**C, D).[31]

Differential diagnosis and pitfalls
Clear cell renal carcinoma can appear cystic and heterogeneous[32] (**Fig. 7**). Metastatic disease such as squamous cell carcinoma also can be necrotic and have cystic features. Renal lymphoma can be hypoenhancing and mimic a cystic mass. These entities present as a potential pitfall when diagnosing an abscess; however, the presence of internal vascularity on Doppler ultrasound and enhancement on CT and MR imaging within the solid components distinguishes a neoplasm from an abscess.[33]

Pyonephrosis
Pyonephrosis is defined as "pus under pressure" and signifies the presence of infected urine within an obstructed urinary collecting system. It commonly develops in the setting of obstruction from a stone or ureteropelvic junction obstruction from extrinsic causes in a young adult. In the elderly, often a malignant ureteral stricture is the underlying etiology.[34] Superinfection of stagnant urine becomes filled with bacteria, debris, and pus. The most common organism is *E coli*.[34] Pyonephrosis can lead to bacteremia and septic shock with a 25% to 50% mortality. A delay in treatment results in irreversible renal parenchymal

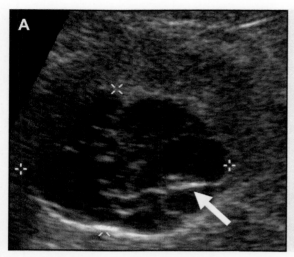
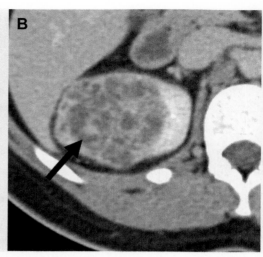

Fig. 7. Cystic renal cell carcinoma mimicking a renal abscess. Transverse ultrasound view of the right kidney (*A*) shows a multiloculated cystic mass with thick internal septations (*arrow*). Axial CT image of the abdomen with intravenous contrast (*B*) demonstrates the same mass with multiple internal septations that are thick and nodular with enhancement (*arrow*) consistent with a cystic renal cell carcinoma. Note the absence of surrounding inflammatory stranding.

damage and renal failure, thus early diagnosis and drainage is essential.[35] Pyonephrosis is one of the few urologic emergencies.

Imaging features
On ultrasound, the renal pelvis is dilated and filled with internal debris and low-level luminal echoes (**Fig. 8A**). Other findings of obstructing renal pelvis stones, urothelial thickening, or even gas within the obstructed collecting system may be present.[36] CT is helpful in long-standing pyonephrosis

and can evaluate for potential complications such as renal parenchymal abscesses and renal atrophy. Sometimes, a fluid and debris level can be identified or air in the renal pelvis.[37] The most classic appearance of pyonephrosis is a peripherally enhancing, thickened and dilated renal pelvis (**Fig. 8B**).[38] However, the clinical presentation of UTI with hydronephrosis on CT is considered a more sensitive indicator of pyonephrosis than most other CT characteristics alone.[31] Diffusion restriction within the dilated collecting system on

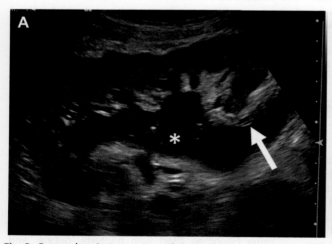
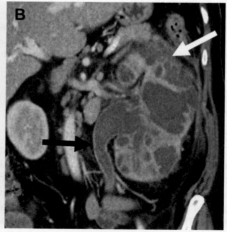

Fig. 8. Pyonephrosis. Long view of the kidney on grayscale sonogram (*A*) shows a markedly dilated renal collecting system with urothelial thickening (*arrow*) and intraluminal low-level echoes representing debris (*asterisk*). Coronal CT of the abdomen with contrast (*B*) shows an enlarged left kidney with hydronephrosis, hydroureter, and smooth urothelial thickening (*black arrow*) secondary to a distal obstructing stone (not shown). Multiple renal parenchymal fluid collections represent abscesses (*white arrow*).

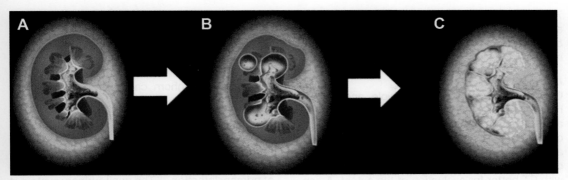

Fig. 9. Schematic diagram shows role of struvite stones in the evolution of chronic pyelonephritis. Obstructing staghorn calculus (*A*) leads to chronic smoldering pyelonephritis and XGP (*B*) that causes severe renal parenchymal atrophy and renal replacement lipomatosis characterized by severe reactive renal sinus and fat proliferation (*C*).

MR imaging is helpful in differentiating pyonephrosis from hydronephrosis.[39]

Chronic Pyelonephritis

Chronic pyelonephritis represents a spectrum of long-standing sequelae of renal infection that encompasses rare but severe variants including xanthogranulomatous pyelonephritis (XGP) and renal replacement lipomatosis. Initially, there is chronic tubulo-interstitial inflammation and often asymmetric cortical atrophy with clubbing of the renal calyces from retraction of the papillae due to scarring.[2] Frequently, the cause is recurrent infections from chronic vesicoureteral reflux or renal stones.[4]

Role of struvite stones in chronic pyelonephritis
Struvite stones are also known as *infectious stones* and develop frequently in patients with urinary stasis or recurrent UTIs. These can occupy and obstruct the entire pelvicalyceal system and serve as a nidus of infection with bacteria colonizing the renal pelvis or calyces and segmentally infiltrating the renal parenchyma.[40] Smoldering infection leads to pseudo tumor formation with lipid-laden foam cells, termed XGP long-standing obstructing urolithiasis and chronic pyelonephritis eventually leads to renal parenchymal destruction and atrophy as well as proliferation of renal sinus and perirenal fat, termed as renal replacement lipomatosis[41] (**Fig. 9**).

Xanthogranulomatous Pyelonephritis

XGP is a chronic form of suppurative pyelonephritis that develops in the setting of chronic obstruction and is thought to be a result of atypical, partial immune response to subacute bacterial infection leading to progressive parenchymal destruction.[2] Most often it is unilateral, and 70% of cases present in women. A staghorn calculus is present in

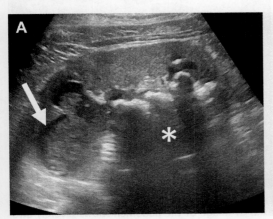
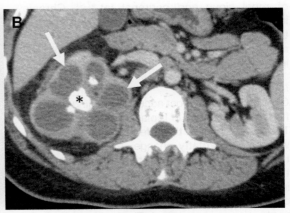

Fig. 10. XGP. Long sonographic view of the kidney (*A*) shows clean shadowing from a staghorn calculus in the calyces and pelvis (*asterisk*). The calyces are dilated with internal echogenic debris (*arrow*). Axial CT of the abdomen with contrast (*B*) shows centrally obstructing staghorn stones (*asterisk*) with surrounding low-attenuation collections, corresponding to the blown-out calyces seen (*arrows*) with XPG.

75% of the cases superimposed on an infection by a urease-positive organism such as *Proteus mirabilis* or *E coli*. There is infiltration with lipid-laden macrophages leading to xanthomas.[42]

Imaging features

On grayscale ultrasound, multiple anechoic to hypoechoic masses are seen with extensive acoustic shadowing from the central staghorn calculus (**Fig. 10**A). There is associated parenchymal atrophy and hydronephrosis.[43] Inflammatory changes can extend to the perinephric region with CT better for evaluation of the extent. A centrally obstructing staghorn stone is commonly seen with replacement of the renal parenchyma by low-attenuation collections, which are in fact lipid-rich xanthogranulomatous tissue. This pattern resembles a bear's paw[44] (**Fig. 10**B). XGP can be either focal or diffuse. Focal XGP is often masslike and can mimic an abscess or even renal cell carcinoma.[45] The inflammatory process can cross renal boundaries and extend into the perirenal space. MR imaging has no advantage over CT and is usually not used because of limited capacity to detect calcifications.[46] Definitive treatment is surgical nephrectomy.

Renal Replacement Lipomatosis

Renal replacement lipomatosis is the end result of severe atrophy of renal parenchyma commonly associated with long-standing inflammation and obstructing stones. Although renal *sinus* lipomatosis involves only prominent fat proliferation in the renal sinuses with mass effect on the intrarenal collecting system without obstruction, in contrast, renal replacement lipomatosis is characterized by marked proliferation and expansion of renal sinus *and* perirenal fat.[47,48] Chronic inflammation leads to fibrosis and retraction of the pelvis with severe parenchymal atrophy, scarring, and replacement of the parenchyma with adipose tissue.

Imaging features

CT is perhaps the most accurate imaging modality for the identification of replacement lipomatosis.[49] The renal sinus of the affected kidney expands with gross fibrofatty change. Although atrophic, the renal cortex maintains the reniform shape of the kidney, and there is typically a staghorn stone in the renal pelvis. Superimposed findings of acute or chronic pyelonephritis such as XGP or pyonephrosis may be present. The hyperplastic fat in the renal sinuses and surrounding the kidney does not permeate into the renal parenchyma (**Fig. 11**).

Differential diagnosis and pitfalls

Replacement lipomatosis can be tumefactive, in which case other focal fatty lesions including a lipoma, angiomyolipoma, or liposarcoma must be considered. The presence of renal parenchymal atrophy and staghorn calculus are useful clues for excluding these entities.

Renal Tuberculosis

Renal tuberculosis (TB) occurs due to hematogenous seeding of the kidney from a pulmonary site of primary infection.[50] The genitourinary system is one of the most common sites of extrapulmonary TB, accounting for 15% to 20% of infections outside the lungs.[51] The bacilli lodge in the glomerular capillaries and proliferate with the end result of destruction and calcification of the entire kidney. Genitourinary TB can manifest 5 to 40 years after the initial pulmonary infection and at the time of diagnosis only 5% patients will have active cavitary pulmonary disease.[52] TB can involve any part of the kidney and collecting system.

Imaging features

CT urogram is the modality of choice for identifying all the manifestations of renal TB.[53] Early stages of the disease are marked by papillary necrosis with caliectasis, which is often nonuniform. Urothelial enhancement may be present. Progressive disease causes parenchymal scarring and multifocal strictures with a preponderance to involve the pelvo-infundibular region that lead to focal or generalized hydronephrosis and poor

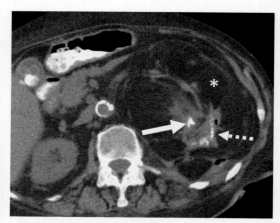

Fig. 11. Renal replacement lipomatosis. Noncontrast axial CT image of the abdomen shows severely atrophic and calcified left renal parenchyma (*dashed arrow*) with a central chronic staghorn stone (*white arrow*). There is extensive perirenal and renal sinus fat hypertrophy (*asterisk*).

enhancement of the renal parenchyma (**Fig. 12A, B**).[54] Coarse parenchymal and urothelial dystrophic calcifications are seen in between 24% and 44% of patients.[55] Sometimes, low-density parenchymal pseudotumoral lesions of varying sizes form, which represent tuberculomas due to caseous necrosis and appear as peripherally enhancing cystic lesions (**Fig. 12C**).[53] With long-standing TB, the kidney loses its morphology and appears as a conglomerate of thin-walled cysts. The end stage of renal TB is a completely atrophic and calcified kidney, which is termed as autonephrectomy or "putty kidney" (**Fig. 12D**).[56]

Differential diagnosis and pitfalls

A tuberculoma can appear masslike and mimic renal cell carcinoma on imaging and can lead to unwanted nephrectomy that can otherwise be treated with anti-tuberculous multidrug therapy.[57]

Renal Hydatid Disease

Renal hydatid disease is a zoonosis caused by the larvae of *Echinococcus granulosus* tapeworm. Dogs are the definitive host with human infection due to ingestion of contaminated water and food that contains eggs of the parasite.[58] In the United

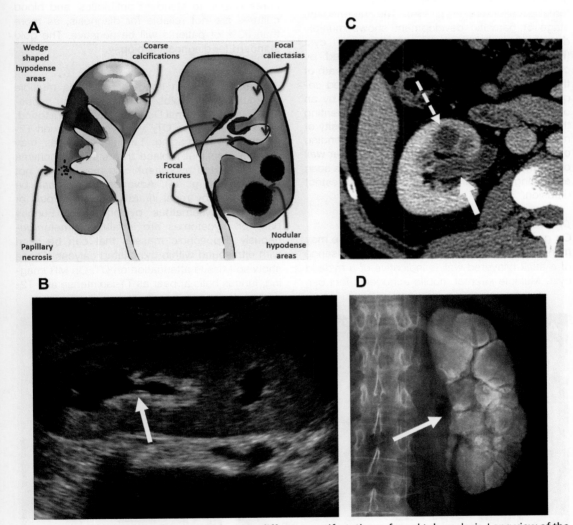

Fig. 12. Renal TB. Schematic diagram (*A*) showing different manifestations of renal tuberculosis. Long view of the kidney on ultrasound (*B*) demonstrates focal urothelial thickening and stricture at the infundibulum of the superior calyx (*arrow*) in a patient with renal TB. Axial CT of the abdomen with contrast (*C*) shows smooth urothelial enhancement (*arrow*) along with tuberculomas (*dashed arrow*) in the right kidney. Abdominal radiograph in another patient (*D*) shows a completely calcified left kidney and proximal ureter (*arrow*) representing autonephrectomy from end stage TB. ([*A*] Courtesy of Eugenio Zalaquett M.D.)

States, most cases present in immigrants from endemic countries. The disease is rare in the kidneys, accounting for approximately 2% to 3% of all hydatids.[59] The parasite passes through the portal system and retroperitoneal lymphatics to reach the kidney. It remains usually asymptomatic for many years. When symptomatic, the patient presents with a flank mass or renal colic.[60]

Imaging features

Renal hydatid cysts are frequently solitary and involve the cortex of the upper or lower pole. These can reach a very large size of up to 10 cm before becoming symptomatic.[33] Early stage of disease may present as unilocular cyst without internal architecture (**Fig. 13**A). The intermediate stage of parasitic development shows multiple daughter cysts within a single large cyst (**Fig. 13**B). End-stage disease is signified by completely calcified cyst and represents death of the parasite.[61] On MR imaging T2-weighted sequences, hydatid cysts are characterized by an outer rim that is low in signal intensity representing the dense fibrous pericyst. The signal intensity of maternal and daughter cysts may differ depending on the matrix contents. Sometimes, the inner wall of the maternal cyst may detach and can be seen as floating membranes. These cysts also restrict diffusion.[58]

Differential diagnosis and pitfalls

On grayscale ultrasound, the unilocular type may mimic a simple renal cyst; however, the presence of a thick bilayered wall is indicative of a hydatid cyst. Multiple internal mobile echogenic foci can be seen that disperse when the patient changes position. These foci represent hydatid sand and are pathognomonic of hydatid cyst, also called the "falling snowflake" or "snow storm sign."[62]

Renal Fungal Infections

Renal fungal infections are commonly seen as part of a disseminated infection in immunocompromised hosts. Fungal UTI is an important cause of morbidity and mortality in renal transplant patients. Organisms such as *Candida* species, *Aspergillus* species, *Histoplasma capsulatum*, *Pneumocystis jirovecii*, *Cryptococcus* species, *Nocardia*, or *Mucor* may be seen in this setting.[63] The fever is unresponsive to standard antibiotics, and blood cultures are not reliable for diagnosis, as more than 80% of patients will be negative. The gold standard for diagnosis is biopsy.[64]

Imaging features

The most common imaging finding is multiple parenchymal microabscesses that appear hypoechoic without internal Doppler flow on ultrasound, hypoattenuating on CT, and hyperintense on T2-weighted MR imaging. Larger abscesses may also develop that replace the renal parenchyma and associated hydronephrosis may or may not be present (**Fig. 14**). Advanced cases can be complicated by renal infarction and necrosis or rarely emphysematous pyelonephritis. Fungus balls or mycetomas are intraluminal heterogeneously hypoechoic masses that can be seen with ultrasound within the dilated calyces. These show soft tissue attenuation on CT. On MR imaging, fungus balls appear as T1-isointense and T2-

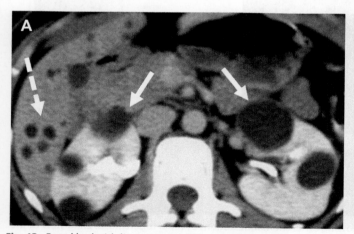
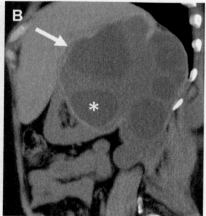

Fig. 13. Renal hydatid disease. Axial CT image of the abdomen with intravenous contrast (*A*) shows multiple bilateral unilocular cysts in both kidneys (*arrows*) as well as the visualized liver parenchyma (*dashed arrow*) representing early developmental stage of the hydatid cyst. Sagittal CT image of the abdomen without contrast (*B*) shows a large cystic lesion in the kidney (*arrow*) with multiple inner daughter cysts (*asterisk*) representing the intermediate stage of hydatid disease.

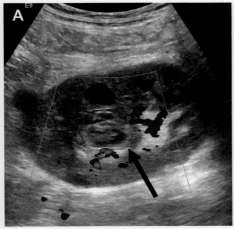
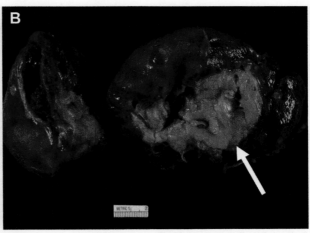

Fig. 14. Renal transplant abscess due to nocardiosis. Ultrasound image of the transplant kidney (*A*) shows a heterogeneously hypoechoic mass in the interpolar region (*arrow*) that does not have internal vascularity. Gross pathologic specimen after transplant nephrectomy (*B*) shows central area of necrosis (*arrow*) consistent with culture positive *Nocardia* infection.

hyperintense filling defects within the collecting system demonstrating diffusion restriction but no internal enhancement.[63] Concomitant thrombophlebitis may be present. Chronic or healed fungal infections lead to parenchymal calcifications.[65]

SUMMARY

A wide spectrum of renal infectious and inflammatory conditions exist ranging from uncomplicated pyelonephritis to obstructed pyonephrosis and renal abscess. Severe renal inflammation and associated complications are primarily assessed via imaging with ultrasound, CT, and MR imaging subsidizing a vital role in the diagnostic process. It is imperative for the radiologist to recognize the various imaging features to direct appropriate management and avoid potential pitfalls.

ACKNOWLEDGMENTS

Image 12A courtesy of Eugenio Zalaquett, MD.

CONFLICTS OF INTEREST

None of the authors have any relevant commercial or financial disclosures.

REFERENCES

1. Schappert SM, Rechtsteiner EA. Ambulatory medical care utilization estimates for 2007. Vital Health Stat 13 2011;(169):1–38.
2. Craig WD, Wagner BJ, Travis MD. Pyelonephritis: radiologic-pathologic review. Radiographics 2008; 28(1):255–76.
3. Chung BI, Sommer G, Brooks J. Anatomy of the lower urinary tract and male genitalia. In: Wein AJ, Kavoussi LR, Novick AC, et al, editors. Campbell-walsh urology. 10th edition. Philadelphia: Saunders Elsevier; 2012. p. 59–60.
4. Flores-Mireles AL, Walker JN, Caparon M, et al. Urinary tract infections: epidemiology, mechanisms of infection and treatment options. Nat Rev Microbiol 2015;13(5):269–84.
5. Roberts JA. Etiology and pathophysiology of pyelonephritis. Am J Kidney Dis 1991;17(1):1–9.
6. Borghi L, Nouvenne A, Meschi T. Nephrolithiasis and urinary tract infections: 'the chicken or the egg' dilemma? Nephrol Dial Transplant 2012;27(11): 3982–4.
7. Moe OW. Kidney stones: pathophysiology and medical management. Lancet 2006;367(9507):333–44.
8. Flannigan R, Choy WH, Chew B, et al. Renal struvite stones—pathogenesis, microbiology, and management strategies. Nat Rev Urol 2014;11:333–41.
9. Scales CD Jr, Smith AC, Hanley JM, et al, Urologic Diseases in America Project. Prevalence of kidney stones in the United States. Eur Urol 2012;62(1):160–5.
10. Singh M, Chapman R, Tresidder GC, et al. The fate of the unoperated staghorn calculus. Br J Urol 1973;45(6):581–5.
11. Vourganti S, Agarwal PK, Bodner DR, et al. Ultrasonographic evaluation of renal infections. Radiol Clin North Am 2006;44(6):763–75.
12. Edell SL, Bonavita JA. The sonographic appearance of acute pyelonephritis. Radiology 1979;132(3): 683–5.
13. Soulen MC, Fishman EK, Goldman SM, et al. Bacterial renal infection: role of CT. Radiology 1989; 171(3):703–7.

14. Wolin EA, Hartman DS, Olson JR. Nephrographic and pyelographic analysis of CT urography: differential diagnosis. Am J Roentgenol 2013;200(6): 1197–203.

15. Oh SJ, Je B-K, Lee SH, et al. Comparison of computed tomography findings between bacteremic and non-bacteremic acute pyelonephritis due to *Escherichia coli*. World J Radiol 2016;8(4): 403–9.

16. Saunders HS, Dyer RB, Shifrin RY, et al. The CT nephrogram: implications for evaluation of urinary tract disease. Radiographics 1995;15(5):1069–85.

17. Wicks JD, Bigongiari LR, Foley WD, et al. Parenchymal striations in renal vein thrombosis: arteriographic demonstration. Am J Roentgenol 1977; 129(1):95–8.

18. Paul GJ, Stephenson TF. The cortical rim sign in renal infarction. Radiology 1977;122(2):338.

19. Browne RFJ, Meehan CP, Colville J, et al. Transitional cell carcinoma of the upper urinary tract: spectrum of imaging findings. Radiographics 2005;25(6): 1609–27.

20. Ubee SS, McGlynn L, Fordham M. Emphysematous pyelonephritis. BJU Int 2011;107(9):1474–8.

21. Evanoff GV, Thompson CS, Foley R, et al. Spectrum of gas within the kidney: emphysematous pyelonephritis and emphysematous pyelitis. Am J Med 1987;83(1):149–54.

22. Huang J-J, Tseng C-C. Emphysematous pyelonephritis: clinicoradiological classification, management, prognosis, and pathogenesis. JAMA Intern Med 2000;160(6):797–805.

23. Stapleton A. Urinary tract infections in patients with diabetes. Am J Med 2002;113(1, Supplement 1): 80–4.

24. Kuo YT, Chen MT, Liu GC, et al. Emphysematous pyelonephritis: imaging diagnosis and follow-up. Kaohsiung J Med Sci 1999;15(3):159–70.

25. Grayson DE, Abbott RM, Levy AD, et al. Emphysematous infections of the abdomen and pelvis: a pictorial review. Radiographics 2002;22(3):543–61.

26. Allen HA 3rd, Walsh JW, Brewer WH, et al. Sonography of emphysematous pyelonephritis. J Ultrasound Med 1984;3(12):533–7.

27. Wan YL, Lee TY, Bullard MJ, et al. Acute gas-producing bacterial renal infection: correlation between imaging findings and clinical outcome. Radiology 1996;198(2):433–8.

28. Nayeemuddin M, Wiseman OJ, Turner AG. Emphysematous pyelonephritis. Nat Clin Pract Urol 2005; 2:108–12.

29. Kawashima A, Sandler CM, Goldman SM, et al. CT of renal inflammatory disease. Radiographics 1997;17(4):851–66.

30. Hoddick W, Jeffrey RB, Goldberg HI, et al. CT and sonography of severe renal and perirenal infections. Am J Roentgenol 1983;140(3):517–20.

31. Brown ED, Brown JJ, Kettritz U, et al. Renal abscesses: appearance on gadolinium-enhanced magnetic resonance images. Abdom Imaging 1996;21(2):172–6.

32. Israel GM, Bosniak MA. Pitfalls in renal mass evaluation and how to avoid them. Radiographics 2008; 28(5):1325–38.

33. Wood CG 3rd, Stromberg LJ 3rd, Harmath CB, et al. CT and MR imaging for evaluation of cystic renal lesions and diseases. Radiographics 2015;35(1): 125–41.

34. Kenney PJ, Breatnach ES, Stanley RJ. Pyonephrosis. In: Pollack HM, editor. Clinical urography. 1st edition. Philadelphia: Saunders; 1990. p. 843–9.

35. Camúñez F, Echenagusia A, Prieto ML, et al. Percutaneous nephrostomy in pyonephrosis. Urol Radiol 1989;11(1):77.

36. Jeffrey RB, Laing FC, Wing VW, et al. Sensitivity of sonography in pyonephrosis: a reevaluation. Am J Roentgenol 1985;144(1):71–3.

37. Fultz PJ, Hampton WR, Totterman SMS. Computed tomography of pyonephrosis. Abdom Imaging 1993;18(1):82–7.

38. Yoder IC, Pfister RC, Lindfors KK, et al. Pyonephrosis: imaging and intervention. Am J Roentgenol 1983;141(4):735–40.

39. Chan JHM, Tsui EYK, Luk SH, et al. MR diffusion-weighted imaging of kidney: differentiation between hydronephrosis and pyonephrosis. Clin Imaging 2001;25(2):110–3.

40. Friedl A, Tuerk C, Schima W, et al. Xanthogranulomatous pyelonephritis with staghorn calculus, acute gangrenous appendicitis and enterocolitis: a multidisciplinary challenge of kidney-preserving conservative therapy. Curr Urol 2015;8(3):162–5.

41. Nicola R, Menias CO. Urinary obstruction, stone disease, and infection. In: Hodler J, Kubik-Huch RA, von Schulthess GK, editors. Diseases of the abdomen and pelvis 2018-2021: diagnostic imaging - IDKD book. Cham (Switzerland): Springer International Publishing; 2018. p. 223–8.

42. Li L, Parwani AV. Xanthogranulomatous pyelonephritis. Arch Pathol Lab Med 2011;135(5):671–4.

43. Tiu CM, Chou YH, Chiou HJ, et al. Sonographic features of xanthogranulomatous pyelonephritis. J Clin Ultrasound 2001;29(5):279–85.

44. Dyer RB, Chen MY, Zagoria RJ. Classic signs in uroradiology. Radiographics 2004;24(suppl_1): S247–80.

45. Bhatt S, MacLennan G, Dogra V. Renal pseudotumors. Am J Roentgenol 2007;188(5):1380–7.

46. Anezinis P, Prassopoulos P, Daskalopoulos G, et al. MRI and CT features in two unusual cases of xanthogranulomatous pyelonephritis. Eur J Radiol 1998;28(1):98–101.

47. Rha SE, Byun JY, Jung SE, et al. The renal sinus: pathologic spectrum and multimodality imaging

approach. Radiographics 2004;24(suppl_1): S117–31.

48. Ambos MA, Bosniak MA, Gordon R, et al. Replacement lipomatosis of the kidney. Am J Roentgenol 1978;130(6):1087–91.

49. Kullendorff B, Nyman U, Aspelin P. Computed tomography in renal replacement lipomatosis. Acta Radiol 1987;28(4):447–50.

50. Leder RA, Low VH. Tuberculosis of the abdomen. Radiol Clin North Am 1995;33(4):691–705.

51. Farer LS, Lowell AM, Meador MP. Extrapulmonary tuberculosis in the United States. Am J Epidemiol 1979;109(2):205–17.

52. Figueiredo AA, Lucon AM. Urogenital tuberculosis: update and review of 8961 cases from the world literature. Rev Urol 2008;10(3):207–17.

53. Jung YY, Kim JK, Cho K-S. Genitourinary tuberculosis: comprehensive cross-sectional imaging. Am J Roentgenol 2005;184(1):143–50.

54. Wong A, Dhingra S, Surabhi VR. AIRP best cases in radiologic-pathologic correlation: genitourinary tuberculosis. Radiographics 2012;32(3):839–44.

55. Kollins SA, Hartman GW, Carr DT, et al. Roentgenographic findings in urinary tract tuberculosis. Am J Roentgenol 1974;121(3):487–99.

56. Gibson MS, Puckett ML, Shelly ME. Renal tuberculosis. Radiographics 2004;24(1):251–6.

57. Panwar A, Ranjan R, Drall N, et al. Pseudotumor presentation of renal tuberculosis mimicking renal cell carcinoma: a rare entity. Turk J Urol 2016;42(3): 206–9.

58. Pedrosa I, Saíz A, Arrazola J, et al. Hydatid disease: radiologic and pathologic features and complications. Radiographics 2000;20(3):795–817.

59. Gossios KJ, Kontoyiannis DS, Dascalogiannaki M, et al. Uncommon locations of hydatid disease: CT appearances. Eur Radiol 1997;7(8):1303–8.

60. Polat P, Kantarci M, Alper F, et al. Hydatid disease from head to toe. Radiographics 2003;23(2):475–94.

61. Ishimitsu DN, Saouaf R, Kallman C, et al. Renal hydatid disease. Radiographics 2010;30(2):334–7.

62. Turgut AT, Ödev K, Kabaalioğlu A, et al. Multitechnique evaluation of renal hydatid disease. Am J Roentgenol 2009;192(2):462–7.

63. Orlowski HLP, McWilliams S, Mellnick VM, et al. Imaging spectrum of invasive fungal and fungal-like infections. Radiographics 2017;37(4):1119–34.

64. Shoham S, Marr KA. Invasive fungal infections in solid organ transplant recipients. Future Microbiol 2012;7(5):639–55.

65. Erden A, Fitoz S, Karagülle T, et al. Radiological findings in the diagnosis of genitourinary candidiasis. Pediatr Radiol 2000;30(12):875–7.

Reporting on Renal Masses, Recommendations for Terminology, and Sample Templates

Patricia Balthazar, MD[a], Hena Joshi, MD[a], Marta E. Heilbrun, MD[b],*

KEYWORDS

- Renal masses • Renal cell carcinoma • Structured reporting • Templates • Bosniak classification
- Nephrometry scoring systems

KEY POINTS

- Incidental renal masses are frequently encountered by radiologists and their management is usually guided by imaging features.
- Reporting of renal masses is improved by the use of structured templates with specific terminology and management guidelines.
- The Society of Abdominal Radiology's Disease Focused Panel on Renal Cell Carcinoma (DFPRCC) published the results of a survey of academic radiologists and urologists to determine the most desired contents of a structured radiology report describing a renal mass.
- A proposed update to the widely used Bosniak classification system aims to improve its specificity through changes, such as providing clearer definitions of descriptors and incorporating MR imaging findings.
- We present sample templates for reporting of renal masses with a glossary of terms by building on templates created by the DFPRCC and incorporating the 2019 Bosniak classification update.

INTRODUCTION

Radiologists have increasingly adopted structured radiology report templates and constrained vocabularies for describing imaging findings.[1–6] There are many arguments in favor of moving in this direction, including a decrease in error rate, improved quality, comprehensiveness, adherence to guidelines, consistency, and revenue capture.[7–9] The body of literature demonstrating a preference for structured radiology reports by referring providers and radiologists is growing.[3,6,7,10] Structured report templates using common data elements facilitate cross-institution collaborations and the creation of radiology registries to support translational and clinical research.[11,12] Such registries could also be used to establish national quality benchmarks and to drive the creation and adoption of artificial intelligence algorithms.[11]

Generally, constrained vocabularies are modality-specific and intended to reduce variability of terminology in reports, improve communication between radiologists and recipients of radiology report data, and create a framework for improving understanding of the diseases imaged. Many constrained vocabularies and scoring systems have been cataloged and developed through the American College of Radiology Reporting and Data Systems initiative.[13,14] Although no specific

[a] Department of Radiology and Imaging Sciences, Emory University School of Medicine, 1364 Clifton Road, Northeast, Atlanta, GA 30322, USA; [b] Department of Radiology and Imaging Sciences, Emory University Healthcare, 1364 Clifton Road, Northeast, Suite CG24, Atlanta, GA 30322, USA
* Corresponding author.
E-mail address: marta.heilbrun@emory.edu
Twitter: @PBalthazarMD (P.B.); @hjoshimd (H.J.); @meh1rad (M.E.H.)

Radiol Clin N Am 58 (2020) 925–933
https://doi.org/10.1016/j.rcl.2020.06.003

vocabulary has been developed for renal masses, the Bosniak system, created more than 30 years ago, with a suggested update in 2019, is commonly used for cystic renal mass classification.[15,16] The advent of minimally invasive techniques for management of solid renal masses, such as partial nephrectomy, has driven the surgical literature to devise scoring rubrics for surgical risk stratification.[17–20] Finally, because of the frequency of detection of renal masses, algorithms for management have been developed.[21]

This article summarizes and describes recent updates and understanding of the critical observations and descriptors of renal masses. A series of template modules are included and a glossary of terms. This article reviews the consensus work out of the Society of Abdominal Radiology Disease Focused Panel on Renal Cell Carcinoma (DFPRCC) (https://www.abdominalradiology.org/page/DFPRCC).

EPIDEMIOLOGY OF RENAL MASSES

More than 330,000 new cases of kidney cancer are diagnosed a year, making it the 13th most common cancer worldwide. The incidence of renal cell carcinoma (RCC) has been increasing steadily since the 1970s.[22] Although changes in lifestyle and exposure to risk factors have been implicated in the increased incidence of RCC, the rise in use of diagnostic imaging is also a factor in detection.[21] Most renal masses are benign cysts, with the prevalence of cysts also increasing with age. In fact, renal cysts are identified in 20% to 45% of a general imaging population, suggesting they may be in the realm of a normal finding.[21,23,24] However, of those incidental renal lesions, a proportion are RCCs and patient prognosis seems to improve if the renal mass was detected incidentally.[25,26] This apparent improvement in outcome may be the consequence of early treatment or increased detection of benign neoplasms or indolent cancers. Because of the role imaging plays in the detection of these masses and the associated epidemiologic impact, it behooves the radiology community to leverage the knowledge and understanding of the features that differentiate malignant and benign renal masses, to mitigate risks associated with potential overtreatment if the disease is overdiagnosed.[27]

INCREASING PRECISION IN THE DESCRIPTION OF RENAL MASSES
Addressing Stakeholder Concerns

Through the leadership and initiative of the DFPRCC, the knowledge and understanding of

the features that radiologists should be describing when characterizing newly discovered renal masses is improving. This improvement is manifest through the radiology report that is generated when a radiologist encounters the incidental renal mass. In 2019, the DFPRCC published the results of their survey of radiologists and urologists from nine tertiary care academic institutions that was designed to determine the most desired contents of a structured report of a computed tomography (CT) or MR imaging performed to evaluate a renal mass.[1]

Davenport and colleagues[1] determined that consensus was reached if 70% of respondents agreed that a particular reporting element was essential or preferred. This threshold was chosen because of the range of opinions and local practice patterns that were elicited in the survey. Features that met this 70% threshold included whether a mass is cystic or solid, including a Bosniak classification of cystic masses with the features used to assign said classification; mass size in comparison with prior imaging, with a desire for mass size to be in the impression if it is a mass that will require surveillance or intervention, such as solid, Bosniak IIF, Bosniak III, and Bosniak IV masses; the presence of fat or enhancement and how much of the mass enhances, whether or not there is necrosis in a solid mass; the features of the margin, whether circumscribed or infiltrative; and finally radiologic staging for solid masses and Bosniak IV cystic masses. Additionally, there were several specific features that assist in surgical planning for patients who might benefit from a nephron-sparing therapy that met the 70% threshold for consensus. These include the axial location of the mass, capsular location of the mass, distance of the mass to the sinus fat, and distance of the mass to the collecting system.

Not surprisingly, there were some differences in opinion between urologists and radiologists as to essential features. The urologists were more likely to want enhancement on CT to be reported quantitatively (eg, Hounsfield units of the precontrast and postcontrast and/or calculated difference) rather than qualitatively (eg, enhancement, no enhancement). Other than a recommendation of the best type and interval of follow-up imaging, most urologists did not want management recommendations included in the report.

Updating the Bosniak Classification

Given the importance of the Bosniak classification in the description of cystic renal masses and known inconsistencies in the application of the original features to classification, another recent development is a proposed update of the Bosniak classification of cystic renal masses.[16] The Bosniak classification is widely used in clinical practice to stratify the risk of malignancy in cystic renal masses based on imaging features on contrast-enhanced CT and to guide management. The Bosniak classification, version 2019, proposes several updates to the original classification system to improve specificity and reduce the number of benign masses that undergo unnecessary treatment. The updated version accomplishes this by providing specific definitions for previously vague imaging features, incorporating MR imaging findings into the classification, expanding the number of masses that can be included in the classification, and increasing the proportion of masses that can be assigned to lower Bosniak classes. In addition, specific management language is included, also with the goals of increasing consistency.

In the updated Bosniak classification, a cystic mass is defined as a mass of which less than 25% is composed of enhancing tissue. A summary of the Bosniak classes follows. The imaging features that differentiate classes are illustrated in **Fig. 1**.

Bosniak I

Bosniak I cysts are simple cysts without septa, solid component, or calcification. A Bosniak I cyst must be well-defined with a smooth, thin wall that may enhance. A "thin" wall is defined as being less than or equal to 2 mm.

The updated version defines enhancement as either clearly visible enhancement or nonvisible enhancement based on established quantitative criteria, which includes increase of 20 HU or more on contrast-enhanced CT when compared with noncontrast study or an increase in signal intensity of 15% or more on contrast-enhanced MR imaging compared with noncontrast MR imaging.

Bosniak I cysts are benign cysts and do not require further work-up or follow-up. When encountered these can be described as "Bosniak I: benign simple cyst requiring no follow-up."[16]

Bosniak II

Bosniak II category includes

1. "Minimally complicated" cysts, which may have few thin and smooth septa with or without any type of calcification. "Few" septa are defined as between one and three, and "thin" is defined as less than or equal to 2 mm.
2. "Benign hyperattenuating" cysts that are homogeneous and 70 HU or greater on noncontrast CT, or 20 HU or greater and do not enhance on renal mass protocol CT.

The updated Bosniak classification, version 2019, also includes in the Bosniak II category those renal masses that are incompletely

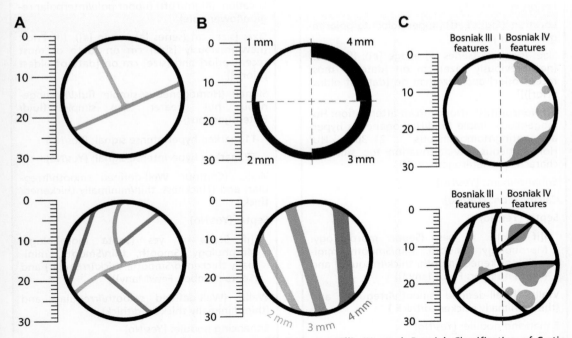

Fig. 1. (*A–C*) The Bosniak classes. (*From* Silverman SG, Pedrosa I, Ellis JH, et al. Bosniak Classification of Cystic Renal Masses, Version 2019: An Update Proposal and Needs Assessment. *Radiology.* 2019;292(2):475-488; with permission.)

characterized but have a high likelihood of being benign fluid-filled lesions. These include homogeneous masses that are

1. Between −9 and 20 HU on noncontrast CT
2. Between 21 and 30 HU on portal venous phase CT
3. Hypoattenuating masses on CT that are too small to characterize
4. Markedly T2 hyperintense masses with signal intensity that is similar to cerebrospinal fluid on noncontrast T2-weighted MR imaging
5. Markedly T1 hyperintense masses, which are defined as approximately 2.5 times renal parenchymal signal intensity, on noncontrast T1-weighted MR imaging

Bosniak II masses are also considered benign with a less than 1% chance of malignancy and do not require further follow-up. Those that are confirmed to be cysts can be reported as "benign Bosniak II renal cyst requiring no follow-up," whereas those that are low-attenuating but too small to characterize can be reported as "likely benign Bosniak II renal mass requiring no follow-up."[16]

Bosniak IIF

Bosniak IIF class includes well-defined cystic masses with more than a few septa. The septa and wall may be thin, or they may be smooth with minimal thickening. The updated Bosniak classification defines "more than a few septa" as greater than four, "thin" as less than or equal to 2 mm, and "minimal thickening" as 3 mm or less. The walls or septa of a Bosniak IIF mass must enhance.

Bosniak IIF also includes cystic masses that are heterogeneously hyperintense on fat-saturated T1-weighted MR imaging without contrast and do not meet the criteria for Bosniak III or IV category. Because this finding is a presentation of papillary RCC, it has been added to Bosniak IIF class in the updated version.

Heterogeneous masses detected on CT that do not enhance are incompletely characterized and are further evaluated with contrast-enhanced MR imaging. If the mass is truly cystic on MR imaging, the Bosniak class may be determined based on its MR imaging features.

Bosniak IIF masses are considered indeterminate and undergo surveillance. The phrase that is recommended by Silverman and colleagues[16] to use in the report is, "Bosniak IIF cystic renal mass. Most Bosniak IIF masses are benign. When malignant, nearly all are indolent. Generally, Bosniak IIF masses are followed by imaging at 6 months and 12 months, then annually for a total of 5 years to assess for morphologic change."

Bosniak III

Bosniak III class includes cystic masses with thick and irregular enhancing wall or septa. The definition of "thick" is greater than 4 mm. "Irregular" is defined as a focal or diffuse convex protrusion measuring 3 mm or less with obtuse margins with the wall or septa. Bosniak III masses have 50% likelihood of malignancy and are treated. The phrase that is recommended by Silverman and colleagues[16] to use in the report is, "Bosniak III cystic renal mass. Bosniak III masses have an intermediate probability of being malignant. If not already obtained, consider urology consultation."

Bosniak IV

Bosniak IV category includes cystic masses with enhancing nodules. A "nodule" is defined as a focal or diffuse convex protrusion of any size that has acute margins with the wall or septa, or a convex protrusion that is 4 mm or greater and has obtuse margins with the wall or septa. These masses have 90% likelihood of malignancy and are also treated. The phrase that is recommended by the Silverman and colleagues[16] to use in the report is, "Bosniak IV cystic renal mass. Most Bosniak IV masses are malignant. If not already obtained, consider urology consultation."

Nephrometry Scoring Systems

According to the American Urologic Association and European Association of Urology guidelines, nephron sparing surgery (NSS), or partial nephrectomy, should be prioritized in the treatment of clinical T1a lesions when technically feasible.[28,29] NSS has equivalent oncologic outcomes when compared with radical nephrectomy in localized small tumors, and robust evidence suggests

---

Box 4
CT and MR imaging reporting module for solid renal mass

Lesion #{number:1/2/3/4/5}:

Location: {Side: Right/Left} kidney {Axial: anterior/posterior/neither anterior nor posterior} {Pole: upper pole/interpolar region/lower pole}.

Size: [size] cm (series [#] image [#]), {if Prior: new/previously [size] cm on [date of most recent prior] and [size] cm on [date of oldest prior]}.

Macroscopic fat: {Yes/No}

Necrosis: {Yes/No}

Solid enhancement: {Yes, entire mass/Yes, a portion of the mass/No/Equivocal}

Mass margins: {Circumscribed/Infiltrative}

Capsular location: {≤50% exophytic/>50% exophytic/endophytic}

Distance to the sinus fat or collecting system: [size] cm

Tumor thrombus (distal extent): {No tumor thrombus/Ipsilateral renal vein (no IVC extension)/IVC <2 cm above renal vein/IVC ≥2 cm above renal vein but below hepatic veins/IVC above hepatic veins but below diaphragm/IVC above diaphragm/Into right atrium}

Bland venous thrombus: {Yes/No}

Nodal metastasis: {Yes/No}, {if Yes: [bidirectional size] cm (series [#] image [#])}

Distant metastasis: {Yes/No}, {if Yes: [free text description]}

---

higher overall survival rates, which may be attributable to favorable functional renal outcome.[30–35]

Tumor size, location, and anatomic factors have decisive influence on the technical feasibility of NSS. Thus, various systems have proposed standard metrics to assess the tumor complexity and predict risk of complications after partial nephrectomy. These systems have been referred to as nephrometry scoring systems. For instance, the R.E.N.A.L. (radius, exophytic/endophytic,

---

Box 5
Management options for incidental renal mass

Recommendation: [Benign. No further work-up./Indeterminate, MR imaging without and with contrast or CT without and with contrast within 6–12 months./Indeterminate, MR imaging without and with contrast or CT without and with contrast.]

Table 1
Glossary of terms

Term/Phrase and Conditions Where Applied	Definition	Source
Cyst	Renal lesions meeting Bosniak I or Bosniak II imaging criteria, unless too small to characterize	Silverman et al,[16] 2019
Cystic renal mass	<25% of the mass is enhancing tissue	Silverman et al,[16] 2019
Enhancement	Unequivocal change, whether visual or measured using established quantitative thresholds, between precontrast and postcontrast imaging	Silverman et al,[16] 2019
Equivocal CT enhancement	>10 to <20 HU	Herts et al,[21] 2018
Measurable CT enhancement	≥20 HU increase in attenuation between precontrast and postcontrast imaging	Silverman et al,[16] 2019
Measurable MR imaging enhancement	≥15% increase in signal intensity between precontrast and postcontrast imaging	Silverman et al,[16] 2019
Nonenhancing on CT	≤10 HU	Herts et al,[21] 2018
Homogeneous	Entire mass contains similar attenuation, signal intensity, or echogenicity throughout; may have a thin wall without septa or calcifications	Silverman et al,[16] 2019
Hyperattenuating renal mass	≥70 HU at noncontrast CT image	Silverman et al,[16] 2019
Incidental renal mass	A renal mass that is initially detected on an imaging study performed for an indication other than the assessment of urinary tract disease	Herts et al,[21] 2018
Indeterminate renal mass	A renal mass that, because of incomplete characterization, requires further evaluation before management is recommended	Herts et al,[21] 2018
Irregular thickening	≤3 mm focal or diffuse convex enhancing protrusions that have obtuse margins with wall or septa	Silverman et al,[16] 2019
Nodule	1. Focal enhancing convex protrusion of any size that has acute margins with the wall or septa 2. Focal enhancing convex protrusion ≥4 mm that has obtuse margins with the wall or septa	Silverman et al,[16] 2019

(continued on next page)

Table 1
(continued)

Term/Phrase and Conditions Where Applied	Definition	Source
Septum/septa	Linear of curvilinear structures that connect two surfaces	Silverman et al,[16] 2019
Few septa	1 to 3	Silverman et al,[16] 2019
Many septa	≥4	Silverman et al,[16] 2019
Thin	≤2 mm	Silverman et al,[16] 2019
Minimally thickened	3 mm	Silverman et al,[16] 2019
Thick	≥4 mm	Silverman et al,[16] 2019
Simple fluid		Silverman et al,[16] 2019
Noncontrast CT	-9 to 20 HU	Silverman et al,[16] 2019
Portal venous phase CT	21 to 30 HU	Silverman et al,[16] 2019
Noncontrast MR imaging T2 signal	Markedly hyperintense, similar to cerebrospinal fluid	Silverman et al,[16] 2019
Noncontrast MR imaging T1 signal	Markedly hyperintense, approximately 2.5 times normal renal parenchyma	Silverman et al,[16] 2019
Ultrasound	Anechoic with increased posterior through-transmission	Silverman et al,[16] 2019
Too small to characterize renal lesion	1. A mass that is less than half the diameter of the section thickness of the imaging 2. Intrarenal mass ≤1.5 cm that, because of adjacency to avidly enhancing renal parenchyma, may be affected by pseudoenhancement	Silverman et al,[16] 2019

nearness to collecting system/sinus, anterior/posterior, and location relative to polar lines)[17] and the Preoperative Aspects and Dimensions Used for an Anatomic (PADUA) classification systems[18] use similar semiquantitative anatomic factors and methodologies. In contrast, centrality index (C-index)[19] and mathematical tumor contact surface area[20] use the geometric relationship between the tumor and kidney. Despite demonstration of external validation and association with perioperative outcomes, the roles of each of these surgical planning scoring systems are still being studied, and clinical adoption is variable.[36,37]

Percutaneous thermal ablation should be considered as an alternate organ-sparing treatment of clinical T1s renal tumors less than 3 cm.[28] Studies have shown that the surgical scoring systems, including R.E.N.A.L. and PADUA, may not have the same predictive efficacy when applied to patients undergoing ablation.[38] This limitation is in part because the percutaneous access approach and ablation technique invoke different periprocedural risks than a surgical approach. For example, a surgeon, whether using open or laparoscopic techniques, is able to physically move adjacent organs, such as bowel or liver, that may be near the tumor, whereas the percutaneous approach relies on hydrodissection to mitigate risk related to adjacency. Thus, interventional radiologists have also advocated for the use of scoring systems to stratify complexity of percutaneous ablation of renal tumors, but with appropriate modifications, including the proximity of the tumor to surrounding anatomic structures.[38]

Management Algorithms

Using the imaging criteria described previously, the incidentally detected renal masses are sorted into several categories for consideration of additional imaging.[2,21,39] As defined by the American College of Radiology Incidental Findings committee, for the purpose of further imaging after incidental detection on CT, the approach to subsequent imaging depends on whether the mass was initially detected on a contrast-enhanced or nonenhanced CT study, the size of the mass, the attenuation pattern, and absolute attenuation values. If the mass cannot be confidently characterized using subjective criteria on the initial examination, it should be classified as indeterminate.

The management recommendations include no further work-up, MR imaging without and with contrast, or CT without and with contrast either within 6 to 12 months or as soon as can be scheduled. Once the lesion is characterized, the cystic lesions fall into management recommendations based on the updated Bosniak criteria manuscript, and the solid renal masses are managed based on size categories of less than 1.0 cm, 1.0 to 4.0 cm, and greater than or equal to 4.0 cm.[16,21,28] The sample phrases to include in the summary of any report describing a cystic renal lesion are discussed previously in the summary of the new Bosniak classification recommendations.

Sample Structured Templates

To facilitate the incorporation of the essential features into radiology reporting workflow, including the new Bosniak classification features, we used a sample template rubric (**Box 1**) to create a series of modules for cystic and solid renal mass reporting (**Boxes 2–4**) and a management recommendation module (**Box 5**). A glossary of terms is also included (**Table 1**). These templates build on those created by the DFPRCC[2] and incorporate the 2019 Bosniak classification update. By building these reports out using Common Data Elements (CDEs) (https://radelement.org/) that encapsulate specific definitions for the terms in the reports, it is possible to have a more streamlined appearing report. Essentially, each pick list presented in the templates is a CDE. Then, the set of CDEs that make up the descriptive module is the rich content that enables the data mining that advances knowledge and understanding about the natural history and risk of these masses, captured when the constrained choices are used for reporting.

SUMMARY

Given the incidence of small renal masses, from benign cysts to malignancy, most radiologists encounter these lesions numerous times during their career. Radiologists have an opportunity to collect attributes of renal masses in standardized reports that further refine the understanding of the impact of these masses on patient outcomes. The templates and glossary of terms presented in this review article facilitate reporting of standard data elements, giving radiologists the opportunity to improve diagnostic accuracy and influence management of small renal masses.

DISCLOSURE

The authors have nothing to disclose.

REFERENCES

1. Davenport MS, Hu EM, Smith AD, et al. Reporting standards for the imaging-based diagnosis of renal masses on CT and MRI: a national survey of academic abdominal radiologists and urologists. Abdom Radiol (NY) 2017;42(4):1229–40.
2. Davenport MS, Hu EM, Zhang A, et al. Standardized report template for indeterminate renal masses at CT and MRI: a collaborative product of the SAR Disease-Focused Panel on Renal Cell Carcinoma. Abdom Radiol (NY) 2019;44(4):1423–9.
3. Eberhardt SC, Heilbrun ME. Radiology report value equation. Radiographics 2018;38(6):1888–96.
4. Juluru K, Heilbrun ME, Kohli MD. Describing disease-specific reporting guidelines: a brief guide for radiologists. Radiographics 2019;39(5):1233–5.
5. Kahn CE Jr, Heilbrun ME, Applegate KE. From guidelines to practice: how reporting templates promote the use of radiology practice guidelines. J Am Coll Radiol 2013;10(4):268–73.
6. Powell DK, Silberzweig JE. State of structured reporting in radiology, a survey. Acad Radiol 2015;22(2):226–33.
7. Goldberg-Stein S, Chernyak V. Adding value in radiology reporting. J Am Coll Radiol 2019;16(9 Pt B):1292–8.
8. Silveira PC, Dunne R, Sainani NI, et al. Impact of an information technology-enabled initiative on the quality of prostate multiparametric MRI reports. Acad Radiol 2015;22(7):827–33.
9. Sahni VA, Silveira PC, Sainani NI, et al. Impact of a structured report template on the quality of MRI reports for rectal cancer staging. AJR Am J Roentgenol 2015;205(3):584–8.
10. Schwartz LH, Panicek DM, Berk AR, et al. Improving communication of diagnostic radiology findings through structured reporting. Radiology 2011;260(1):174–81.
11. Kohli M, Alkasab T, Wang K, et al. Bending the artificial intelligence curve for radiology: informatics tools from ACR and RSNA. J Am Coll Radiol 2019;16(10):1464–70.
12. Rubin DL, Kahn CE Jr. Common data elements in radiology. Radiology 2017;283(3):837–44.
13. ACR. Reporting and data systems. Available at: https://www.acr.org/Clinical-Resources/Reporting-and-Data-Systems. Accessed November 15, 2019.

14. An JY, Unsdorfer KML, Weinreb JC. BI-RADS, C-RADS, CAD-RADS, LI-RADS, Lung-RADS, NI-RADS, O-RADS, PI-RADS, TI-RADS: reporting and data systems. Radiographics 2019;39(5):1435–6.

15. Bosniak MA. The current radiological approach to renal cysts. Radiology 1986;158(1):1–10.

16. Silverman SG, Pedrosa I, Ellis JH, et al. Bosniak classification of cystic renal masses, version 2019: an update proposal and needs assessment. Radiology 2019;292(2):475–88.

17. Kutikov A, Uzzo RG. The R.E.N.A.L. nephrometry score: a comprehensive standardized system for quantitating renal tumor size, location and depth. J Urol 2009;182(3):844–53.

18. Ficarra V, Novara G, Secco S, et al. Preoperative aspects and dimensions used for an anatomical (PADUA) classification of renal tumours in patients who are candidates for nephron-sparing surgery. Eur Urol 2009;56(5):786–93.

19. Simmons MN, Ching CB, Samplaski MK, et al. Kidney tumor location measurement using the C index method. J Urol 2010;183(5):1708–13.

20. Hsieh PF, Wang YD, Huang CP, et al. A mathematical method to calculate tumor contact surface area: an effective parameter to predict renal function after partial nephrectomy. J Urol 2016;196(1):33–40.

21. Herts BR, Silverman SG, Hindman NM, et al. Management of the incidental renal mass on CT: a white paper of the ACR incidental findings committee. J Am Coll Radiol 2018;15(2):264–73.

22. Scelo G, Larose TL. Epidemiology and risk factors for kidney cancer. J Clin Oncol 2018;36. JCO2018791905.

23. Carrim ZI, Murchison JT. The prevalence of simple renal and hepatic cysts detected by spiral computed tomography. Clin Radiol 2003;58(8): 626–9.

24. Mensel B, Kuhn JP, Kracht F, et al. Prevalence of renal cysts and association with risk factors in a general population: an MRI-based study. Abdom Radiol (NY) 2018;43(11):3068–74.

25. Volpe A, Panzarella T, Rendon RA, et al. The natural history of incidentally detected small renal masses. Cancer 2004;100(4):738–45.

26. Patard JJ, Rodriguez A, Rioux-Leclercq N, et al. Prognostic significance of the mode of detection in renal tumours. BJU Int 2002;90(4):358–63.

27. Sohlberg EM, Metzner TJ, Leppert JT. The harms of overdiagnosis and overtreatment in patients with small renal masses: a mini-review. Eur Urol Focus 2019;5(6):943–5.

28. Campbell S, Uzzo RG, Allaf ME, et al. Renal mass and localized renal cancer: AUA guideline. J Urol 2017;198(3):520–9.

29. Ljungberg B, Bensalah K, Canfield S, et al. EAU guidelines on renal cell carcinoma: 2014 update. Eur Urol 2015;67(5):913–24.

30. Van Poppel H, Da Pozzo L, Albrecht W, et al. A prospective, randomised EORTC intergroup phase 3 study comparing the oncologic outcome of elective nephron-sparing surgery and radical nephrectomy for low-stage renal cell carcinoma. Eur Urol 2011;59(4):543–52.

31. Pierorazio PM, Johnson MH, Patel HD, et al. Management of renal masses and localized renal cancer: systematic review and meta-analysis. J Urol 2016;196(4):989–99.

32. Huang WC, Elkin EB, Levey AS, et al. Partial nephrectomy versus radical nephrectomy in patients with small renal tumors: is there a difference in mortality and cardiovascular outcomes? J Urol 2009; 181(1):55–61 [discussion: 61–2].

33. Krebs RK, Andreoni C, Ortiz V. Impact of radical and partial nephrectomy on renal function in patients with renal cancer. Urol Int 2014;92(4):449–54.

34. Thompson RH, Boorjian SA, Lohse CM, et al. Radical nephrectomy for pT1a renal masses may be associated with decreased overall survival compared with partial nephrectomy. J Urol 2008; 179(2):468–71 [discussion: 472–3].

35. Weight CJ, Lieser G, Larson BT, et al. Partial nephrectomy is associated with improved overall survival compared to radical nephrectomy in patients with unanticipated benign renal tumours. Eur Urol 2010;58(2):293–8.

36. Wang YD, Huang CP, Chang CH, et al. The role of RENAL, PADUA, C-index, CSA nephrometry systems in predicting ipsilateral renal function after partial nephrectomy. BMC Urol 2019;19(1):72.

37. Gupta R, Tori M, Babitz SK, et al. Comparison of RENAL, PADUA, CSA, and PAVP nephrometry scores in predicting functional outcomes after partial nephrectomy. Urology 2019;124:160–7.

38. Mansilla AV, Bivins EE Jr, Contreras F, et al. CT-guided microwave ablation of 45 renal tumors: analysis of procedure complexity utilizing a percutaneous renal ablation complexity scoring system. J Vasc Interv Radiol 2017;28(2):222–9.

39. Kang SK, Huang WC, Pandharipande PV, et al. Solid renal masses: what the numbers tell us. AJR Am J Roentgenol 2014;202(6):1196–206.

Use of Contrast Ultrasound for Renal Mass Evaluation

Kevin G. King, MD

KEYWORDS

- Renal masses • Contrast-enhanced ultrasound • RCC subtypes

KEY POINTS

- Contrast-enhanced ultrasound is useful for the identification and characterization of renal masses, and its use in this regard is increasing.
- Clear cell renal cell carcinoma is typically a hypervascular and heterogeneous mass, enhancing earlier and to a greater degree than renal cortex.
- Papillary renal cell carcinoma is hypoenhancing throughout, and shows a later peak than clear cell renal cell carcinoma.
- Oncocytoma and lipid-poor angiomyolipoma remain difficult to distinguish from clear cell renal cell carcinoma with contrast-enhanced ultrasound.

INTRODUCTION

The evaluation of renal masses with contrast has typically been performed with computed tomography (CT) scans or MR imaging in the United States, but the use of contrast-enhanced ultrasound (CEUS) for this purpose is expanding, and will likely continue to increase as familiarity with CEUS and its advantages grow.

With the extensive use of cross-sectional imaging in medicine, incidental renal masses have become a commonly encountered entity; some 13% to 27% of imaging studies of the abdomen will demonstrate an incidental renal lesion.[1] Most of these incidentally detected lesions will be cysts, and many can be confidently diagnosed as such on the imaging study on which they are initially detected. For indeterminate lesions, US has long been used to verify the simple nature of a renal cyst, or alternatively to show its complexity, owing to the high specificity of US for fluid content in general. However, CEUS provides a relatively new addition to the toolkit available when evaluating a renal lesion by US and can be added to the same examination when needed.

ADVANTAGES, DISADVANTAGES, AND SAFETY OF CONTRAST-ENHANCED ULTRASOUND

The advantages of US in general are well-known, such as low cost, real-time imaging, portability, and lack of ionizing radiation, but there are several additional advantages specific to CEUS. US contrast is not nephrotoxic, and therefore not only does not require preadministration laboratory testing, but also can be given multiple times during a study. Additionally, much finer detail of the enhancement characteristics of a lesion over time is shown with CEUS. For example, it is commonplace to acquire 1000 images during a 2-minute observation of a lesion after a contrast bolus, outperforming the number of images acquired during even perfusion studies obtained with CT scans or MR imaging.

US does have disadvantages, however, including operator dependence, habitus-related limitations, and obscuration by bowel gas or dense calcification. Rapid respiratory rate can also at times create difficulty for CEUS.

Keck School of Medicine, University of Southern California, Norris Cancer Center, 1500 San Pablo Street, 2nd Floor Imaging, Los Angeles, CA 90033, USA
E-mail address: kingk@med.usc.edu

Radiol Clin N Am 58 (2020) 935–949
https://doi.org/10.1016/j.rcl.2020.05.002
0033-8389/20/© 2020 Elsevier Inc. All rights reserved.

radiologic.theclinics.com

Table 1
UCAs

Agent	Gas	Shell
Definity	Octafluoropropane	Phospholipid
Optison	Octafluoropropane	Albumin
Lumason (Sonovue in Europe)	Sulfur hexafluoride	Phospholipid

CEUS maintains an excellent safety profile. In the past there had been some concern over the safety of CEUS in patients with certain cardiovascular diseases such as intracardiac shunts or pulmonary hypertension, but large studies have shown CEUS to be safe even in these populations.[2–5] Hypersensitivity to an US contrast agent (UCA) or one of its components is currently considered the only contraindication to the use of a UCA.

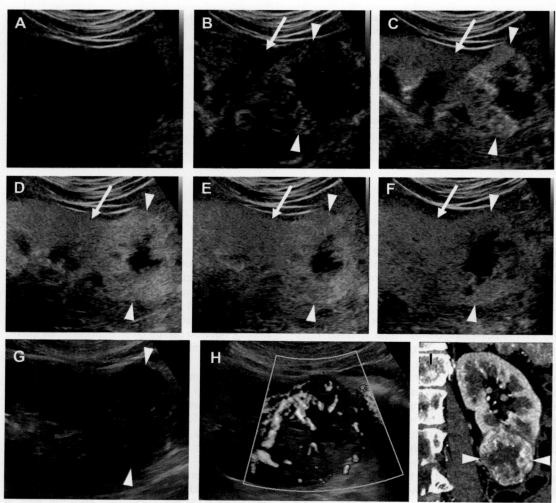

Fig. 1. Longitudinal CEUS (*A–F*), longitudinal grayscale and Doppler US (*G, H*), and coronal contrast-enhanced CT (CECT) scan (*I*) of a left renal ccRCC (*arrow* = cortex; *arrowheads* = tumor). Images obtained just before (*A*) and just after (*B*) the arrival of contrast (8 seconds) show that a portion of the tumor begins enhancing before the adjacent cortex. At early corticomedullary phase (*C*) (11 seconds), the tumor is hyperenhancing compared with cortex, and heterogeneous, with central necrosis. At late corticomedullary phase (*D*) (20 seconds), cortical enhancement has increased, but the tumor remains hyperenhancing relative to cortex, and will peak before cortex. (*E*) At nephrographic phase (35 seconds) the tumor is still slightly hyperenhancing, though it has peaked and is de-enhancing. (*F*) At delayed phase (90 seconds) the tumor and cortex have become nearly isoenhancing. The tumor has a typical heterogeneous, solid appearance at grayscale US (*G*) with internal Doppler flow (*H*), and a typical appearance at CECT scanning (*I*).

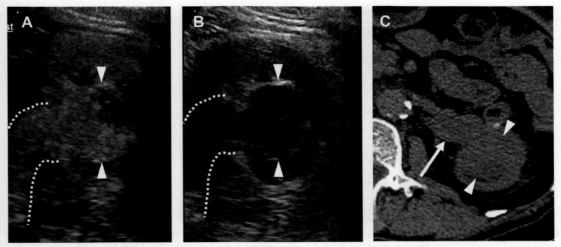

Fig. 2. Transverse CEUS (*A*), transverse grayscale US (*B*), and axial noncontrast CT (*C*) images show a central ccRCC in the left kidney (*arrowheads*), contiguous with tumor invading the renal vein (*dotted lines* in *A* and *B*, *arrow* in *C*) that is seen to be enhancing on CEUS. The patient could not receive CT contrast because of renal failure.

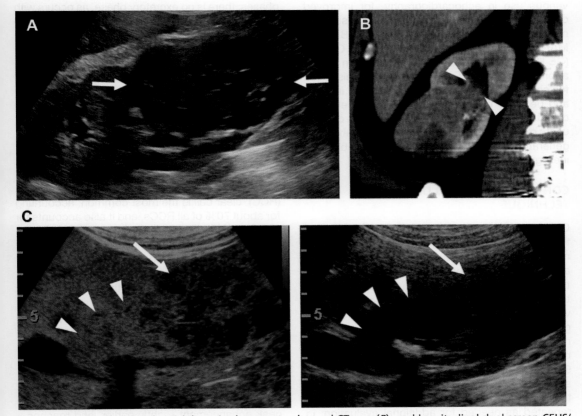

Fig. 3. Longitudinal grayscale US (*A*), sagittal contrast-enhanced CT scan (*B*), and longitudinal dual-screen CEUS/grayscale imaging (*C*) of the right kidney at delayed phase. A large, heterogeneously enhancing ccRCC is seen at the lower pole of the kidney (*arrows* in *A* and *C*). A portion of the tumor invades the collecting system, with enhancement of this invasive extension also seen (*arrowheads* in *C*). Tumor invasion of the collecting system is corroborated on the CT scan (*arrowheads* in *B*).

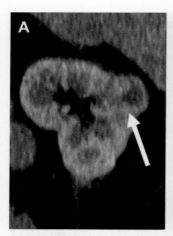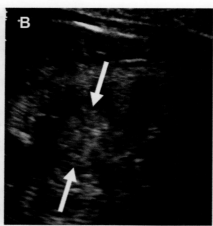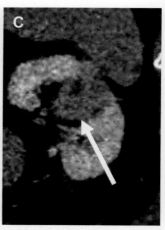

Fig. 4. Preoperative sagittal contrast-enhanced CT (CECT) scan (*A*), and postoperative longitudinal CEUS (*B*) and sagittal CECT scan (*C*) 2 years after surgery. Partial nephrectomy was performed for a left renal 3.5 cm ccRCC (*arrow in A*). Two years later at surveillance CEUS an avidly enhancing mass was seen more centrally in the kidney (*arrows in B*), and also shown at subsequent CECT (*arrow in C*). Recurrent ccRCC was confirmed at re-resection.

At the time of this writing, 3 UCAs are approved by the US Food and Drug Administration for intravenous use in echocardiography, for improved delineation of the endocardial border in suboptimal studies: Definity (Lantheus, North Billerica, MA), Lumason (Bracco, Milan, Italy), and Optison (GE Healthcare, Oslo, Norway).[6] Lumason is also approved by the US Food and Drug Administration for characterization of focal liver lesions in adult and pediatric patients. However, "off-label" uses of CEUS are widespread and growing. The constituents of these 3 agents are provided in **Table 1**; in general, UCAs are composed of microbubbles of inert gas surrounded by a stabilizing shell.

CONTRAST-ENHANCED ULTRASOUND TECHNIQUE

CEUS is performed with a low mechanical index, typically less than 0.1. The low mechanical index minimizes microbubble destruction, and also creates nonlinear echoes from microbubble oscillations, which are detected when a phase inversion technique is used. After establishing an optimal view of the lesion of interest, a contrast bolus is given intravenously, and followed by a 10-mL normal saline flush. Cine acquisition is usually begun with the flush, and typically continues for 90 to 120 seconds. After this, additional cines or still images can be obtained for any length of time desired. Contrast administration can be repeated as needed for additional evaluation; in between in each contrast bolus, bubble destruction is achieved by high mechanical index pulses ("flashes"), or continuous Doppler imaging (for its higher mechanical index).

For renal imaging, it is worth noting that CEUS produces only corticomedullary and nephrographic phases; there is no excretory phase, as occurs with CT scans and MR imaging with contrast. This is due to the size of the UCA microbubbles. Because they are roughly one-half the size of a red blood cell, they remain completely intravascular, and never pass into the extracellular space. Eventually the microbubbles break down, with the gas component excreted by the lungs, and the shell portion typically metabolized by the liver.

IMAGING FINDINGS
Clear Cell Renal Cell Carcinoma

Of the many subtypes of renal cell carcinoma (RCC), clear cell is the most common, accounting for about 70% of all RCCs, and it also accounts for the majority of metastatic disease from RCC. About 60% of all sporadic clear cell RCCs (ccRCCs) are associated with mutations of the tumor suppressor gene VHL on chromosome 3p, and an inherited mutation of this gene produces Von Hippel Lindau disease.[7]

A ccRCC is typically a heterogeneous hypervascular mass, and may demonstrate internal necrosis, hemorrhage, or cystic change. Consequently, at CEUS examination ccRCC typically shows avid hyperenhancement, which is heterogeneous. Compared with normal renal cortex, ccRCC normally begins enhancing slightly earlier, reaches peak enhancement slightly earlier, and reaches a higher peak intensity of enhancement (**Fig. 1**).[7–13] Washout of ccRCC is more variable, but at delayed phase is usually either isoenhancing or hypoenhancing relative to cortex.

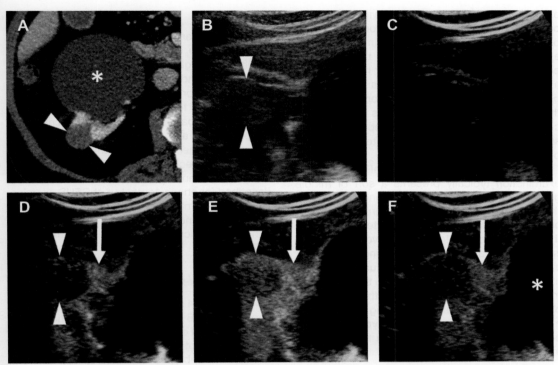

Fig. 5. Axial contrast-enhanced CT (CECT) scan (*A*), transverse grayscale US (*B*), and transverse CEUS at precontrast (*C*), corticomedullary (*D*), nephrographic (*E*), and delayed (*F*) phases of a type 1 pRCC in the right kidney. The mass (*arrowheads*) is hypoenhancing on the CECT scan, and slightly hyperechoic on US compared with the cortex. At corticomedullary phase (*D*), the mass shows slight enhancement, less than the cortex (*arrow*). Its enhancement increases, showing greater enhancement by nephrographic phase (*E*), although still less than the cortex. This figure demonstrates the later peak of pRCC compared with ccRCC (compare with **Fig. 1**). By delayed phase, the mass has de-enhanced, and remains hypoenhancing to cortex. A large renal cyst (*asterisk*) seen on CT scanning is also partially imaged during CEUS (*asterisk* on *F*).

Evaluation for local invasion is key for ccRCC staging, and often in advanced tumors CEUS examination can demonstrate invasion of the renal vein (**Fig. 2**) or renal collecting system (**Fig. 3**). However, there may be instances where depth limits evaluation for invasion of these structures at US examination. Furthermore, with more extensive invasion of the renal vein and inferior vena cava, CT scan or MR imaging is preferred to ensure complete coverage for surgical planning.

Partial nephrectomy has become more commonly performed for RCC in general in recent years, and the rates of local recurrence are low.[14,15] Evaluation for local recurrence can be performed with CEUS examination, with recurrent masses of ccRCC tending to show more avid enhancement (**Fig. 4**) than postoperative fibrosis, which is typically hypoenhancing.

Papillary Renal Cell Carcinoma

Papillary RCC (pRCC) is the second most common RCC subtype, constituting about 15% of all

RCCs.[16] There are 2 histologically distinct types of pRCCs, and most are type 1, a more indolent tumor with infrequent metastatic disease, and a 5-year survival rate of 95%.[17] The less common type 2 pRCC is a more aggressive tumor with a 5-year survival rate of 66%, a rate more similar to ccRCC.

Distinguishing pRCC from ccRCC by enhancement pattern is straightforward with CEUS. Whereas ccRCC enhances earlier, peaks earlier, and reaches a greater peak enhancement than renal cortex, pRCC reaches its peak enhancement later than cortex, and always remains hypoenhancing compared with cortex (**Fig. 5**). Whether or not the 2 types of pRCC can be distinguished by CEUS examination is currently unknown.

Chromophobe Renal Cell Carcinoma

The third most common subtype, chromophobe RCC (chRCC) represents 5% to 8% of all RCCs,[16,18] and is usually a low-grade neoplasm with a better prognosis than ccRCC. chRCC is 1 of 3 renal oncocytic neoplasms, with the other 2 being oncocytoma and hybrid oncocytic/chromophobe tumor.[19,20] That this spectrum exists poses a problem for needle biopsy of these lesions; because of the potential for tumor heterogeneity, needle biopsies of these tumors are often interpreted as an "oncocytic renal neoplasm" at pathology, with a definitive diagnosis deferred until complete resection. Essentially, biopsy of these lesions may not always be able to differentiate benign from malignant.

The enhancement pattern of chRCC at CEUS examination typically presents a sort of middle ground between the hyperenhancing ccRCC and the hypoenhancing pRCC. In general, chRCC enhances very similar to renal cortex throughout the contrast bolus (Fig. 6).[7] However, this finding is not actually a helpful distinguishing appearance at CEUS examination, mainly because of the relative rarity of chRCC compared with the fairly common ccRCC. In everyday practice, the observation of a renal tumor that is isoenhancing with cortex is more likely to be a slightly atypical ccRCC, because of its commonness, than the less common chRCC (Fig. 7).

Oncocytoma

Oncocytomas are benign tumors that are difficult to differentiate from RCC radiologically, often resulting in surgical resection; 5% to 7% of renal tumors that undergo partial nephrectomy prove to be oncocytoma at pathology.[21,22] Classically, the radiologic features of a central scar or a spoke-wheel pattern have been described for oncocytomas, and when seen may be of use. However, neither of these features is sufficiently sensitive or specific for oncocytoma diagnosis.[23] Variable enhancement patterns have been described for oncocytoma, but at CEUS examination oncocytomas most commonly show early hyperenhancement followed by washout (Fig. 8), hence the difficulty in distinguishing them from ccRCC.[10,24]

Other Subtypes of Renal Cell Tumors

Aside from the 4 most common subtypes reviewed above, the 2016 World Health Organization classification of renal cell tumors includes multiple other uncommon subtypes (Box 1).[25] Most of the other uncommon subtypes are rare (<1% or renal

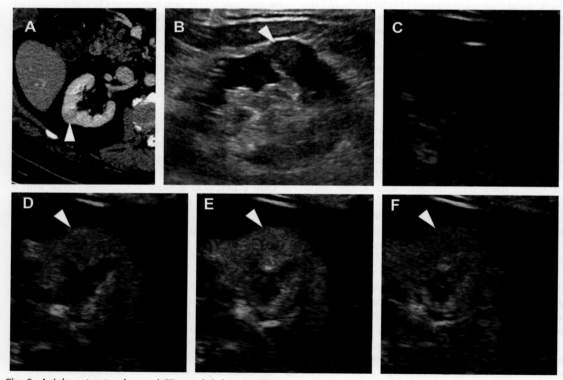

Fig. 6. Axial contrast-enhanced CT scan (A), longitudinal grayscale US examination (B), and longitudinal CEUS examination at the precontrast (C), corticomedullary (D), nephrographic (E), and delayed (F) phases of a chRCC in the right kidney. The mass (arrowheads) shows only subtle hypoenhancement compared with cortex at CT scanning, and is slightly hyperechoic at US examination. At CEUS examination, the mass is nearly isoenhancing to cortex at all phases.

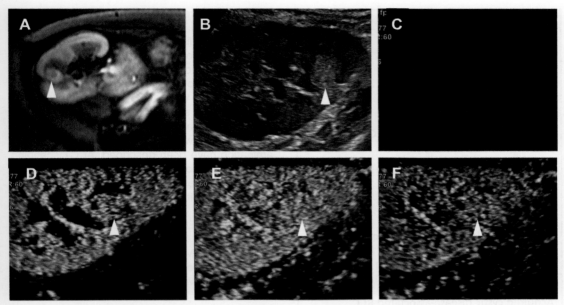

Fig. 7. Axial contrast-enhanced MR imaging (*A*), longitudinal grayscale US examination (*B*), and longitudinal CEUS examination at the precontrast (*C*), corticomedullary (*D*), nephrographic (*E*), and delayed (*F*) phases of a ccRCC in a transplanted kidney. The mass (*arrowheads*) is slightly hyperenhancing at MR imaging, and is slightly hyperechoic at US examination. At CEUS the mass is nearly isoenhancing to cortex at all phases. The isoenhancing pattern of enhancement of chRCC (see Fig. 6) is not specific to chRCC; it is more common to see isoenhancement in a slightly atypical ccRCC, because of the commonness of this subtype.

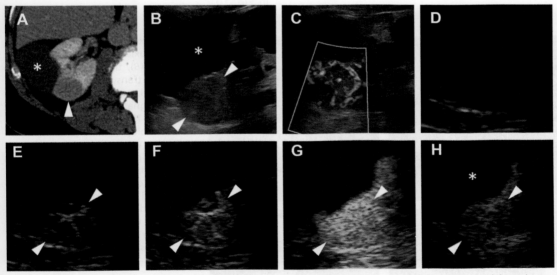

Fig. 8. Axial contrast-enhanced CT scan (*A*), transverse grayscale US (*B*), transverse color Doppler US (*C*), and transverse CEUS at the precontrast (*D*), contrast arrival (*E*), corticomedullary (*F*), nephrographic (*G*), and delayed (*H*) phases of an oncocytoma in the right kidney. The mass (*arrowheads*) shows homogenous enhancement at CT scanning; a cyst (*asterisk*) abuts the tumor. The mass is slightly hyperechoic at grayscale US, and color Doppler shows a spoke-wheel pattern, with vessels radiating from the center, and vessels at the rim. At CEUS examination, the spoke-wheel pattern is again seen at contrast arrival (*E*) and at corticomedullary phase (*F*). By nephrographic phase (*G*) the mass is homogenously enhancing, followed by washout at delayed phase (*H*). The near-field anechoic structure is the abutting cyst (*asterisk* in *H*).

Box 1
2016 World Health Organization classification of renal cell tumors

ccRCC

Multilocular cystic renal neoplasm of low malignant potential

pRCC

Hereditary leiomyomatosis and RCC-associated RCC

chRCC

Collecting duct carcinoma

Renal medullary carcinoma

MiT family translocation RCCs

Succinate dehydrogenase-deficient renal carcinoma

Mucinous tubular and spindle cell carcinoma

Tubulocystic RCC

Acquired cystic disease-associated RCC

Clear cell pRCC

RCC, unclassified

Papillary adenoma

Oncocytoma

tumors), and are the subject of few reports in the CEUS literature. However, some of these subtypes will be briefly discussed. Multilocular cystic renal neoplasm of low malignant potential is a rare low-grade tumor, and has been considered by some to exist on a spectrum with predominantly cystic ccRCC, which also has a more favorable prognosis than standard ccRCC.[26,27] Few reports of the appearance of multilocular cystic renal neoplasm of low malignant potential at CEUS examination have been described. At CT scanning, this tumor is most commonly a Bosniak III lesion, and at CEUS examination the definite enhancement of the multiple internal septations will usually be even more obvious, owing to the increased sensitivity of CEUS for enhancement of septations in general (Fig. 9).

Most of the MiT family translocation RCCs are RCCs characterized by varieties of translocations that involve the *TFE3* gene located on chromosome Xp11.2.[28] A much rarer variant in this family is the t(6;11) RCC, involving the TFEB gene on chromosome 6. The MiT family of RCCs accounts for a large number (20%–75%) of RCCs in childhood, although they can occur in adults as well. A report on the CEUS appearance of 22 cases of Xp11.2-RCC described them as usually mixed solid/cystic tumors, but without a characteristic enhancement pattern for the solid component.[29] An example is shown in Fig. 10.

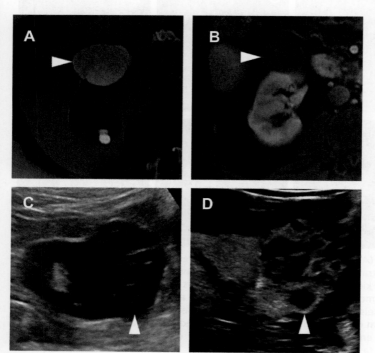

Fig. 9. Axial T2-weighted MR imaging (*A*), axial contrast-enhanced MR imaging (*B*), transverse grayscale US (*C*), and transverse CEUS (*D*) of an multilocular cystic renal neoplasm of low malignant potential of the right kidney. The lesion (*arrowheads*) shows multiple fine septations at MR imaging, which show faint enhancement. At grayscale US the septations seem to be thickened, and at CEUS there is clear enhancement of the thickened and nodular septations. Compared with CT scanning and MR imaging, CEUS often shows greater sensitivity for enhancement of septations.

Mucinous tubular and spindle cell carcinoma of the kidney is a rare subtype that is usually low grade, with a generally favorable outcome and infrequent metastatic disease.[30] They are thought to arise from either the loop of Henle or the collecting duct. Two small case series of these tumors (2 and 6 cases) both describe them as heterogeneously hypoechoic masses that are hypoenhancing on CEUS examination.[31,32]

Clear cell papillary RCC (ccpRCC) is another relatively indolent carcinoma that accounts for 1% to 4% of renal epithelial neoplasms.[33] Although it shares features with other RCC subtypes, it is considered a unique histologic entity with distinct morphologic and immunophenotypic features.[34] Tordjman and colleagues[33] studied the CT appearance of 44 ccpRCCs, and found that about one-half were solid lesions, whereas the other one-half were predominantly cystic. An example of a cystic-type ccpRCC at CEUS is shown in **Fig. 11**.

Urothelial Carcinoma

Urothelial carcinoma is about twice as common in men as in women, is commonly associated with

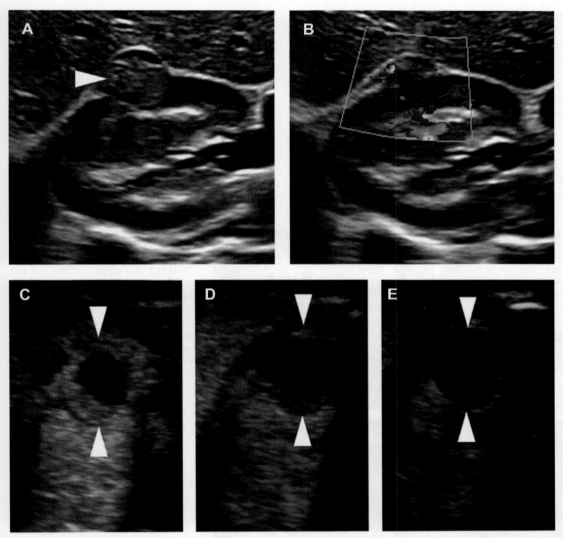

Fig. 10. Transverse grayscale US (*A*), transverse color Doppler US (*B*), and transverse CEUS at the corticomedullary (*C*), nephrographic (*D*), and delayed (*E*) phases of an Xp11.2 translocation RCC in a 30-year-old woman. The mass (*arrowheads*) seems to be mostly solid at grayscale US with small internal cystic spaces, and has small foci of internal Doppler flow. At CEUS the mass is centrally cystic and has a thick enhancing rim that avidly enhances at corticomedullary phase (*C*), followed by washout at later phases.

cigarette smoking, and commonly presents with gross hematuria. Most of these carcinomas occur in the bladder, with only 5% to 7% arising in the upper urinary tract (ureter and renal collecting system).[35] Urothelial carcinomas presenting as kidney masses can appear as small focal areas of urothelial thickening or nodularity (often multifocal), or alternatively as large infiltrative masses. If a portion of the collecting system is obstructed by tumor, upstream calyceal dilatation can be seen.

Reports on upper tract urothelial carcinoma at CEUS examination are few,[36,37] but as with other imaging modalities, at CEUS urothelial carcinomas are typically hypoenhancing tumors (Fig. 12). However, enhancement patterns of urothelial carcinomas at CEUS can show some variability, which may depend on the tumor grade.[38,39] One downside of evaluating urothelial tumors with CEUS is the lack of UCA excretion into the collecting system after intravenous administration. Unlike with CT scans or MR imaging, no urographic phase can be obtained, and so there is no possibility of also visualizing tumors as intraluminal filling defects.

Lymphoma

Primary renal lymphoma is rare, and more commonly renal involvement in lymphoma is secondary, often in the setting of extensive extranodal non-Hodgkin lymphoma.[40] Lymphomatous involvement of the kidney can take variable forms, with renal enlargement from diffuse infiltration, multifocal discrete intrarenal masses, and diffuse perirenal involvement all observed. Discrete lymphomatous masses in the kidney are typically very hypoechoic, a characteristic of lymphomatous masses in general. At CEUS examination, renal lymphoma is usually hypoenhancing[41] (Fig. 13).

Angiomyolipoma

Angiomyolipoma (AML) is the most common benign solid renal mass, and is classified among the perivascular epithelioid cell family of mesenchymal tumors. Classic AMLs are composed of 3 elements, namely, smooth muscle components, macroscopic fat, and dysmorphic blood vessels, and it is the identification of macroscopic fat by CT scan or MR imaging that typically allows for the confident imaging diagnosis of AML. However, it is not rare for the fat component to be minimal or absent, which can lead to diagnostic difficulty. These types of AMLs are often termed lipid poor or minimal fat. Additionally, because of the intralesional fat, AMLs are typically hyperechoic on grayscale US examination, but RCC can occasionally

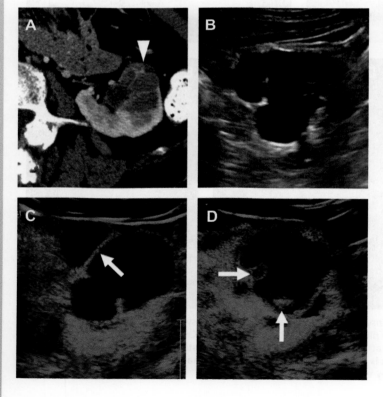

Fig. 11. Axial contrast-enhanced CT scan (A), transverse grayscale US (B), transverse CEUS (C), and longitudinal CEUS (D) of a ccpRCC of the left kidney. At CT scan, the lesion (arrowhead) is mostly cystic, but has multiple internal enhancing septations. Grayscale US also shows a complex appearance, and at CEUS the lesion shows thick enhancing septations (arrow in C) and enhancing mural nodularity (arrows in D).

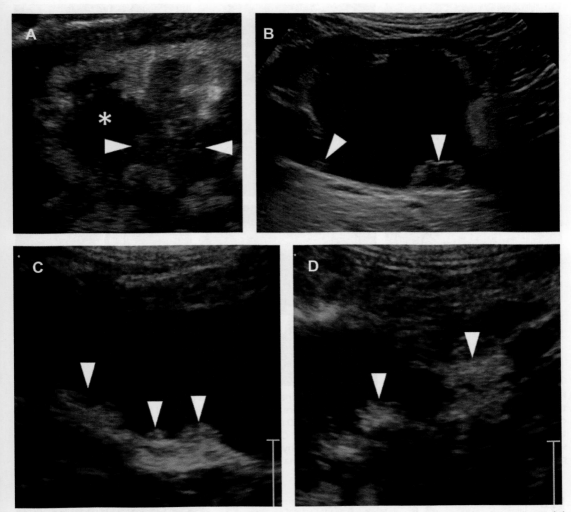

Fig. 12. Upper tract urothelial carcinoma in 2 patients. Longitudinal CEUS examination in the first patient (*A*) shows a hypoenhancing mass (*arrowheads*) centrally in the left kidney, with dilatation of the upper pole collecting system (*asterisk*). Multifocal urothelial tumors (*arrowheads*) are seen in a second patient on longitudinal gray-scale US examination (*B*), and CEUS examination shows multiple enhancing nodular urothelial tumors in the dilated renal pelvis (*C*) and near the ureteropelvic junction (*D*).

be hyperechoic as well, also contributing to diagnostic difficulty.

At CEUS examination, AML usually shows early hyperenhancement (**Fig. 14**), another feature it shares with ccRCC. At the peak of enhancement, AML usually enhances more homogenously than ccRCC,[9,11,12,42] although this differentiation can be difficult in practice, especially with small lesions. Additionally, it has been reported that AMLs de-enhance more slowly than ccRCC,[12,42] although this characteristic is not always observed consistently. Li and colleagues[43] have reported that the quantitative parameters of the enhancement curve may be of use in differentiating AML

and RCC, namely, peak intensity, mean transit time, and area under the curve.

Infection

CEUS examination in pyelonephritis has been reported to show wedge-shaped or rounded focal areas of parenchymal hypoenhancement, best depicted at later phases.[44] In the proper clinical setting, and especially if multifocal, these findings can allow for the diagnosis of pyelonephritis. However, if the clinical findings are ambiguous, and especially if the renal lesion is single and has a masslike appearance, focal infection can be

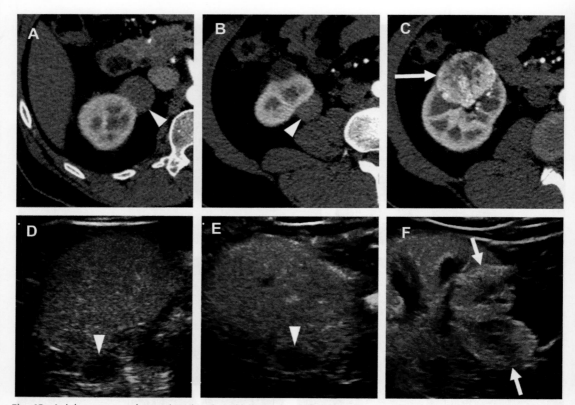

Fig. 13. Axial contrast-enhanced CT (*A–C*) and longitudinal CEUS (*D–F*) in a patient with lymphoma and ccRCC of the right kidney. Hypoenhancing masses (*arrowheads*) are seen at the upper (*A*) and lower (*B*) poles of the kidney on CT scan, and these are also hypoenhancing at CEUS (*D* and *E*, respectively). Also in the mid to lower portion of the kidney is a larger mass, which is hyperenhancing at CT scan (*C*) (*arrow*) and CEUS (*F*) (*arrows*). Nephrectomy showed the hyperenhancing mass to be ccRCC, and the hypoenhancing masses to be 2 foci of marginal zone lymphoma. The patient did not have evidence of lymphoma elsewhere.

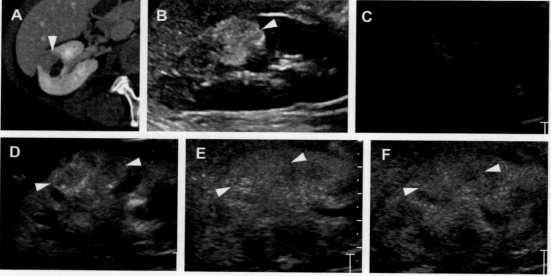

Fig. 14. Axial contrast-enhanced CT (*A*), grayscale longitudinal US (*B*), and longitudinal CEUS at the precontrast (*C*), corticomedullary (*D*), nephrographic (*E*), and delayed (*F*) phases of an AML of the right kidney. The mass (*arrowheads*) shows macroscopic fat at its medial portion on CT scanning, and is very hyperechoic on grayscale US examination. At CEUS it is hyperenhancing at corticomedullary phase (*C*), and then fairly isoenhancing to cortex at later phases.

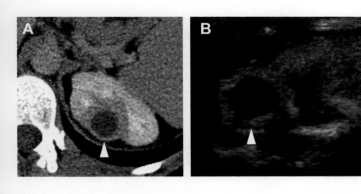

Fig. 15. Axial contrast-enhanced CT scan (*A*) and longitudinal CEUS at the corticomedullary phase (*B*) of a left renal abscess. The patient was a 33-year-old woman being treated for a urinary tract infection. An upper pole lesion (*arrowheads*) shows rim enhancement and central nonenhancement on CT scanning and CEUS examination. After a course of antibiotics, follow-up imaging 4 months later showed resolution of the abscess.

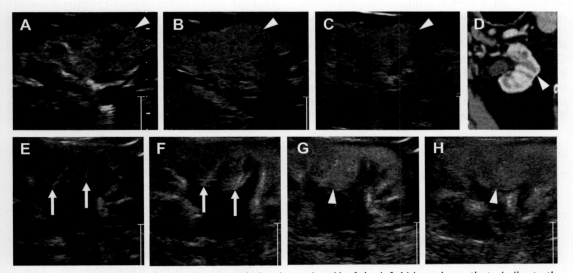

Fig. 16. Longitudinal CEUS of a lateral contour bulge (*arrowheads*) of the left kidney shows that, similar to the parenchyma around it, the area of bulging shows enhancing cortex and hypoenhancing medulla at corticomedullary phase (*A*). Medullary enhancement increases by nephrographic phase (*B*), and the entire bulge remains isoenhancing with parenchyma through the delayed phase (*C*), confirming a dromedary hump. Contrast-enhanced CT obtained 2 years later for other reasons redemonstrates the bulge (*D*). In a separate patient, longitudinal CEUS examination of a masslike area in the left kidney demonstrates internal vessels (*arrows*) at contrast arrival (*E*) and corticomedullary phase (*F*), with the masslike area (*arrowheads*) becoming isoenhancing with adjacent cortex at nephrographic (*G*) and delayed (*H*) phases, indicating a column of Bertin.

confused with tumor. If infection is suspected, confirmation with a short-term follow-up showing a decrease in size or resolution is helpful. However, some indeterminate lesions may undergo biopsy. Pyelonephritis may be complicated by renal abscess, which typically shows avid rim enhancement, and a nonenhancing center (**Fig. 15**).

Pseudolesions

One of the most effective ways to diagnose a pseudolesion is to demonstrate an identical appearance of the lesion in question to adjacent parenchyma. The advantage of CEUS in this regard goes back to a fundamental advantage of the modality, namely, that CEUS allows the observation of hundreds of timepoints over the course of a contrast bolus. Observing that a bulge in the expected location of a dromedary hump, or masslike tissue in the expected location of a column of Bertin, shows enhancement identical to parenchyma throughout the entire period of enhancement allows for confident diagnosis (**Fig. 16**).

SUMMARY

The ongoing expansion of the use of CEUS in the United States is likely to continue, and one area where CEUS is of great usefulness is in the identification and characterization of renal masses. Although complete subtyping of renal masses is not currently known to be possible by CEUS examination, much helpful information can be gained through CEUS; furthermore, knowledge of this modality is still increasing.

A ccRCC is typically a hypervascular and heterogeneous mass, enhancing earlier and to a greater degree than the renal cortex. However, there remains difficulty in distinguishing ccRCC from oncocytoma and lipid-poor AML, which can lead to surgery for benign lesions. A pRCC is clearly distinguishable from a ccRCC, being a hypoenhancing tumor with a later peak of enhancement. A chRCC is uncommon and shows an intermediate curve of enhancement, although this characteristic can overlap somewhat with the appearance of ccRCC. For cystic lesions, CEUS is often more sensitive for enhancement of septations than CT scans or MR imaging. Many other renal tumors and tumorlike conditions can be evaluated with CEUS and experience with these entities is increasing.

DISCLOSURE

The author has nothing to disclose.

REFERENCES

1. Gill IS, Aron M, Gervais DA, et al. Clinical practice. Small renal mass. N Engl J Med 2010;362(7): 624–34.
2. Kalra A, Shroff GR, Erlien D, et al. Perflutren-based echocardiographic contrast in patients with right-to-left intracardiac shunts. JACC Cardiovasc Imaging 2014;7(2):206–7.
3. Parker JM, Weller MW, Feinstein LM, et al. Safety of ultrasound contrast agents in patients with known or suspected cardiac shunts. Am J Cardiol 2013; 112(7):1039–45.
4. Wei K, Mulvagh SL, Carson L, et al. The safety of deFinity and Optison for ultrasound image enhancement: a retrospective analysis of 78,383 administered contrast doses. J Am Soc Echocardiogr 2008;21(11):1202–6.
5. Wever-Pinzon O, Suma V, Ahuja A, et al. Safety of echocardiographic contrast in hospitalized patients with pulmonary hypertension: a multi-center study. Eur Heart J Cardiovasc Imaging 2012;13(10): 857–62.
6. Chang EH. An introduction to contrast-enhanced ultrasound for nephrologists. Nephron 2018;138(3): 176–85.
7. King KG, Gulati M, Malhi H, et al. Quantitative assessment of solid renal masses by contrast-enhanced ultrasound with time-intensity curves: how we do it. Abdom Imaging 2015;40(7):2461–71.
8. Aoki S, Hattori R, Yamamoto T, et al. Contrast-enhanced ultrasound using a time-intensity curve for the diagnosis of renal cell carcinoma. BJU Int 2011;108(3):349–54.
9. Fan L, Lianfang D, Jinfang X, et al. Diagnostic efficacy of contrast-enhanced ultrasonography in solid renal parenchymal lesions with maximum diameters of 5 cm. J Ultrasound Med 2008;27(6):875–85.
10. Gerst S, Hann LE, Li D, et al. Evaluation of renal masses with contrast-enhanced ultrasound: initial experience. AJR Am J Roentgenol 2011;197(4): 897–906.
11. Lu Q, Xue LY, Huang BJ, et al. Histotype differentiation of hypo-echoic renal tumors on CEUS: usefulness of enhancement homogeneity and intensity. Abdom Imaging 2015;40(6):1675–83.
12. Xu ZF, Xu HX, Xie XY, et al. Renal cell carcinoma and renal angiomyolipoma: differential diagnosis with real-time contrast-enhanced ultrasonography. J Ultrasound Med 2010;29(5):709–17.
13. Lu Q, Huang BJ, Xue LY, et al. Differentiation of renal tumor histotypes: usefulness of quantitative analysis of contrast-enhanced ultrasound. AJR Am J Roentgenol 2015;205(3):W335–42.
14. Kreshover JE, Richstone L, Kavoussi LR. Renal cell recurrence for T1 tumors after laparoscopic partial nephrectomy. J Endourol 2013;27(12):1468–70.
15. Lane BR, Gill IS. 7-year oncological outcomes after laparoscopic and open partial nephrectomy. J Urol 2010;183(2):473–9.
16. Young JR, Coy H, Douek M, et al. Type 1 papillary renal cell carcinoma: differentiation from Type 2 papillary RCC on multiphasic MDCT. Abdom Radiol (NY) 2017;42(7):1911–8.
17. Mejean A, Hopirtean V, Bazin JP, et al. Prognostic factors for the survival of patients with papillary renal cell carcinoma: meaning of histological typing and multifocality. J Urol 2003;170(3):764–7.
18. Prasad SR, Humphrey PA, Catena JR, et al. Common and uncommon histologic subtypes of renal cell carcinoma: imaging spectrum with pathologic correlation. Radiographics 2006;26(6):1795–806 [discussion: 806–10].
19. Kryvenko ON, Jorda M, Argani P, et al. Diagnostic approach to eosinophilic renal neoplasms. Arch Pathol Lab Med 2014;138(11):1531–41.
20. Ruiz-Cordero R, Rao P, Li L, et al. Hybrid oncocytic/chromophobe renal tumors are molecularly distinct from oncocytoma and chromophobe renal cell carcinoma. Mod Pathol 2019;32(11):1698–707.
21. Bauman TM, Potretzke AM, Wright AJ, et al. Partial nephrectomy for presumed renal-cell carcinoma: incidence, predictors, and perioperative outcomes of benign lesions. J Endourol 2017;31(4): 412–7.

22. Secin FP, Castillo OA, Rozanec JJ, et al. American Confederation of Urology (CAU) experience in minimally invasive partial nephrectomy. World J Urol 2017;35(1):57–65.

23. Ishigami K, Jones AR, Dahmoush L, et al. Imaging spectrum of renal oncocytomas: a pictorial review with pathologic correlation. Insights Imaging 2015; 6(1):53–64.

24. Wu Y, Du L, Li F, et al. Renal oncocytoma: contrast-enhanced sonographic features. J Ultrasound Med 2013;32(3):441–8.

25. Moch H, Cubilla AL, Humphrey PA, et al. The 2016 WHO classification of tumours of the urinary system and male genital organs-part a: renal, penile, and testicular tumours. Eur Urol 2016;70(1):93–105.

26. Tretiakova M, Mehta V, Kocherginsky M, et al. Predominantly cystic clear cell renal cell carcinoma and multilocular cystic renal neoplasm of low malignant potential form a low-grade spectrum. Virchows Arch 2018;473(1):85–93.

27. Li T, Chen J, Jiang Y, et al. Multilocular cystic renal cell neoplasm of low malignant potential: a series of 76 cases. Clin Genitourin Cancer 2016;14(6): e553–7.

28. Calio A, Segala D, Munari E, et al. MiT family translocation renal cell carcinoma: from the early descriptions to the current knowledge. Cancers (Basel) 2019;11(8).

29. Ling W, Ma X, Luo Y, et al. Ultrasonographic findings of renal cell carcinomas associated with Xp11.2 translocation/TFE3 gene fusion. Contrast Media Mol Imaging 2017;2017:2958357.

30. Ged Y, Chen YB, Knezevic A, et al. Mucinous tubular and spindle-cell carcinoma of the kidney: clinical features, genomic profiles, and treatment outcomes. Clin Genitourin Cancer 2019;17(4):268–74.e1.

31. Yan L, Huang B, Xue L, et al. Contrast-enhanced ultrasound characterization of renal mucinous tubular and spindle cell carcinoma: report of two cases. J Clin Ultrasound 2015;43(1):55–8.

32. Zhang Q, Wang W, Zhang S, et al. Mucinous tubular and spindle cell carcinoma of the kidney: the contrast-enhanced ultrasonography and CT features of six cases and review of the literature. Int Urol Nephrol 2014;46(12):2311–7.

33. Tordjman M, Dbjay J, Chamouni A, et al. Clear cell papillary renal cell carcinoma: a recent entity with distinct imaging patterns. AJR Am J Roentgenol 2020;214(3):579–87.

34. Patel S, Asarian A, Xiao P. Clear cell papillary renal cell carcinoma: a case report and literature review. J Surg Case Rep 2019;2019(6):rjz177.

35. Ali O, Fishman EK, Sheth S. Upper urinary tract urothelial carcinoma on multidetector CT: spectrum of disease. Abdom Radiol (NY) 2019;44(12):3874–85.

36. Drudi FM, Di Candio G, Di Leo N, et al. Contrast-enhanced ultrasonography in the diagnosis of upper urinary tract urothelial cell carcinoma: a preliminary study. Ultraschall Med 2013;34(1):30–7.

37. Xue LY, Lu Q, Huang BJ, et al. Evaluation of renal urothelial carcinoma by contrast-enhanced ultrasonography. Eur J Radiol 2013;82(4):e151–7.

38. Drudi FM, Di Leo N, Malpassini F, et al. CEUS in the differentiation between low and high-grade bladder carcinoma. J Ultrasound 2012;15(4):247–51.

39. Guo S, Xu P, Zhou A, et al. Contrast-enhanced ultrasound differentiation between low- and high- grade bladder urothelial carcinoma and correlation with tumor microvessel density. J Ultrasound Med 2017; 36(11):2287–97.

40. Sheth S, Ali S, Fishman E. Imaging of renal lymphoma: patterns of disease with pathologic correlation. Radiographics 2006;26(4):1151–68.

41. Trenker C, Neesse A, Gorg C. Sonographic patterns of renal lymphoma in B-mode imaging and in contrast-enhanced ultrasound (CEUS)–a retrospective evaluation. Eur J Radiol 2015;84(5):807–10.

42. Lu Q, Li CX, Huang BJ, et al. Triphasic and epithelioid minimal fat renal angiomyolipoma and clear cell renal cell carcinoma: qualitative and quantitative CEUS characteristics and distinguishing features. Abdom Imaging 2015;40(2):333–42.

43. Li CX, Lu Q, Huang BJ, et al. Quantitative evaluation of contrast-enhanced ultrasound for differentiation of renal cell carcinoma subtypes and angiomyolipoma. Eur J Radiol 2016;85(4):795–802.

44. Fontanilla T, Minaya J, Cortes C, et al. Acute complicated pyelonephritis: contrast-enhanced ultrasound. Abdom Imaging 2012;37(4):639–46.

Update on Hereditary Renal Cancer and Imaging Implications

Stephanie M. Walker, BS[a], Rabindra Gautam[b], Baris Turkbey, MD[a],
Ashkan Malayeri, MD[c], Peter L. Choyke, MD[a,*]

KEYWORDS

- Renal cell carcinoma • Hereditary renal cancer syndrome • Von Hippel-Lindau disease
- Hereditary leiomyomatosis and renal cell cancer • Tuberous sclerosis

KEY POINTS

- Hereditary renal tumors are diagnosed at a younger age than sporadic tumors and are often multiple and multifocal.
- All known subtypes of renal cancer have been identified in hereditary syndromes.
- Most hereditary cancers are low grade and therefore less aggressive. However, some hereditary renal cancers are highly aggressive.
- Radiologist awareness of extrarenal findings associated with hereditary renal cancer syndromes is helpful for early diagnosis.

INTRODUCTION

Renal cell carcinoma is the eighth most common type of cancer, with an estimated 73,820 new diagnoses in 2019 in the United States.[1] About one-fifth of patients with renal cell carcinoma have metastases at the time of presentation.[2] Hereditary renal cancers (HRNs) account for an estimated 5% to 8% of renal cancers, although this may be an underestimate because of genetic factors not yet characterized.[3] The diagnosis of a hereditary renal tumor has important implications for the patient and their family. For the patient, knowledge of a germline mutation can play a pivotal role in the future management and treatment of the cancer. Patients with a possible hereditary component to their renal cancer should be referred for genetic testing, which can help guide disease management and inform whether family members could be at risk. Patients with a family history, unique personal history, bilateral or multifocal disease, or early age at diagnosis are at increased risk and therefore, may benefit from genetic testing. Recognition of clinical and imaging features associated with hereditary renal carcinoma is an important part of diagnosis. Imaging findings outside the kidneys may be the first indication of a possible hereditary cancer syndrome. Therefore, knowledge of not only renal tumors but other visceral manifestations of hereditary cancer syndromes is important for a radiologist to have, to recognize HRC syndromes.

Several known genetic mutations are associated with HRC. There are mutations that cause

This research was made possible through the National Institutes of Health (NIH) Medical Research Scholars Program, a public-private partnership supported jointly by the NIH and contributions to the Foundation for the NIH from the Doris Duke Charitable Foundation, Genentech, the American Association for Dental Research, the Colgate-Palmolive Company, and other private donors.
[a] Molecular Imaging Program, National Cancer Institute, National Institutes of Health, 9000 Rockville Pike, Bethesda, MD 20892, USA; [b] Center for Cancer Research, National Cancer Institute, National Institutes of Health, 9000 Rockville Pike, Bethesda, MD 20892, USA; [c] Radiology and Imaging Sciences, Clinical Center, National Institutes of Health, 9000 Rockville Pike, Bethesda, MD 20892, USA
* Corresponding author.
E-mail address: pchoyke@mail.nih.gov

well-characterized renal-epithelial syndromes including von Hippel-Lindau (VHL) syndrome, Birt-Hogg-Dube syndrome (BHD), hereditary leiomyomatosis and renal cell cancer syndrome (HLRCC), tuberous sclerosis complex (TSC), and hereditary nonpolyposis colorectal cancer syndrome (HNPCC). Other genetic mutations associated with HRC are emerging but are less well characterized, including chromosome 3 translocations, BAP1 cancer syndrome, PTEN mutation (Cowden syndrome), succinate dehydrogenase complex subunit B (SDHB), MITF predisposition, and CDCJ3 (hyperparathyroidism jaw tumor syndrome). HRCs are described by their frequency, type of tumor produced, treatments, and aggressiveness among others. This review discusses HRCs from a radiologist's perspective, focusing on imaging features and known associations.

VON HIPPEL-LINDAU SYNDROME

VHL syndrome has a frequency of approximately 1:36,000, making it the most common identified cause of HRC.[4] VHL is an autosomal-dominant hereditary disease caused by mutations in the VHL tumor suppressor gene. There is 90% penetrance by age 60. Nonetheless, up to 20% of cases are caused by sporadic mutations first occurring in the index patient with no antecedent family history.[5,6] Nonrenal manifestations include pancreatic neuroendocrine tumors (pNET), pancreatic cysts, central nervous system (CNS) hemangioblastomas, endolymphatic sac tumors, retinal angiomas, pheochromocytomas, epididymal papillary cystadenomas, and cystadenomas of the broad ligament. Clear cell renal cell cancer (ccRCC) is the main malignant neoplasm in VHL affecting 24% to 45% of patients.[7] Additionally, of these findings, ccRCC has historically been associated with the highest mortality, but because of improved surveillance and earlier diagnosis ccRCC mortality has been superseded by VHL-related CNS diseases.[8,9] Tumor cells lacking a functional VHL tumor suppressor gene overproduce the downstream products of hypoxia-inducible factor target genes, such as vascular endothelial growth factor. This predisposes patients to developing hypervascular masses in various organs.[10]

Renal Imaging Findings

The renal cancer type associated with VHL is virtually always ccRCC, although the precise pathogenesis is not completely understood. Most frequently, it manifests as a hyperplastic or metaplastic clear cell lining of multiple renal cysts from which ccRCC can develop. Later in the progression, solid and cystic components are also seen. All renal cysts in a patient with VHL should be considered premalignant and followed by imaging, although variable behavior is expected, including spontaneous involution.

On computed tomography (CT), lesions have a water attenuation initially because of their cystic nature. On MR imaging, lesions are T1-hypointense and T2-hyperintense. Fat-suppressed T1-weighted MR imaging with contrast can help to differentiate complex cystic components from solid enhancing components.[11] Lesions are characterized as mostly cystic or mostly solid-enhancing, because they are commonly heterogeneous (Fig. 1). ccRCC progression is marked by enlarging solid components, enhancing septations, and solid nodules. As solid components grow, they take over cystic components until the renal masses are comprised of nearly all solid tumor. Because of this, the amount of solid rather than cystic disease determines which lesions warrant treatment.

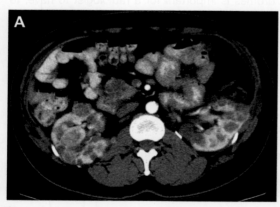
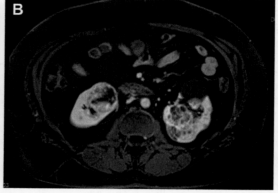

Fig. 1. Postcontrast-enhanced CT (*A*) and MR imaging (*B*) axial images of two different patients with VHL. (*A*, *B*) Bilateral renal lesions with solid and cystic components.

Solid components of renal masses often demonstrate avid enhancement on contrast-enhanced imaging. The clear cell subtype of RCC shows stronger enhancement in the cortico-medullary phase of contrast media enhancement than other tumor subtypes and has more persistent enhancement in the nephrogenic and excretory phase. MR imaging can be substituted for CT in detecting VHL tumors and is superior to ultrasound. MR imaging reduces the radiation burden to patients undergoing multiple studies over their life. VHL tumors are generally T2 bright and T1 hypointense with avid enhancement on different phases of postcontrast T1 similar to CT. The VHL tumors are generally low grade, and demonstrate higher mean apparent diffusion coefficient values than other more aggressive subtypes, such as papillary and chromophobe RCC.[12,13]

Extrarenal Manifestations

In addition to renal lesions, abdominal imaging studies may reveal pancreatic cysts, serous cystadenomas of the pancreas, and solid enhancing nonfunctional pNET. Pancreatic lesions are often multiple and are distributed throughout the pancreas, although solid pNET tumors typically are more concentrated in the head and uncinate process. The most common histologic subtype of cystic pancreatic lesions in VHL is serous cystadenoma that typically has a benign course, although pancreatic insufficiency may be seen. On imaging, pancreatic cystadenomas typically display a central scar with cysts arranged in a rosette pattern around it. Calcification is frequently seen. Serous cystadenomas can grow larger but are not malignant. Patients with VHL with pNET are more likely to have missense mutations in the VHL gene[14] and can develop metastatic disease. An association between pNET metastasis and exon 3 mutations in patients with VHL has been suggested but further studies are needed.[15] On CT they are typically highly vascular and are detected during the arterial phase of contrast administration. Fluorodeoxyglucose (FDG)-PET/CT has been shown to increase sensitivity for detecting pNET over anatomic imaging.[16] 68Ga-Dotatate PET/CT had a significantly higher detection rate for pNET when compared with anatomic imaging for all lesions, and comparable detection rate for pancreatic lesions in patients with VHL.[17] When small, pNET are well circumscribed and hypervascular and often found in the uncinate process. Larger pNETs may become necrotic and appear more heterogeneous. These tumors are bounded by a capsule and thus, displace rather than invade surrounding structures.[18] However, as the tumor grows its margins may become less distinct.

In men, VHL is characterized by multiple hyper-enhancing papillary cystadenomas in the epididymis, occurring in up to 40% of patients, whereas in women cystadenomas may be present in the broad ligament of the uterus.[19] In the adrenals and paraganglia, pheochromocytomas occur. These are bilateral and/or multifocal, subclinical or highly symptomatic.[20] In addition to biochemical evidence of excess catecholamine production, abdominal CT and MR imaging with contrast are sensitive in detecting adrenal and extra-adrenal pheochromocytomas in these patients. These lesions are typically hypervascular. Paragangliomas (extrarenal pheochromocytomas) can vary in appearance on cross-sectional imaging but typically show strong arterial enhancement. If rapidly growing, a necrotic core may be present. The presence of multiple paragangliomas suggests a particular subtype of VHL called type 2 VHL, which is associated with point mutations in the VHL gene.

Within the CNS, the most common lesion is the hemangioblastoma, typically located in the posterior fossa of the brain. On CT or MR imaging these lesions demonstrate avidly enhancing solid and cystic components. Hemangioblastomas in the CNS typically present as mural enhancing nodules on MR imaging with adjacent cystic spaces and can lead to multiple symptoms, particularly difficulty with balance. A similar lesion is found in the retina where they are named retinal capillary angiomas. Diagnosing these retinal lesions early can prevent blindness. This is done with careful eye examinations, and often they are the first manifestation of VHL. Patients with VHL also may develop endolymphatic sac tumors in the inner ear, which can cause deafness if left untreated. They have the potential to invade surrounding bone and infiltrate into the extradural space. On T2-weighted MR imaging, endolymphatic sac tumors are heterogeneous hyperintense masses with avid enhancement.[21]

Screening and Management

Lifelong surveillance is necessary in patients with VHL given the ongoing risks for tumor development with increasing age. Longitudinal surveillance has been shown to decrease morbidity and mortality.[22] Multiple groups have developed surveillance guidelines. The most recent comes from the VHL Alliance last updated in 2017, which recommends screening for retinal hemangioblastoma with ophthalmoscopy starting in infancy because of the noninvasive nature of the examination.[23] Starting at age 5, plasma free metanephrines or 24-hour urinary fractionated metanephrines should be checked annually. In families with a strong history of pheochromocytoma/paraganglioma, this is initiated in patients at 2 years old. Patients with VHL should be screened for RCC, pheochromocytoma, and pNET with abdominal ultrasound annually up to age 16, and then yearly thereafter with alternating ultrasound/MR imaging gradually switching to MR imaging in adulthood. CNS hemangioblastomas should be screened for with biennial MR imaging of the brain and spine starting at age 16, but it may be desirable to begin MR imaging screening as soon as the patient is old enough to tolerate MR imaging without sedation.[24] Pancreatic cysts, pNETs, renal cancers, and pheochromocytomas should all be followed typically with MR imaging, which avoids the radiation associated with CT. Although pancreatic cysts do not necessitate treatment unless they are symptomatic, pNETs have metastatic potential and should be monitored for growth. Although it was once thought that intravenous contrast could induce hypertensive crisis in patients with paraganglioma and pheochromocytoma, there is no evidence for this and so there is no contraindication.[25] There is some concern in the VHL community regarding the cumulative effect of gadolinium after many years of screening MR imaging with contrast. It is known that gadolinium may accumulate in the brain and other organs, although no adverse neurologic effect has been reported. Using gadolinium contrast agents with strong chemical chelates (ie, macrocyclic agent) reduces the potential risk of gadolinium deposition. Gadolinium enhancement provides useful diagnostic information in many VHL cases so the issue needs to be carefully discussed with concerned patients.

If a patient with VHL is diagnosed with RCC, nephron-sparing surgery is the recommended management for tumors greater than or equal to 3 cm because of the risk of metastasis, whereas smaller lesions are monitored safely with imaging surveillance. Improved imaging modalities have led to the detection of more renal cancers at an early stage. Solid tumors less than 3 cm are thought to have near zero metastatic potential and are safely monitored until they reach the 3 cm threshold for surgery. Partial nephrectomy has been shown to be as effective as total nephrectomy for early stage RCC, and other nephron-sparing approaches, such as cryofrequency and radiofrequency ablation, may be appropriate for small tumors while minimizing damage to healthy parts of kidney.[26] Laparoscopic surgery has greatly reduced the recovery period from treatment.

BIRT-HOGG-DUBE SYNDROME

BHD syndrome is an autosomal-dominant condition caused by an inactivating germline mutation in the folliculin (FLCN) tumor suppressor gene. The syndrome presents with lung cysts; pneumothorax; fibrofolliculomas of the skin; and the most threatening potential complication, RCC. Although the penetrance of renal cancer is low, patients with BHD have up to seven times the risk of renal cancer compared with the general population. Approximately 13% to 34% of patients have renal tumors, but unlike VHL, the tumors vary in histologic subtype with the most common being oncocytic-chromophobe type.[27] Major criteria for BHD are greater than five cutaneous fibrofolliculomas or a confirmed germline mutation in FLCN. Minor criteria include family history of BHD, early onset or multifocal renal cancer, and lung cysts.[28] One major or two minor criteria establish a diagnosis.

Renal Imaging Findings

Renal tumors in BHD syndrome are noted at an earlier age than sporadic RCC, with an average age of 50.4 years.[29] The tumors range in histology from oncocytomas (benign) to chromophobe carcinomas (malignant). Oncocytic-chromophobe renal cell carcinoma tend to exhibit homogenous enhancement on CT and MR imaging with scant if any cystic components distinguishing them from VHL (Fig. 2). Central necrosis is not usually seen, but calcifications are common, and the tumors are notable for their uniformity and absence of radiographic necrosis.[30] Compared with other hereditary RCC syndromes, the tumors associated with BHD are somewhat less aggressive and can be monitored for longer; however, aggressive tumors have been documented.[27,31]

Extrarenal Manifestations

Lung cysts affect more than 80% of patients with BHD and are usually multiple and found predominantly in the lower lobes (see Fig. 2). The cysts can grow to be >7 cm, and are frequently multiseptated when large.[32] Spontaneous pneumothoraxes secondary to pulmonary cysts are commonly seen, occurring in 23% to 30% of patients younger than age 40.[33] Cutaneous findings affect 90% of patients and include fibrofolliculomas, trichodiscomas, and acrochordons. Additional cancers that may be associated with the

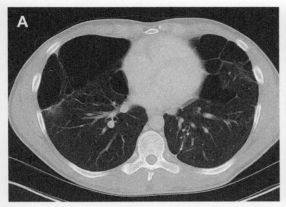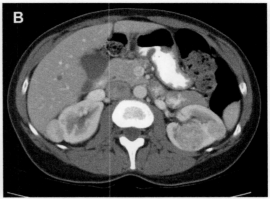

Fig. 2. Axial CT images of a patient with BHD syndrome at the level of the lungs (*A*) and kidneys (*B*). (*A*) Bilateral lung parenchyma includes multiple cysts. (*B*) Multiple chromophobe carcinomas are present bilaterally.

FLCN suppressor gene mutation include clear cell thyroid carcinoma and colorectal carcinoma.[34,35]

Screening and Management

Surveillance is recommended for these patients, but the optimal imaging method and interval remain to be defined. It has been proposed that all patients should undergo high-resolution CT of the chest and MR imaging of the abdomen at diagnosis. At-risk BHD family members should also undergo baseline surveillance with abdominal MR imaging. Screening for renal tumors is recommended starting at age 20, either annually or biannually with MR imaging. When the largest tumor reaches 3 cm, surgical intervention, typically laparoscopic partial nephrectomy, is recommended. Nephron-sparing surgery to preserve renal function is preferred, because patients with BHD may develop more tumors and require repeated surgeries during their lifetime.[36,37]

TUBEROUS SCLEROSIS COMPLEX

TSC, also historically known as Bourneville-Pringle disease, affects an estimated 1 million people worldwide with a frequency of 1:10,000.[38] TSC is caused by germline mutations in TSC1 or TSC2, which encode hamartin and tuberin, respectively. Mutations in TSC2 result in more severe disease manifestations. TSC is acquired as a spontaneous mutation, which occurs in approximately 70% of cases, or by hereditary autosomal-dominant transmission accounting for the remainder. The absence of family history in most cases can make early diagnosis more challenging.[39] TSC is characterized by the presence of multiple hamartomas, primarily on the skin and in the CNS. The risk of renal cancer in patients with TSC is estimated to be 1% to 4%,[40,41] but 70% to 90% of

patients with TSC develop one or more benign renal angiomyolipomas (AMLs).[42] Although they have no malignant potential, AMLs are at risk for spontaneous hemorrhage when they grow larger than 4 cm in diameter and may need to be treated with transarterial embolization.

Renal Imaging Findings

AMLs are by far the most common lesion in the kidney in patients with TSC. AMLs are a benign neoplasm composed of dysmorphic blood vessels, smooth muscle, and adipose tissue. Typical AMLs involve the renal cortex and have a macroscopic fat component (**Fig. 3**), but AMLs without gross visible fat occur in approximately one-third of patients with TSC and can mimic cancer. The AMLs without gross fat demonstrate higher attenuation than normal renal parenchyma and enhance homogenously. AMLs can also mimic cancer by extending into local lymph nodes and the inferior vena cava.[43] The next most common renal lesions in TSC are benign renal cysts, which occur in up to 47% of patients.[44] The cysts are not considered premalignant as they are in VHL.

Although there are a plethora of nonmalignant findings associated with TSC that can help a radiologist identify it, the only cancer patients with TSC are at increased for is RCC and even then, the risk is low. Clear-cell, chromophobe, or papillary subtypes of RCC have all been associated with TSC.[45] Differentiating renal cell carcinoma from an AML without gross fat is often challenging, but MR imaging is useful in differentiating the two. Intratumoral necrosis and larger size are associated with RCC, whereas low SI index on T2-weighted images relative to renal parenchyma and smaller size are associated with AML.[46] Specifically, it has been found that T2 SI ratio less

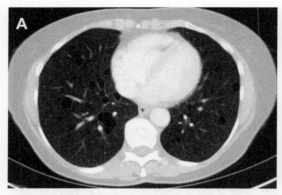
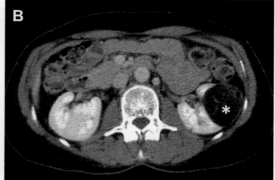

Fig. 3. Postcontrast-enhanced axial CT images in two different patients with tuberous sclerosis. (*A*) Multiple bilateral pulmonary cysts are seen. (*B*) The left kidney contains a lipid-rich angiomyolipoma (*asterisk*).

than 0.9 or an arterial/delayed enhancement ratio greater than 1.5 favor a diagnosis of AML with 99% sensitivity and 73% specificity.[47] AMLs without gross fat also tend to enhance more uniformly than RCC. Despite these suggestive findings, biopsy of the lesion may be desirable before any treatment is contemplated.

Extrarenal Manifestations

TSC is characterized by benign hamartomas, especially in the brain. Ninety percent of patients are affected by subependymal nodules and cortical tubers.[48] They are multiple and can result in neurologic manifestations, such as epilepsy and cognitive disability. On CT of the head, subependymal nodules are seen along ventricular walls, often appearing as calcified foci. On MR imaging, they are isointense to hyperintense on T1- and T2-weighted images. In the frontal lobes, cortical tubers are hypointense lesions on T1-weighted images, and hyperintense on T2 and FLAIR images. Unlike cortical tubers, cerebellar tubers are wedge-shaped and not epileptogenic. Giant cell astrocytomas, a larger variant of subependymal tubers, affect 5% to 15% of patients with TSC and can cause hydrocephalus because of their rapid growth and location adjacent to the interventricular foramen of Monro. They are heterogeneous on CT and MR imaging and may have intratumoral hemorrhage and calcification. Other less common extrarenal manifestations include rectal polyps, bone islands, thyroid adenomas, and lymphangioleiomyomatosis (LAM). LAM, affecting 26% to 49% of women with TSC, causes cystic lung destruction and potential pneumothorax and chylous pleural effusions (see **Fig. 3**).[49] Cardiac rhabdomyomas occur in 50% to 70% of infants with TSC but usually spontaneously resolve in the perinatal period.[50]

Screening and Management

There are limited guidelines available for screening and management of this disease because of a lack of available evidence and low risk. Because of antenatal detection of cardiac rhabdomyomas on ultrasound, the median age at diagnosis is only 6 months.[51] In general, CNS involvement and seizures followed by dermatologic manifestations are the leading features at presentation. LAM has a reported prevalence of 27% in females with TSC aged less than 21 years, thus it is recommended to begin screening with high-resolution CT at age 18 in females with TSC.[49,52] LAM is treated pharmacologically with mTORC1 inhibitors, such as sirolimus, which is Food and Drug Administration approved for the treatment of LAM.[53] Imaging surveillance with abdominal MR imaging or CT is recommended at least every 3 years, although yearly abdominal MR imaging has been recommended by several groups mainly to monitor AML growth.[28,54] Renal imaging is typically dictated by the presence of AMLs but radiologists should remain alert for malignant lesions. Once renal cancers reach about 3 cm in diameter, surgical intervention is recommended, typically nephron sparing or by focal ablation. Renal function should be monitored in patients who undergo repeat surgeries.

HEREDITARY PAPILLARY RENAL CANCER

Hereditary papillary renal cancer (HPRC) is a rare familial cancer syndrome (approximate incidence of 1 in 10 million) caused by an activating mutation in the MET protooncogene. It is an autosomal-dominant disorder with high penetrance. HPRC is associated with an increased risk of type 1 papillary renal carcinoma, with two-thirds of patients developing the cancer by age 60% and 90% by age 80.[5,39] Type 1 papillary renal carcinoma is less aggressive than type 2, and patients can often be placed on active surveillance for their renal lesions. Unlike other HRC syndromes, the only known manifestation of this disease is papillary renal cancer. Renal tumors associated with HPRC generally appear after the age of 30, but an early onset phenotype has been identified that presents in the second decade of life.[55] The disease is limited to a small number of family clusters.

Renal Imaging Findings

HPRC produces multiple bilateral tumors that may number in the hundreds or even thousands, most of which are microscopic. Type I papillary tumors tend to be slow growing and often do not present until later in life. The lesions are hypovascular with minimal enhancement on MR imaging and CT. Enhancement may be so low that it is difficult to qualitatively differentiate the lesions from cysts. For this reason, a quantitative cutoff of 10 to 30 HU increase on contrast-enhanced CT or 15% increase in signal intensity on T2-weighted MR imaging has been previously defined.[43] Ultrasound is not recommended for detection or follow-up of renal lesions in HPRC because they are isoechoic with background and difficult to see.[43] However, ultrasound is used to confirm that a poorly enhancing lesion on CT or MR imaging is solid and not cystic. MR imaging is the most accurate modality in differentiating papillary RCC from other types of RCC with low enhancement, T2 signal hypointensity, and homogenous restricted diffusion on diffusion-weighed imaging (**Fig. 4**).[13,56]

Extrarenal Manifestations

There are no known extrarenal manifestations of HPRC aside from type 1 papillary renal carcinoma.

Screening and Management

Although frequent surveillance is not necessary because tumors are slow growing, shorter imaging intervals are recommended in the early years after diagnosis and can be extended once the lesions are shown to be stable or slowly growing. MR imaging and CT are viable options, but MR imaging generally should be used for surveillance to reduce radiation exposure.[57] Imaging is recommended every 2 to 4 years with MR imaging but may be less frequent if growth patterns are slow.

HEREDITARY LEIOMYOMA RENAL CELL CARCINOMA (REED SYNDROME)

This syndrome results in type II papillary renal cancer, which is a much more aggressive phenotype than type I. Indeed, it is the most aggressive phenotype of all the HRCs and therefore, it is of greater importance that a correct diagnosis be made. It is caused by a mutation in the fumarate hydratase (FH) gene, resulting in an interruption in the Krebs cycle in cells where both alleles are damaged (so-called loss of heterozygosity). The downstream effects of this cause a pseudohypoxic state that promotes cell growth. The mutation is transmitted in an autosomal-dominant pattern with high penetrance. Patients can also present with soft tissue and uterine leiomyomas at an early age. Approximately 20% of those with an FH mutation develop renal cancer, and the average age at diagnosis is 36 to 39 years. Most newly diagnosed patients die of metastasis within 5 years of diagnosis making it the most aggressive of the HRCs.[39] However, family members positively screened may be diagnosed with this aggressive subtype of RCC at an early stage, which results in better outcomes.[58]

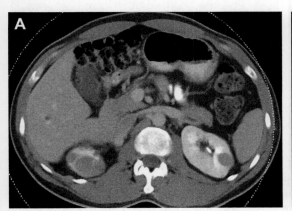
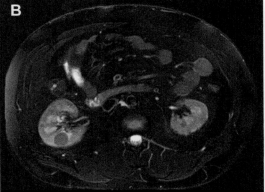

Fig. 4. Postcontrast-enhanced axial CT (*A*) and MR imaging (*B*) images at the level of the kidneys in two different patients with HPRC. CT and MR imaging both demonstrate multiple bilateral renal masses.

Renal Imaging Findings

In contrast to other hereditary cancer syndromes, patients with HLRCC typically have higher grade unilateral and solitary tumors (**Fig. 5**). Initially these tumors appear as small solid or cystic tumors with a nodular component. The solid portion of the tumor demonstrates avid restricted diffusion and low enhancement on MR imaging, although they are more heterogeneous than typical type I papillary cancers. These tumors show lymphovascular metastatic spread, and even small tumors can show microscopic invasion and local lymph node involvement. This contrasts with typical clear cell carcinomas that metastasize later, lymphatically and hematogenously. Fifty percent of cases present with metastases, often to lymph nodes and perinephric spaces.[59] Peritoneal dissemination, unusual with other renal cancers, is not uncommon. Because FH is a key enzyme in the Krebs cycle, these tumors are highly glycolytic and FDG-PET avid. Combined with CT or MR imaging, FDG-PET is a useful imaging modality for staging and detecting metastases (**Fig. 6**).[58]

Extrarenal Manifestations

Patients present with cutaneous leiomyomas in the second to fourth decade of life, which are skin-colored or brownish red nodules measuring up to 2 cm on the trunk and limbs. These are benign tumors and their presentation is variable even within families. Uterine leiomyomas are seen in more than 90% of women with HLRCC, leading to menorrhagia and frequently requiring hysterectomies before 30 years of age.[60] Although these lesions in the skin and uterus are considered benign, malignant transformation has been reported.[39]

Screening and Management

In contrast to VHL, HPRC, and BHD, the aggressive nature of type 2 papillary renal carcinoma requires prompt surgical intervention rather than surveillance. Surveillance with serial imaging is warranted to detect renal tumors early. Expert guidelines have recommended biannual imaging or even annual imaging based on the aggressiveness of the tumor.[54,61] The 3-cm threshold for surgical intervention does not apply in HLRCC, and thin slices (<3 mm) when imaging the kidneys is recommended to improve the detection of smaller tumors. Once a tumor is identified, either radical or partial nephrectomy is warranted, and wide surgical margins are recommended.[62]

HEREDITARY NONPOLYPOSIS COLON CANCER (LYNCH SYNDROME)

Although HNPCC is characterized by colorectal cancers, patients with this disease are also at increased risk for endometrial, renal, pancreatic, ovarian, and biliary cancers. HNPCC is caused by an autosomal-dominant germline mutation in one of four DNA mismatch repair genes (MSH1, MSH2, MSH6, and PMS2). MSH1 and MSH2 account for 90% of patients.[63] These mutations result in a high frequency of microsatellite instability. Urinary tract cancers are the third most common cancer associated with the syndrome and most involve the upper urinary tract, that is, the renal pelvis and ureter as urothelial malignancies.[64]

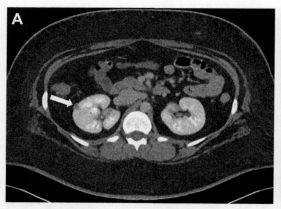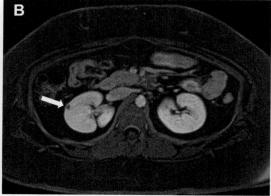

Fig. 5. Postcontrast-enhanced axial CT (*A*) and MR imaging (*B*) images at the level of the kidneys in the same patient with HLRCC. CT and MR imaging demonstrate a small lesion in the right kidney that is poorly vascularized, consistent with HLRCC-associated papillary RCC (*arrow*). Note that this lesion is only considered suspicious because the patient was part of a family with known HLRCC and early detection is of paramount importance in preventing metastasis.

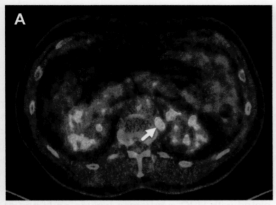
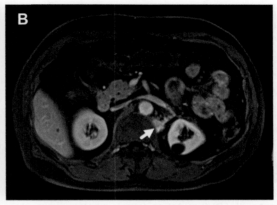

Fig. 6. Axial view on FDG PET/CT showing uptake in a left retrocrural node (*arrow*) represents metastasis (*A*). Enlarged retrocural lymph node (*arrow*) is seen in axial postcontrast-enhanced MR imaging correlating with the FDG PET/CT positive node (*B*).

Renal Imaging Findings

Cystoscopy is the reference standard for detecting urothelial cancer of the bladder. CT or MR urography are the preferred first-line examinations for upper tract evaluations and surveillance in patients with hematuria.[65] Upper tract malignancies appear as a filling defect in the renal pelvis or ureter, with or without obstruction. Tumors are contrast enhancing and the wall of the renal pelvis/ureter may be thickened. Urothelial malignancies arising in the renal pelvis and intrarenal collecting structures can be polypoid or if more aggressive can infiltrate the renal parenchyma and preserve the reniform shape of the kidney rather than forming discrete mass.[66]

Extrarenal Manifestations

Upper tract urothelial cancer is the third most common malignancy in HNPCC, whereas HNPCC most commonly results in colorectal cancer, and second most commonly endometrial cancer. Patients are also at an increased risk for other genitourinary and gastrointestinal cancers compared with the general population. Family history of multiple malignancies should raise concern for HNPCC (Lynch syndrome).

Screening and Management

It is most important that these patients are screened for colorectal cancers with colonoscopy annually beginning around age 25, but this can be tailored to the mutation type and family history. Female patients should be screened for endometrial cancer with routine pelvic examination and biopsy beginning at age 30. The US Multi-Society Task Force recommends screening for urothelial cancer with urinalysis and urine cytology annually beginning at age 30 to 35 because it is noninvasive and inexpensive.[67] Screening for neoplasia of the ureter, renal pelvis, and kidney may involve CT, MR imaging, or ultrasound; however, MR imaging has the desirable feature of tumor detection similar to CT (whereas ultrasound often misses small tumors) without the use of ionizing radiation. Because there is the highest risk among MSH2 mutation carriers for upper urinary tract malignancy, it has been suggested to focus screening on these patients.[68,69]

SUCCINATE DEHYDROGENASE SUBUNIT B

Succinate dehydrogenase is another enzyme involved in the Krebs cycle. Mutations in this enzyme cause 0.1% to 0.2% of all renal cancers. The mean age at presentation is 40 years, and there is also an association with gastrointestinal stromal tumors and pheochromocytoma/paraganglioma.[70] Tumors have been reported to be solid or solid with cystic components, and early metastases can occur, making SDHB tumors more aggressive among HRCs (**Fig. 7**). The masses are generally classified as carcinomas, but may be a unique histologic type.[70] FDG/PET is helpful in imaging these lesions for similar reasons to HLRCC tumors.[71] SDHB tumors should be managed with surgery similarly to HLRCC because of their aggressive nature; active surveillance is not an option in these patients.

CHROMOSOME 3 TRANSLOCATIONS

Translocations of the third chromosome (1:3, 2:3, 3:8, 3:6) are associated with tumors that express mutations in the VHL gene.[39] Families that have these chromosomal translocations have higher rates of clear cell RCC and hypervascular renal

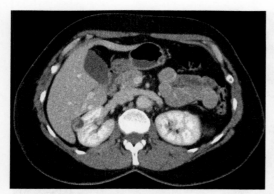

Fig. 7. Postcontrast-enhanced axial CT image of a patient with SDHB mutation reveals a heterogeneously enhancing mass in the right kidney with features of a malignant lesion.

lesions but lack the other syndromic findings associated with VHL. The radiologic findings associated with the renal tumors in these patients are like those of ccRCC identified in patients with VHL. The tumors are managed similarly with nephron-sparing surgery used when tumors under surveillance become large.

PHOSPHATASE AND TENSIN HOMOLOGUE LOSS (COWDEN DISEASE)

Mutation in the phosphatase and tensin homologue gene (PTEN), or Cowden syndrome, results in a hamartoma-tumor syndrome that increases the risk of RCC among other malignancies. The incidence of PTEN mutations is 1:200,000 and these patients have a 34% lifetime risk of RCC with a mean age at diagnosis of 40.[72] Papillary, clear cell, and chromophobe subtypes have all been reported. Additionally, patients are at an increased risk of breast, endometrial, and thyroid cancers.[73]

MiTF-ASSOCIATED CANCER SYNDROME

Microphthalmia-associated transcription factor (MiTF) is a melanoma oncogene. A germline missense variant of MiTF is associated with malignant melanoma and RCC. Patients with this mutation often develop both cancer types but the syndrome is rare.[74]

HEREDITARY HYPERPARATHYROIDISM–JAW TUMOR SYNDROME

Hereditary hyperparathyroidism–jaw tumor syndrome is a rare autosomal-dominant disorder that predisposes patients to primary hyperparathyroidism, caused by parathyroid adenomas

(solitary or multiple), and parathyroid carcinoma in 15% of patients. Renal manifestations of hereditary hyperparathyroidism–jaw tumor syndrome include polycystic kidneys, renal hamartomas, late-onset Wilms tumors, renal cortical adenomas, and RCCs.[39] Benign and malignant uterine tumors are identified in up to 75% of women.[75]

SUMMARY

HRCs represent a diverse group of cancer syndromes from genetic disorders that result in development of various subtypes of renal cell carcinoma. Common trends in renal cancers associated with HRC syndromes include early age at diagnosis, and multiple and bilateral lesions. Early diagnosis of HRC is frequently based on recognition of extrarenal findings associated with each syndrome. Renal lesions are often not the first symptom of an HRC syndrome, and diagnosis of the syndrome before the renal cancer develops or advances allows implementation of renal cancer screening and surveillance, which can prevent mortality.

The list of mutations causing HRC syndromes will probably expand in the future with increased knowledge of genomics. It is also likely that combinations of genes contributing to renal cancer will be discovered that are inherited but not in typical autosomal-dominant patterns. Radiologists play an important role in recognizing and suggesting diagnoses when imaging findings associated with HRC syndromes are encountered. Diagnosis of an inherited cancer syndrome is not only important for the patient but also for close family members who may be affected.

REFERENCES

1. Siegel RL, Miller KD, Jemal A. Cancer statistics, 2019. CA Cancer J Clin 2019;69(1):7–34.
2. Dabestani S, Thorstenson A, Lindblad P, et al. Renal cell carcinoma recurrences and metastases in primary non-metastatic patients: a population-based study. World J Urol 2016;34(8):1081–6.
3. Shuch B, Vourganti S, Ricketts CJ, et al. Defining early-onset kidney cancer: implications for germline and somatic mutation testing and clinical management. J Clin Oncol 2014;32(5):431–7.
4. Lonser RR, Glenn GM, Walther M, et al. von Hippel-Lindau disease. Lancet 2003;361(9374):2059–67.
5. Adeniran AJ, Shuch B, Humphrey PA. Hereditary renal cell carcinoma syndromes: clinical, pathologic, and genetic features. Am J Surg Pathol 2015;39(12):e1–18.
6. Tarade D, Ohh M. The HIF and other quandaries in VHL disease. Oncogene 2018;37(2):139–47.

7. Choyke PL, Glenn GM, Walther MM, et al. von Hippel-Lindau disease: genetic, clinical, and imaging features. Radiology 1995;194(3):629–42.

8. Dornbos D III, Kim HJ, Butman JA, et al. Review of the neurological implications of von Hippel–Lindau disease. JAMA Neurol 2018;75(5):620–7.

9. Binderup MLM, Jensen AM, Budtz-Jørgensen E, et al. Survival and causes of death in patients with von Hippel-Lindau disease. J Med Genet 2017; 54(1):11.

10. Leung SK, Ohh M. Playing tag with HIF: the VHL story. J Biomed Biotechnol 2002;2(3):131–5.

11. Kawashima A, Young SW, Takahashi N, et al. Inherited renal carcinomas. Abdom Radiol (NY) 2016;41(6):1066–78.

12. Wang H, Cheng L, Zhang X, et al. Renal cell carcinoma: diffusion-weighted MR imaging for subtype differentiation at 3.0 T. Radiology 2010;257(1): 135–43.

13. Paschall AK, Mirmomen SM, Symons R, et al. Differentiating papillary type I RCC from clear cell RCC and oncocytoma: application of whole-lesion volumetric ADC measurement. Abdom Radiol (NY) 2018;43(9):2424–30.

14. Libutti SK, Choyke PL, Alexander HR, et al. Clinical and genetic analysis of patients with pancreatic neuroendocrine tumors associated with von Hippel-Lindau disease. Surgery 2000;128(6): 1022–8.

15. Chung DC, Smith AP, Louis DN, et al. A novel pancreatic endocrine tumor suppressor gene locus on chromosome 3p with clinical prognostic implications. J Clin Invest 1997;100(2):404–10.

16. Sadowski SM, Weisbrod AB, Ellis R, et al. Prospective evaluation of the clinical utility of 18-fluorodeoxyglucose PET CT scanning in patients with von Hippel-Lindau-associated pancreatic lesions. J Am Coll Surg 2014;218(5):997–1003.

17. Shell J, Tirosh A, Millo C, et al. The utility of 68Gallium-DOTATATE PET/CT in the detection of von Hippel-Lindau disease associated tumors. Eur J Radiol 2019;112:130–5.

18. Dick EA, M C Hugh K, Kimber C, et al. Imaging of non-central nervous system primitive neuroectodermal tumours: diagnostic features and correlation with outcome. Clin Radiol 2001;56(3):206–15.

19. Cox R, Vang R, Epstein JI. Papillary cystadenoma of the epididymis and broad ligament: morphologic and immunohistochemical overlap with clear cell papillary renal cell carcinoma. Am J Surg Pathol 2014;38(5):713–8.

20. Lenders JWM, Eisenhofer G, Mannelli M, et al. Phaeochromocytoma. Lancet 2005;366(9486):665–75.

21. Ganeshan D, Menias CO, Pickhardt PJ, et al. Tumors in Von Hippel–Lindau syndrome: from head to toe—comprehensive state-of-the-art review. Radiographics 2018;38(3):849–66.

22. Rednam SP, Erez A, Druker H, et al. Von Hippel–Lindau and hereditary pheochromocytoma/paraganglioma syndromes: clinical features, genetics, and surveillance recommendations in childhood. Clin Cancer Res 2017;23(12):e68–75.

23. VHLA suggested active surveillance guidelines. 2017. 2019. Available at: https://www.vhl.org/wp-content/uploads/2017/07/Active-Surveillance-Guidelines.pdf. Accessed May 18, 2020.

24. Alliance TV. The VHL handbook. 5th edition. Boston (MA): VHL Alliance; 2015.

25. Bessell-Browne R, O'Malley ME. CT of pheochromocytoma and paraganglioma: risk of adverse events with IV administration of nonionic contrast material. AJR Am J Roentgenol 2007;188(4):970–4.

26. Allasia M, Soria F, Battaglia A, et al. Radiofrequency ablation for renal cancer in Von Hippel–Lindau syndrome patients: a prospective cohort analysis. Clin Genitourinary Cancer 2018;16(1): 28–34.

27. Linehan WM. Evaluation and screening for hereditary renal cell cancers. Can Urol Assoc J 2013; 7(9–10):324–5.

28. Menko FH, van Steensel MAM, Giraud S, et al. Birt-Hogg-Dubé syndrome: diagnosis and management. Lancet Oncol 2009;10(12):1199–206.

29. Pavlovich CP, Grubb RL 3rd, Hurley K, et al. Evaluation and management of renal tumors in the Birt-Hogg-Dube syndrome. J Urol 2005;173(5): 1482–6.

30. Adley BP, Smith ND, Nayar R, et al. Birt-Hogg-Dube syndrome: clinicopathologic findings and genetic alterations. Arch Pathol Lab Med 2006;130(12): 1865–70.

31. Khoo SK, Giraud S, Kahnoski K, et al. Clinical and genetic studies of Birt-Hogg-Dube syndrome. J Med Genet 2002;39(12):906–12.

32. Agarwal PP, Gross BH, Holloway BJ, et al. Thoracic CT findings in Birt-Hogg-Dubé syndrome. AJR Am J Roentgenol 2011;196(2):349–52.

33. Zbar B, Alvord WG, Glenn G, et al. Risk of renal and colonic neoplasms and spontaneous pneumothorax in the Birt-Hogg-Dube syndrome. Cancer Epidemiol Biomarkers Prev 2002;11(4):393–400.

34. Benusiglio PR, Gad S, Massard C, et al. Case report: expanding the tumour spectrum associated with the Birt-Hogg-Dube cancer susceptibility syndrome. F1000Res 2014;3:159.

35. Nahorski MS, Lim DH, Martin L, et al. Investigation of the Birt-Hogg-Dube tumour suppressor gene (FLCN) in familial and sporadic colorectal cancer. J Med Genet 2010;47(6):385–90.

36. Stamatakis L, Metwalli AR, Middelton LA, et al. Diagnosis and management of BHD-associated kidney cancer. Fam Cancer 2013;12(3):397–402.

37. Schmidt LS, Linehan WM. Genetic predisposition to kidney cancer. Semin Oncol 2016;43(5):566–74.

38. Yang P, Cornejo KM, Sadow PM, et al. Renal cell carcinoma in tuberous sclerosis complex. Am J Surg Pathol 2014;38(7):895–909.

39. Verine J, Pluvinage A, Bousquet G, et al. Hereditary renal cancer syndromes: an update of a systematic review. Eur Urol 2010;58(5):701–10.

40. Axwijk PH, Kluijt I, de Jong D, et al. Hereditary causes of kidney tumours. Eur J Clin Invest 2010; 40(5):433–9.

41. Washecka R, Hanna M. Malignant renal tumors in tuberous sclerosis. Urology 1991;37(4):340–3.

42. Froemming AT, Boland J, Cheville J, et al. Renal epithelioid angiomyolipoma: imaging characteristics in nine cases with radiologic-pathologic correlation and review of the literature. AJR Am J Roentgenol 2013;200(2):W178–86.

43. Choyke PL, Glenn GM, Walther MM, et al. Hereditary renal cancers. Radiology 2003;226(1):33–46.

44. Gupta P, Mukund A, S.H.C., et al. Tuberous sclerosis complex: imaging findings. Indian J Pediatr 2012; 79(1):127–9.

45. Peron A, Vignoli A, La Briola F, et al. Do patients with tuberous sclerosis complex have an increased risk for malignancies? Am J Med Genet A 2016;170(6): 1538–44.

46. Hindman N, Ngo L, Genega EM, et al. Angiomyolipoma with minimal fat: can it be differentiated from clear cell renal cell carcinoma by using standard MR techniques? Radiology 2012;265(2): 468–77.

47. Sasiwimonphan K, Takahashi N, Leibovich BC, et al. Small (<4 cm) renal mass: differentiation of angiomyolipoma without visible fat from renal cell carcinoma utilizing MR imaging. Radiology 2012;263(1): 160–8.

48. Srigley JR, Delahunt B, Eble JN, et al. The International Society of Urological Pathology (ISUP) Vancouver classification of renal neoplasia. Am J Surg Pathol 2013;37(10):1469–89.

49. Gupta N, Henske EP. Pulmonary manifestations in tuberous sclerosis complex. Am J Med Genet C Semin Med Genet 2018;178(3):326–37.

50. Gupta S, Kang HC, Ganeshan DM, et al. Diagnostic approach to hereditary renal cell carcinoma. AJR Am J Roentgenol 2015;204(5):1031–41.

51. Ebrahimi-Fakhari D, Mann LL, Poryo M, et al. Incidence of tuberous sclerosis and age at first diagnosis: new data and emerging trends from a national, prospective surveillance study. Orphanet J Rare Dis 2018;13(1):117.

52. Cudzilo CJ, Szczesniak RD, Brody AS, et al. Lymphangioleiomyomatosis screening in women with tuberous sclerosis. Chest 2013;144(2):578–85.

53. McCormack FX, Gupta N, Finlay GR, et al. Official American Thoracic Society/Japanese Respiratory Society clinical practice guidelines. Lymphangioleiomyomatosis 2016;194(6):748–61.

54. Ho TH, Jonasch E. Genetic kidney cancer syndromes. J Natl Compr Canc Netw 2014;12(9): 1347–55.

55. Schmidt LS, Nickerson ML, Angeloni D, et al. Early onset hereditary papillary renal carcinoma: germline missense mutations in the tyrosine kinase domain of the met proto-oncogene. J Urol 2004;172(4 Part 1): 1256–61.

56. Cornelis F, Tricaud E, Lasserre AS, et al. Routinely performed multiparametric magnetic resonance imaging helps to differentiate common subtypes of renal tumours. Eur Radiol 2014;24(5):1068–80.

57. Corral de la Calle MÁ, Encinas de la Iglesia J, Martín López MR, et al. Carcinoma papilar de células renales: el papel del radiólogo en su manejo. Radiología 2017;59(2):100–14.

58. Grubb RL 3rd, Franks ME, Toro J, et al. Hereditary leiomyomatosis and renal cell cancer: a syndrome associated with an aggressive form of inherited renal cancer. J Urol 2007;177(6):2074–80 [discussion: 2079—80].

59. Northrup BE, Jokerst CE, Grubb RL, et al. Hereditary renal tumor syndromes: imaging findings and management strategies. AJR Am J Roentgenol 2012; 199(6):1294–304.

60. Badeloe S, Frank J. Clinical and molecular genetic aspects of hereditary multiple cutaneous leiomyomatosis. Eur J Dermatol 2009;19(6):545–51.

61. Smit D, Mensenkamp A, Badeloe S, et al. Hereditary leiomyomatosis and renal cell cancer in families referred for fumarate hydratase germline mutation analysis. Clin Genet 2011;79(1):49–59.

62. Linehan WM. Genetic basis of kidney cancer: role of genomics for the development of disease-based therapeutics. Genome Res 2012;22(11):2089–100.

63. Duraturo F, Liccardo R, De Rosa M, et al. Genetics, diagnosis and treatment of Lynch syndrome: old lessons and current challenges. Oncol Lett 2019;17(3): 3048–54.

64. Bernstein IT, Myrhøj T. Surveillance for urinary tract cancer in Lynch syndrome. Fam Cancer 2013; 12(2):279–84.

65. Wolfman DJ, Marko J, Nikolaidis P, et al. ACR Appropriateness Guidelines. Hematuria J Am Coll Radiol 2020;17(5S):S138–47.

66. Vikram R, Sandler CM, Ng CS. Imaging and staging of transitional cell carcinoma: part 2, upper urinary tract. AJR Am J Roentgenol 2009;192(6): 1488–93.

67. Giardiello FM, Allen JI, Axilbund JE, et al. Guidelines on genetic evaluation and management of Lynch syndrome: a consensus statement by the US Multi-Society Task Force on Colorectal Cancer. Gastroenterology 2014;147(2):502–26.

68. Vasen HFA, Stormorken A, Menko FH, et al. MSH2 mutation carriers are at higher risk of cancer than MLH1 mutation carriers: a study of hereditary

nonpolyposis colorectal cancer families. J Clin Oncol 2001;19(20):4074–80.

69. Dominguez-Valentin M, Sampson JR, Seppälä TT, et al. Cancer risks by gene, age, and gender in 6350 carriers of pathogenic mismatch repair variants: findings from the Prospective Lynch Syndrome Database. Genet Med 2020;22(1):15–25.

70. Gill AJ, Hes O, Papathomas T, et al. Succinate dehydrogenase (SDH)-deficient renal carcinoma: a morphologically distinct entity: a clinicopathologic series of 36 tumors from 27 patients. Am J Surg Pathol 2014;38(12):1588–602.

71. Ricketts CJ, Shuch B, Vocke CD, et al. Succinate dehydrogenase kidney cancer: an aggressive example of the Warburg effect in cancer. J Urol 2012;188(6):2063–71.

72. Nelen MR, Padberg GW, Peeters EA, et al. Localization of the gene for Cowden disease to chromosome 10q22-23. Nat Genet 1996;13(1):114–6.

73. Mester JL, Zhou M, Prescott N, et al. Papillary renal cell carcinoma is associated with PTEN hamartoma tumor syndrome. Urology 2012;79(5):1187.e1-7.

74. Bertolotto C, Lesueur F, Giuliano S, et al. A SUMOylation-defective MITF germline mutation predisposes to melanoma and renal carcinoma. Nature 2011;480(7375):94–8.

75. Newey PJ, Bowl MR, Thakker RV. Parafibromin: functional insights. J Intern Med 2009;266(1):84–98.

Review of Multimodality Imaging of Renal Trauma

Ling-Chen Chien, MD[a], Keith D. Herr, MD[b],*, Krystal Archer-Arroyo, MD[b], Mona Vakil, MD[b], Tarek N. Hanna, MD[b]

KEYWORDS

• Renal • Kidney • Trauma • Injury • Imaging • Computed tomography

KEY POINTS

- The kidneys are the most commonly injured organ in the genitourinary system, with blunt injury accounting for the vast majority of these injuries.
- Multiphasic contrast-enhanced computed tomography (CT) is the imaging modality of choice for the detection of renal trauma. Both arterial and portal venous phase acquisitions are recommended to optimize sensitivity for the range of injury. The use of other imaging modalities, including ultrasound, dual-energy CT, MR imaging and conventional angiography, may be indicated in special situations but are much less common in practice.
- Excretory phase CT is important for the detection of collecting system injury and is selectively used based on findings from the arterial- and portal venous phase images.
- The American Association for the Surgery of Trauma (AAST) Organ Injury Scale (OIS), the most commonly used grading system for renal trauma, was updated in 2018 and incorporates imaging findings from contrast-enhanced CT, including parenchymal, collecting system, and vascular injury.
- The primary goal in the management of acute renal trauma is to optimize patient survival and preserve renal function. Imaging has played a pivotal role in a paradigm shift away from invasive surgical diagnosis and treatment toward nonoperative management.

INTRODUCTION

The kidneys are the most commonly injured organ in the genitourinary system, although renal injuries occur in only 1.2% to 3.25% of all trauma patients.[1,2] Renal trauma occurs at a mean patient age of 20 to 30 years and affects men at 3 times the rate of women.[1,2] The vast majority (71%–95%) of renal injuries occur secondary to a blunt mechanism, such as motor vehicle crashes and falls, and a minority are due to penetrating trauma, most commonly gunshot and stab wounds.[1,2] Due to their retroperitoneal location, bounded anteriorly by peritoneal organs and posteriorly by paraspinal musculature, thoracolumbar vertebrae, and ribs, the kidneys are relatively resistant to injury. Injury in blunt trauma likely results from shear forces from differential deceleration of vital structures, particularly around the relatively fixed renal hilum, or from crush injury against the spine and ribs.[3] Most renal injuries are minor and clinically insignificant. More significant renal trauma usually occurs concomitantly with injuries to other abdominal organs.[3]

In recent decades, there has been a steady and continuing paradigm shift from surgical intervention to nonoperative management for renal

[a] Department of Radiology and Imaging Sciences, Emory University, Emory University School of Medicine, 550 Peachtree Street, Atlanta, GA 30308, USA; [b] Division of Emergency and Trauma Imaging, Department of Radiology and Imaging Sciences, Emory University School of Medicine, Emory University, 550 Peachtree Street, Atlanta, GA 30308, USA
* Corresponding author.
E-mail address: kherr@emory.edu
Twitter: @KeithHerrmd (K.D.H.); @krystal_archer (K.A.-A.); @MonaVakil (M.V.); @ER_Rad_Hanna (T.N.H.)

Radiol Clin N Am 58 (2020) 965–979
https://doi.org/10.1016/j.rcl.2020.05.005
0033-8389/20/© 2020 Elsevier Inc. All rights reserved.

trauma. This trend has been facilitated by the widespread availability of computed tomography (CT) for the evaluation of trauma patients,[4] improvements in conservative management approaches, and evidence that conservative management is safe and effective. The development of a validated renal injury scoring system based on surgical findings, the American Association for the Surgery of Trauma Organ Injury Scale (AAST OIS), has helped to standardize research and clinical treatment of renal injuries. As contrast-enhanced CT (CECT) findings have demonstrated a relatively strong correlation with intraoperative findings,[5,6] CECT has been largely relied on as a nonoperative proxy for estimating OIS grade and is now the modality of choice for the initial evaluation of clinically stable patients with suspected renal trauma.

MULTIPHASIC CONTRAST-ENHANCED COMPUTED TOMOGRAPHY IN RENAL TRAUMA

The main goals of imaging in the setting of suspected renal trauma are to accurately stage and differentiate injuries requiring early operative versus conservative management, distinguish traumatic from preexisting renal pathology, assess the integrity and function of the contralateral kidney, and identify other associated abdominal organ injuries.[1] Approximately 95% of patients with renal injury present with at least microscopic hematuria ($\geq$5 red blood cells per high-powered field). It is important to note, however, that patients with disruption of the renal vascular pedicle or the ureteropelvic region may not present with hematuria. Accordingly, the degree of hematuria does not always correlate with the severity of renal injury.[7–9] Generally accepted indications for imaging to evaluate for blunt renal injury include macroscopic hematuria, microscopic hematuria with either shock or coexisting abdominal organ injuries, and severe mechanism of injury with documented factors associated with renal trauma, such as posterior flank hematoma and rib or spinal fractures detected on radiography. In penetrating injury with a trajectory likely to involve the kidneys, CECT is indicated in hemodynamically stable patients regardless of the presence of hematuria.[6]

CECT is readily available in essentially all institutions providing emergency services and can quickly, safely, and accurately depict renal and other injuries in the abdomen and pelvis. Radiology departments in trauma centers are increasingly adopting the use of arterial and portal venous phases in the evaluation of abdominal trauma, including renal trauma.

Dual-phase imaging can be achieved by either 2 separate CT acquisitions of the initial intravenous contrast bolus (conventional technique) or by a split-bolus technique that requires 2 separate intravenous contrast administrations and a single CT acquisition. which then contains simultaneous arterial and portal venous phase imaging information. Using a fixed-time delay protocol with the conventional technique, the arterial phase is acquired 15 to 20 seconds after the administration of intravenous contrast. This phase provides excellent delineation of arterial injury and, along with the portal venous phase acquisition, can help to differentiate active bleeding from contained vascular injury (pseudoaneurysm and arteriovenous fistulas [AVFs]). Renal parenchymal injury, however, is poorly evaluated on the arterial phase as it typically corresponds to a corticomedullary enhancement pattern of renal parenchyma. The portal venous phase acquisition (with a 70- to 80-second delay from the time of the contrast bolus administration), which corresponds to the nephrogenic or late corticomedullary enhancement pattern in most instances, is needed to optimize the detection of the range of renal parenchymal injuries, which are hypoattenuating on a background of the uniformly enhancing renal soft tissue.

The detection of renal collecting system disruption requires the addition of an excretory phase, which occurs between 5 and 10 minutes following the administration of intravenous contrast. The decision to proceed with an excretory phase is made on a case-by-case basis after a provisional review of the arterial and portal venous data set, and optimally while the patient is still in the scanner. Deep lacerations that appear to extend to the renal calyces or renal pelvis, or the presence of a significant volume of perinephric or periureteral simple or nonsimple fluid, are imaging findings that justify rescanning the patient in the excretory phase to assess for urinary extravasation.[10]

GRADING TRAUMATIC RENAL INJURIES

The most widely used classification system for renal trauma is the AAST OIS, first devised in 1989.[11] This scale assigns a numerical score from 1 to 5, from least to most severe injury. Research has demonstrated that AAST renal grade correlates well with patient mortality and the need for nephrectomy.[12,13] Because the original version was published before the widespread use of CECT in the evaluation of trauma, scoring was based solely on operative findings. Since the first iteration, however, CECT has largely supplanted surgical exploration as the diagnostic standard for renal and other abdominal organ trauma. Furthermore, CECT is able to detect clinically relevant injuries that were not included in the original OIS. These include pseudoaneurysms, AVFs, active bleeding, and collecting system disruption, for which advances in minimally invasive management have been developed, particularly image-guided endovascular embolization. Recognizing the impact of these injuries on patient outcomes and the reliability of CECT for their detection, the AAST OIS Patient Assessment Committee convened in 2015 to revise the OIS, publishing the first revised version in 2018.[14] The revised OIS encourages the use of CECT for grading renal trauma and sets out specific CECT-based criteria for this purpose. As in the original version, the new OIS advises to upgrade coexisting grade 1 or 2 injuries by 1 point (up to grade 3), when assigning the final organ injury grade. The 2018 AAST OIS for the kidney is summarized in **Table 1** and **Fig. 1**.

Contrast-Enhanced Computed Tomography

The full range of renal parenchymal, vascular, and urinary collecting system injury have characteristic features on CECT, and are described as follows:

- *Contusion*: Renal contusions are the most minor form of parenchymal injury and represent focal areas of bruising. On CECT in the portal venous (or nephrogenic) phase, contusions appear as focal, indistinctly marginated, subtly hypodense regions, reflecting areas of hemorrhage intermixed with uninjured tissue (**Fig. 2**). Clotted blood in a contusion may appear isodense to normally enhancing parenchyma and, therefore, may be missed. A contusion is often inapparent on the arterial phase due to the suboptimal enhancement of background renal parenchyma, again underscoring the importance of a portal venous phase for the detection of tissue injury. On the excretory phase, a focal "delayed nephrogram" of retained contrast may be demonstrated, indicating impaired localized parenchymal function. *A contusion reflects an AAST grade 1 injury.*
- *Laceration*: A laceration appears as an irregular or branching linear hypoattenuation on the portal venous phase of CECT (**Fig. 3**). Lacerations are classified by length and whether they extend to the renal collecting system. Although collecting system involvement can often be inferred when the deepest portion of a laceration extends to a calyx or the renal pelvis (and/or when there is an associated adjacent fluid collection suspicious for

extravasated urine), an excretory phase is required for confirmation. *Lacerations can be a feature of AAST grades 2 to 5.*
- *Subcapsular hematoma*: A subcapsular hematoma is contained by the renal capsule peripherally and exerts mass effect on the underlying renal parenchyma. This results in a characteristic eccentric, crescentic, or biconvex appearance of the hematoma on CT (**Fig. 4**). The hemorrhage within a subcapsular hematoma may be unclotted (30–50 Hounsfield units [HU]) or clotted (50–70 HU). *A subcapsular hematoma represents an AAST grade 2 injury.*
- *Perirenal hematoma*: A perirenal, or perinephric, hematoma represents accumulated blood products around the kidney, and is further classified as being contained by Gerota (perirenal or perinephric) fascia or extending beyond Gerota fascia within the retroperitoneum or into the peritoneal cavity. A perirenal hematoma is characterized by a poorly marginated, hyperattenuating collection superficial to renal capsule. This finding is rarely present in isolation and more commonly occurs in association with parenchymal lacerations and/or vascular injury (**Fig. 5**). *A perirenal hematoma can be a feature of grades 2 to 5.*
- *Renal collecting system injury*: Recognizing the presence of renal collecting system injury is important because it reflects high-grade injury that may require intervention with urinary diversion. Lacerations that appear to extend to the collecting system on nephrographic phase of imaging raise the suspicion of collecting system injury and should be further evaluated with excretory phase imaging. The presence of a significant amount of perirenal hemorrhage or simple fluid is an additional imaging feature that is concerning for collecting system injury. On excretory phase, collecting system injury is confirmed by the presence of excreted contrast beyond the collecting system (**Fig. 6**). In complete ureteropelvic disruption, excreted contrast will accumulate in the region of wall injury but will not be present in the ureter distal to the injury. In partial pelvic or ureteropelvic tears, contrast may opacify the entire ureter because a portion remains intact. *Collecting system injury may be a feature of AAST grade 4 or 5 injuries.*
- *Renal infarction*: Renal infarction is characterized as either *segmental* or *complete*. A segmental infarct reflects injury to a segmental renal artery and results in a

Table 1
2018 revision of American Association for the Surgery of Trauma renal Organ Injury Scale, CT characteristics[1]

Grade	Type	CECT Imaging Features
1	Contusion Hematoma	Isolated parenchymal contusion Subcapsular hematoma
2	Laceration Hematoma	Laceration <1 cm *without* extension to collecting system Perinephric hematoma *contained by Gerota fascia*
3	Laceration Vascular	Laceration >1 cm *without* extension to collecting system Any grade 1–3 with PSA/AVF or active bleeding *contained by Gerota fascia*
4	Laceration Vascular	Laceration *with* extension to collecting system Renal pelvis laceration or complete ureteropelvic laceration Segmental renal artery or vein intimal injury/thrombosis Active bleeding *beyond* Gerota fascia Segmental or complete renal infarction from vessel thrombosis *without* active bleeding
5	Laceration Vascular	Shattered kidney Main renal artery or vein laceration or avulsion from renal hilum Complete organ devascularization *with* active bleeding

From Kozar RA, Crandall M, Shanmuganathan K, et al. Organ injury scaling 2018 update: Spleen, liver, and kidney. *J Trauma Acute Care Surg.* 2018;85(6):1119-1122; with permission.

characteristic wedge-shaped region of parenchymal hypoattenuation with the apex directed toward the hilum (**Fig. 7**). A segmental infarct will remain hypoattenuating on all phases of imaging, which aids in distinguishing it from a contusion. Complete renal infarction occurs as a result of severe vascular injury (main renal artery or vein avulsion or thrombosis) and is characterized by the absence of enhancement of the affected kidney on all phases (see **Fig. 7**). Complete infarction, particularly when associated with active bleeding from the main renal vessels, may necessitate emergent nephrectomy. *A segmental renal infarct is currently classified as AAST grade 4*; however, there is some controversy over assigning it such a high grade because these types of injury generally heal with conservative management and without clinically significant sequela.[15] *Complete renal infarction without active bleeding reflects an AAST grade 4 injury, whereas with active bleeding, it is classified as grade 5.*

• *Vascular injury*: As in other abdominal organs, renal vascular injury is further classified as either *contained* or *uncontained vascular injury* or *arterial or venous thrombosis*. *Contained vascular injury* consists of *pseudoaneurysm* and *AVFs*. It should be noted that the 2018 revision of the AAST renal OIS equates "vascular injury" to pseudoaneurysms and

AVFs exclusively and treats other forms of vascular damage as separate entities.[14] For the purposes of this review and to reflect the meaning typically reported in the radiology literature, the term "vascular injury" includes the range of vessel injury that is detectable on CECT.[16] Pseudoaneurysms and AVFs are usually indistinguishable on CECT except in the unusual circumstance in which an affected adjacent artery and vein enhance simultaneously on the arterial phase, reflecting a fistulous communication between the 2 in AVF. More typically, pseudoaneurysm and AVFs manifest as a rounded focus of extravascular contrast with constant morphology on all phases of contrast and attenuation similar to aortic blood pool, diminishing in density over subsequent phases (**Fig. 8**). Uncontained vascular injury, also referred to as *active extravasation* or *active bleeding*, appears as an irregular focus of extravascular contrast with attenuation similar to that of the aortic blood pool on the arterial phase that subsequently increases in size and changes in morphology on portal venous and later phases (**Fig. 9**). Its attenuation will typically remain the same or become only slightly less dense as it mixes with less concentrated extravasated intravascular contrast. Venous bleeding will not be apparent on the arterial phase but will manifest on the portal venous

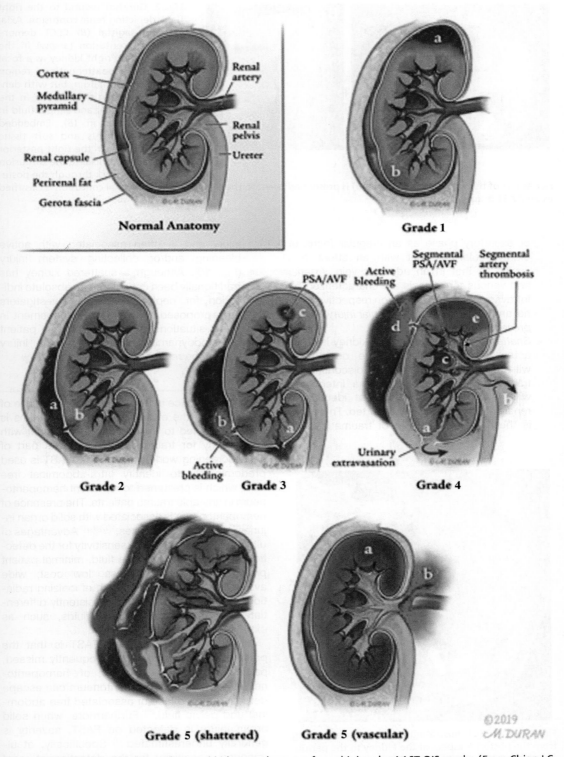

Fig. 1. Graphical representation of normal kidney and range of renal injury by AAST OIS grade. (*From* Chien LC, Vakil M, Nguyen J, et al. The American Association for the Surgery of Trauma Organ Injury Scale 2018 update for computed tomography-based grading of renal trauma: a primer for the emergency radiologist. *Emerg Radiol.* 2019; with permission.)

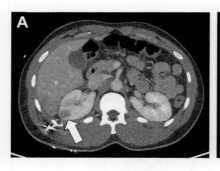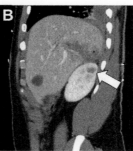

Fig. 2. Gunshot wound to the right flank depicting renal contusion. Axial (*A*) and sagittal (*B*) CECT demonstrating a contusion (*arrow*) in the posterolateral right kidney as a focal relatively hypoattenuating region with indistinct margin, but with density greater than that of bile in the gallbladder in (*A*) and simple fluid in a hepatic cyst in (*B*). Embedded metallic fragments and soft tissue gas are present in the right posterior chest wall superficial to the contusion in (*A*). Bullet track through the posterior aspect of the right hepatic lobe in (*B*) is present adjacent to the renal contusion. A renal contusion is classified as an AAST grade 1 injury.

or excretory phase as an irregular focus of extravascular contrast with an attenuation similar to that in an adjacent vein. Arterial and venous thrombosis are characterized by intravascular filling defects on respective arterial and venous phases. *Vascular injury can be present in grades 3 to* 5.

• *Shattered kidney*: A shattered kidney is characterized by extensive tissue destruction with the formation of multiple discontinuous fragments of renal parenchyma intermixed with blood products such that identifiable renal anatomy is severely distorted. This entity is the most severe form of traumatic renal

injury and is often associated with active bleeding and/or collecting system injury (**Fig. 10**). Although a shattered kidney has traditionally been considered an absolute indication for nephrectomy, the investigators have proposed conservative management in select situations, notably[17] when the patient is hemodynamically stable and the injury spares the renal pedicle vasculature.[18]

Ultrasound

In current practice in the United States, the use of ultrasound in the evaluation of trauma victims is mostly confined to the focused assessment with sonography for trauma (FAST) scan as part of initial screening workup and triage. FAST is used predominately to identify intra-abdominal free fluid, which is presumed to represent hemoperitoneum in unstable trauma patients. The presence of hemoperitoneum is associated with solid organ injuries in up to 90% of cases.[10,19,20] Advantages of ultrasound include its high sensitivity for the detection of intra-abdominal free fluid, minimal patient preparation, noninvasiveness, low cost, wide availability, portability, and lack of ionizing radiation; however, FAST cannot consistently differentiate blood from other body fluids, such as extravasated urine.[10,21]

A significant drawback to FAST is that the presence of organ injuries is frequently missed, particularly in the absence of hemoperitoneum.[22–27] Injury to retroperitoneum can escape detection due to lack of associated free abdominal and pelvic fluid.[28] Furthermore, when solid organ injury is detected on FAST, severity is generally underestimated.[10] Specifically, at ultrasound, sensitivity for the detection of renal injury ranges from 22% to 59%,[10,17,22,26,27,29] while specificity is excellent (98%–99%).[22,29–31] Unlike excretory phase CECT imaging with its

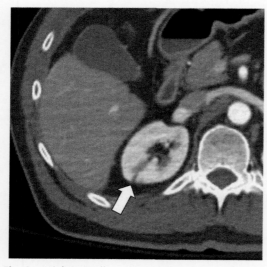

Fig. 3. Axial CECT illustrating a laceration extending from the posterior aspect of the kidney to the periphery of a renal pyramid (*arrow*). Because this laceration measures less than 1 cm in length and clearly does not extend to a calyx or pelvis, this injury would be classified as AAST grade 2.

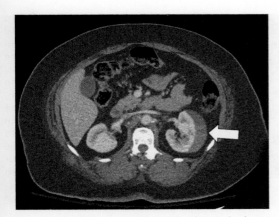

Fig. 4. Axial CECT demonstrating a subcapsular hematoma along the lateral aspect of the left kidney (*arrow*). The renal contour is maintained and there is no perinephric hemorrhage, consistent with a subcapsular hematoma with an intact capsule. This injury is consistent with an AAST grade 1 injury.

excellent depiction of urinary collecting system injury, ultrasound cannot reliably detect such injury.[32] Sonographic renal evaluation in trauma may be technically limited by overlying rib

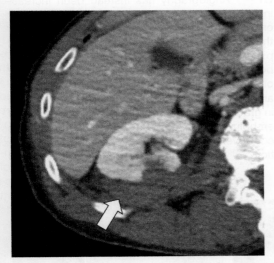

Fig. 5. Axial CECT depicting a perirenal hematoma (*arrow*). The edges of a perirenal hematoma are ill-defined and do not exhibit significant mass effect on the kidney, in contrast to a subcapsular hematoma. Perirenal hematomas are further classified as either contained by Gerota fascia (present case) or extending beyond Gerota fascia. Most perirenal hematomas occur along with other renal injuries, as in this instance, in which a laceration along the posteromedial aspect of the kidney is present. Ordinarily, an isolated perirenal hematoma would be classified as AAST grade 2; however, because in this case it is associated with a low-grade laceration (grade 2), the injury complex would advance 1 grade from grade 2 to 3.

fractures and subcutaneous emphysema, ileus, and patient immobility. Because ultrasound requires patient cooperation (for example, the need to follow breathing instructions), patient discomfort and diminished sensorium often emerge as limiting factors in trauma. Although the right kidney is generally technically easier to evaluate on ultrasound, the left kidney is frequently obscured by bowel gas and ribs. Finally, ultrasound performance is operator-dependent, provides a smaller diagnostic field of view compared with CT, and can be limited in obese patients.[26]

On ultrasound, renal parenchymal injuries present as hyper- or hypoechoic areas with distortion of normal renal echotexture.[17,26] Renal contusions appear as subtle hypoechoic areas. Subcapsular hematomas present as heterogeneous, round or elliptical fluid collections subjacent to the intact renal capsule and may flatten the normally rounded renal contour, as on CT or other cross-sectional imaging (**Fig. 11**). Higher grade injuries are often diagnosed by associated perirenal hematomas, which may vary in echogenicity, and/or extravasated urine, which may appear as simple or complex fluid in the perirenal space.[33] Blood and urine cannot be reliably distinguished on ultrasound. Renal lacerations appear as a hypoechoic linear region, usually perpendicular to the organ surface, with loss of normal Power Doppler flow in the affected region.[33,34]

Recent literature has shown improved solid organ injury detection with the use of contrast-enhanced ultrasound (CEUS) compared with conventional ultrasonography,[35] with an ability to characterize lesion size, extent, margins, and relationship with the renal capsule and vascular pedicle similar to that of CECT.[17] For the detection of solid organ injuries including liver, spleen, and kidney, compared with CT as the gold standard, CEUS has a sensitivity of 82% to 100% and specificity of 89% to 99%[35] CEUS can be particularly helpful in cases in which conventional ultrasound detects intra-abdominal free fluid but fails to identify the source of bleeding.[27] These improvements in performance compared with conventional ultrasound notwithstanding, CEUS is not commonly used in the setting of trauma in the United States.

MR Imaging

MR imaging is not routinely used in the emergent trauma setting due to its relatively long imaging time when compared with CT, variable availability in emergency departments, and certain limiting patient factors, such as the need for intensive

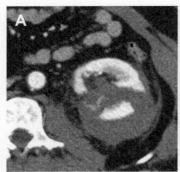
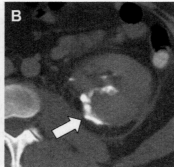

Fig. 6. Urinary extravasation from renal collecting system injury. Axial CECT in the portal venous/nephrographic phase (A) and excretory phase (B). In (A), extensive lacerations traverse the inferior pole of the left kidney. A perinephric hematoma is present along the posterior margin of the kidney. In (B), excreted contrast leaks out of the collecting system and accumulates along the inferomedial aspect of the kidney (arrow). Urinary collecting system involvement is a feature of only AAST grade 4 or 5 injury.

monitoring and contraindications from certain implanted medical devices or embedded metallic foreign bodies. In certain circumstances, such as in patients with contraindication to iodinated contrast or in pregnant women, MR imaging may demonstrate some value. In general, the findings in renal trauma on MR imaging are similar to those of CT.[36] Renal lacerations appear as irregular, linear hypointense regions on a background of enhancing parenchyma, and infarcts will appear as hypoenhancing regions with a characteristic wedge shape when subsegmental. The signal characteristics of intraparenchymal, subcapsular, and perinephric hematomas depend predominately on the oxidative state of hemoglobin at the time of imaging, which varies in a time-dependent fashion (Fig. 12). The appearance of vascular and collecting system injury on contrast-enhanced MR imaging parallels that of multiphasic CECT. A urinoma will appear as a T1 hypointense and T2 hyperintense perinephric fluid collection.[36]

Angiography

Angiography is now seldom used for the initial diagnosis and evaluation of trauma patients because CECT performs similarly with respect to the detection of vascular injury.[9,10] Selective renal arteriography or venography can occasionally provide more detailed anatomy of vascular injury in cases in which suspected vascular injuries are not sufficiently characterized on CT.[9,21] Angiography has instead been increasingly used in conjunction with transcatheter embolization, stenting, and/or thrombolysis for the treatment of active bleeding, posttraumatic pseudoaneurysms, AVFs, renal arterial thrombosis, and/or segmental arterial injuries detected on CECT.[1,10,28,37,38] In particular, transcatheter arterial embolization has become more common in grades 4 and 5 renal injury, although the use of embolization in grade 5 renal injury remains controversial and is an area of ongoing investigation.[39,40] In clinical practice, CECT is often used

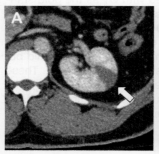
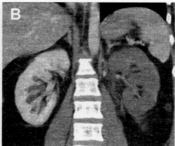
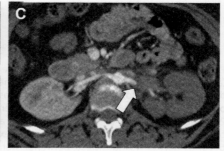

Fig. 7. Renal infarcts. (A) Axial CECT demonstrates the typical appearance of a segmental infarct as a wedge-shaped hypoattenuating area spanning the full thickness of the kidney, with apex at the hilum (arrow). A segmental renal infarct reflects an AAST grade 4 injury. Coronal (B) and axial (C) CECT of complete left renal infarction in a different patient who sustained a motor vehicle collision. In (C), abrupt left main renal artery occlusion is noted (arrow). A faintly enhancing artery in the renal hilum represents a small intact accessory renal artery. Complete renal infarction due to vessel thrombosis without active bleeding is classified as an AAST grade 4 injury. The patient was successfully treated with renal artery stenting.

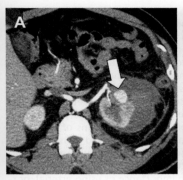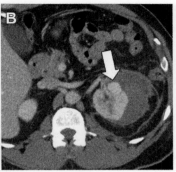

Fig. 8. Axial CECT in the arterial (*A*) and portal venous/nephrogenic phase (*B*) demonstrating an arterial pseudoaneurysm. In (*A*), a lobulated focus of contrast is present within the anterior aspect of the interpolar region of the left kidney (*arrow*) with attenuation similar to that of the aorta. A perinephric hematoma is also present. In (*B*), the focus of contrast in the later phase retains its rounded morphology (*arrow*) but has a diminished attenuation when compared with the arterial phase, but similar to that of the aortic blood pool. A pseudoaneurysm contained to Gerota fascia is consistent with an AAST 4 injury.

to determine the grade of renal injury and location/severity of arterial injury before endovascular intervention.[41] An analysis of 9145 trauma patients admitted for abdominopelvic injuries from 1996 to 2010 showed significantly decreased diagnostic angiography use and increased embolization rates in patients who underwent angiography, reflecting the current role of angiography as predominately used in the setting of therapeutic interventions.[42]

The appearance of renal trauma on angiography depends on the grade and location of injury. In the case of active bleeding, an amorphous blush of contrast is seen, which dissipates slowly after injection (**Fig. 13**). In the case of a traumatic pseudoaneurysm, a focal, discrete, lobular, or rounded pool of contrast will be seen, which follows arterial opacification. Finally, in a case of traumatic arterial occlusion (whether segmental or main artery), the arterial contrast column will abruptly cut off without perfusion of the supplied parenchyma. Contusions and small lacerations appear on angiography as focal, minimal perfusion defects (**Fig. 14**), whereas more extensive parenchymal injuries present as frank disruption of the normal renal nephrogram. Subcapsular hematomas appear as renal parenchymal compression,

whereas perinephric collections are less confined and produce renal displacement rather than renal deformity. Large perinephric fluid collection can elevate the ipsilateral hemidiaphragm, and because perinephric fluid tends to collect in the dorsolateral aspect of the kidney, the kidney is displaced anteriorly and appears magnified. Devitalized segments of renal parenchyma from thrombosis or vasospasm show absent perfusion in nephrographic phase. An absent nephrogram or just a "rim" nephrogram indicates main renal artery injury and/or occlusion.[21]

Intravenous Urogram

Intravenous urography (IVU), also known as "one-shot intravenous pyelography," once a mainstay in the evaluation of renal collecting system injury, is now primarily used intraoperatively in patients who are too unstable to undergo CT. Rapid bolus of intravenous contrast is given with plain abdominal radiography obtained 10 minutes after injection. IVU can exclude life-threatening renal injury, assess gross function of the uninjured contralateral kidney, and detect delayed excretion or urinary extravasation.[9,28,43] If a deformed renal contour, urinary contrast extravasation, or

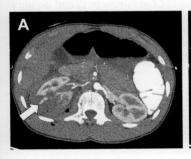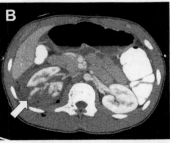

Fig. 9. Active bleeding on CECT from gunshot wound. Irregular focus of contrast (*arrow*) within the right kidney on the arterial phase (*A*), which expands on the portal venous phase (*arrow*) in (*B*). Note additional findings of lacerations, perinephric hematoma, and gas. Due to uncontrollable blood loss, the patient underwent nephrectomy. Active bleeding contained to Gerota fascia corresponds to an AAST grade 4 injury.

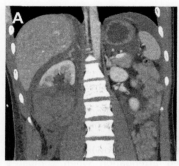
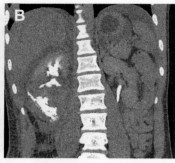

Fig. 10. Shattered kidney. Coronal portal venous (A) and excretory (B) phase CECT demonstrates complete destruction of the interpolar region and inferior pole of the right kidney, whereas a portion of the upper appears more intact. No areas of vascular injury were detected. In (B), there is extensive urinary extravasation within the regions of destroyed renal tissue. Shattered kidney is often associated with vascular and/or collecting system injury, underscoring the importance of using arterial, portal venous, and excretory phases of contrast. These injuries are classified as AAST grade 5.

nonvisualization of the renal pelvis and/or ureter is demonstrated, further evaluation with CECT, angiography, or surgical exploration should be considered.[43]

FOLLOW-UP IMAGING IN RENAL TRAUMA

Follow-up CT imaging in patients with renal trauma can lead to early identification of treatment failure following nonoperative management and identification of complications following initial conservative or invasive management; however, only in a fraction of cases does it lead to a change in patient treatment, and there is insufficient evidence to make concrete recommendations regarding the necessity for and timing of follow-up imaging in renal trauma, particularly for high-grade injury. Follow-up

imaging has not been shown to affect outcomes in AAST grade 1 or 2 injury, and is not indicated.[3,32,44] Breen and colleagues[44] noted that selective reimaging only in patients who have had a clinical deterioration would detect the vast majority of complications. In a study by Aldiwani and colleagues,[45] 12% of repeat imaging demonstrated a relevant finding (eg, urinoma, pseudoaneurysm) that altered management in 3 of the 49 patients who received follow-up imaging after known renal trauma (6.1%). Accordingly, in grades 1 to 3 injury, no follow-up imaging is needed except in cases of clinical deterioration. In grade 4 injury without urinary extravasation, no follow-up imaging is needed. In grade 4 injury with urinary extravasation or in grade 5 injury, the decision to pursue follow-up

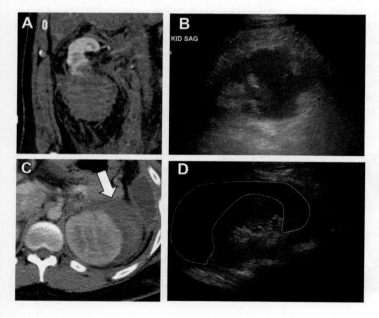

Fig. 11. Shattered kidney in a patient injured in a motor vehicle collision on CECT (A) and ultrasound (B). The shattered portion of the lower pole on CECT is depicted on ultrasound as an irregular hypoechoic region. Intact medullary pyramids are characterized by hyperechoic regions subjacent to the cortex. A subcapsular hematoma in a separate patient is demonstrated on CECT in (arrow in C) and on ultrasound in (dashed outline in D) as a hypoechoic collection contained by the renal capsule and exerting mass effect on the renal parenchyma.

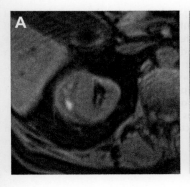
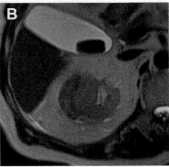

Fig. 12. Subcapsular hematoma on MR imaging. T1-weighted (*A*) and T2-weighted (*B*) MR imaging demonstrating a subcapsular hematoma with mixed signal characteristics on T1 and predominately hypointense on T2. Note the curvilinear T1-hypointensity and T2-hypointensity along the medial aspect of the hematoma reflecting hemosiderin staining, consistent with a subacute time course.

imaging is dependent on clinical parameters, patient status (including renal failure), and the proposed intervention[44,45] (**Fig. 15**). Of note, the 2013 European Association of Urology guidelines on urologic trauma advocate no repeat imaging for injury grades 1 to 4 in the absence of clinical deterioration.[46]

CLINICAL MANAGEMENT OF RENAL TRAUMA

Low-grade (AAST grades 1 and 2) renal injuries heal fully without intervention and without loss of renal function; as such, grade 1 and 2 renal injuries are treated nonoperatively, and in isolation may not even warrant admission for observation.[8,47] Hydration and analgesia are recommended as supportive measures.[48–50] On follow-up imaging, low-grade renal lacerations may result in focal cortical scarring but are not clinically detectable or relevant.

In contemporary practice, approximately 80% of grades 3 to 5 injuries are also treated nonoperatively.[51] These patients are often admitted for observation, analgesia, and hydration for their renal injuries, but they frequently require management for concomitant injuries. McClung and colleagues[52] reported nephrectomy rates to be 4.5% for grade 3 injuries using 2002 to 2007 data; in 2018, Keihani and colleagues[51] reported an even lower rate of nephrectomy (0.4%) for patients with grade 3 injuries. These data support an ongoing shift to renal-sparing and nonoperative management in grade 3 injuries. Ultimately, nephrectomy for grade 3 injury is dependent on overall patient status and the presence of active bleeding and concomitant injuries. Even in the presence of vascular injury, including active bleeding, a trial of endovascular embolization may be considered if the patient is hemodynamically stable.

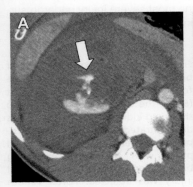
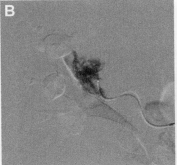
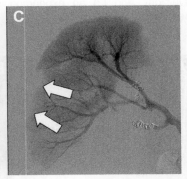

Fig. 13. Active arterial bleeding. Axial CECT in (*A*) in the portal venous phase demonstrates irregular pooling of contrast (*arrow*) from the kidney with attenuation similar to that of aortic blood pool, consistent with active bleeding (or extravasation). Multiple parenchymal lacerations and a large perinephric hematoma are also present. Digital subtraction angiography with selective catheterization of an upper pole segmental renal arterial branch in (*B*) depicts an irregular "blush" of contrast that increased in size in real-time over the course of the injection. Areas of vascular injury were successfully treated with coil embolization in (*C*). Note perfusion defects along the lateral aspect of the kidney in (*C*) corresponding to lacerations (*arrows*).

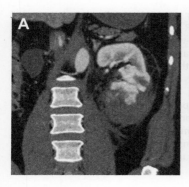
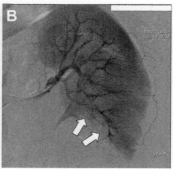

Fig. 14. Angiographic correlate of multiple lacerations disrupting the inferior renal pole. Coronal CECT (*A*) and digital subtraction angiography (*B*) demonstrating multiple lacerations of the inferior pole and perinephric hematoma in (*A*). On the angiogram, confluence of lacerations has the appearance of perfusion defects (*B, arrows*).

Not surprisingly, surgical management for grades 4 and 5 renal injury is more frequently pursued than for lower-grade injuries. The New England Trauma Consortium reported an overall nephrectomy rate of 21% for grades 4 and 5 renal injuries. The decision to proceed to nephrectomy in high-grade injury is dictated by specific clinical or imaging factors, often reserved for unstable patients with uncontrollable hemorrhage or severe/untreatable collecting system injury. Active contrast extravasation and large perirenal hematomas have been shown to be highly associated with the need for endovascular or open procedures to control bleeding.[53] Specifically, Keihani and colleagues[51] demonstrated that a perirenal hematoma thickness ≥3.5 cm and a laceration depth ≥2.5 cm can be used as thresholds for endovascular or surgical intervention, with an additional 15% increased likelihood of an intervention for every inch of increase in hematoma thickness beyond 3.5 cm. Three generally accepted absolute indications for surgical exploration for renal injury include (1) life-threatening hemorrhage, (2) renal pedicle avulsion (including ureteropelvic avulsion), and (3) an expanding retroperitoneal hematoma.[1,8]

Nephrectomy is the most common surgical procedure performed in the management of renal trauma, but only 8% of all renal injuries are managed in this way,[54] and many still are increasingly managed conservatively (Fig. 16). Grade 5 injuries are the mostly likely injury grade to require nephrectomy. Indeed, attempts at vascular repair in grade 5 injuries have been associated with a nearly 100% failure rate as well as a 15-fold increase in death, need for delayed nephrectomy, and hypertension, and as such, nephrectomy is the treatment of choice.[1] It is important to recognize that the retroperitoneal location of the kidneys confers a unique tamponade effect on renal injury, such as active bleeding or urinary extravasation, which is released on surgical exploration. Accordingly, surgical exploration may paradoxically exacerbate these underlying injuries, potentially leading to uncontrollable hemorrhage or urinary extravasation, in some cases necessitating emergent nephrectomy. The interpreting radiologist should bear this fact in mind when staging renal injury to help the trauma surgeon ensure that only those individuals with the most severe injury undergo surgical exploration.

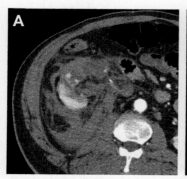
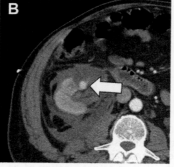

Fig. 15. Axial CECT on the date of blunt injury (*A*) and 5 weeks following conservative management (*B*). At the time of initial imaging, a shattered kidney (AAST grade 5) was demonstrated with extensive retroperitoneal hematoma in this arterial phase with hematoma extending beyond Gerota fascia, but no arterial injury was detected. Portal venous and excretory phase imaging confirmed the absence of vascular or collecting system injury. On repeat imaging at 5 weeks (*B*) for new-onset gross hematuria, an intrarenal arterial pseudoaneurysm was identified (*arrow*), new since the initial imaging. The patient underwent successful endovascular coil embolization.

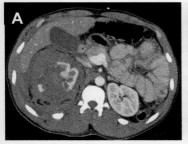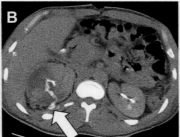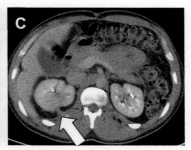

Fig. 16. Axial CECT in the late-arterial (*A*) and excretory (*B*) phase demonstrating a shattered right kidney with extensive perinephric hematoma in (*A*) and urinary extravasation (*arrow*) in (*B*). 5 weeks after nonoperative management, a focal area of scarring is present along the posteromedial aspect, but the urinary extravasation had resolved (*arrow* in *C*). Depending on patient and imaging factors, even high-grade injury can be managed nonoperatively.

SUMMARY

Nonoperative management has essentially replaced surgical exploration in the evaluation and management of renal trauma in recent years, largely owing to the widespread adoption of CECT in the initial workup of abdominal trauma in hemodynamically stable patients. CECT can rapidly and safely depict the full range of renal parenchymal, vascular, and collecting system injury with a high degree of precision. In fact, the imaging features of these injuries are now included in the AAST OIS, the most widely used injury classification system for solid organ injury. Ultrasound and MR imaging have limited value in the image-based diagnosis of renal injury, but may be useful in select clinical circumstances. Angiography is typically reserved for those patients in whom catheter-directed therapy, such as embolization for arterial injury, is being considered. Owing to advances in imaging and nonoperative management options, most renal injury is treated conservatively, sometimes supplemented by angiographic endovascular treatment. Nephrectomy is necessary in only the most severe forms of injury. The radiologist plays a pivotal role in the detection and subsequent management of renal trauma by assisting the treating clinician at arriving at a clinically relevant renal injury grade as well as detecting any concomitant abdominal injury.

DISCLOSURE

Authors have nothing to disclose.

REFERENCES

1. Santucci RA, Wessells H, Bartsch G, et al. Evaluation and management of renal injuries: consensus statement of the renal trauma subcommittee. BJU Int 2004;93(7):937–54.

2. Wessells H, Suh D, Porter JR, et al. Renal injury and operative management in the United States: results of a population-based study. J Trauma 2003;54(3):423–30.

3. Erlich T, Kitrey ND. Renal trauma: the current best practice. Ther Adv Urol 2018;10(10):295–303.

4. Santucci RA. 2015 William Hunter Harridge lecture: how did we go from operating on nearly all injured kidneys to operating on almost none of them? Am J Surg 2016;211(3):501–5.

5. Lee YJ, Oh SN, Rha SE, et al. Renal trauma. Radiol Clin North Am 2007;45(3):581–92, ix.

6. Santucci RA, McAninch JW, Safir M, et al. Validation of the American Association for the Surgery of Trauma organ injury severity scale for the kidney. J Trauma 2001;50(2):195–200.

7. Alsikafi NF, Rosenstein DI. Staging, evaluation, and nonoperative management of renal injuries. Urol Clin 2006;33(1):13–9.

8. Bonatti M, Lombardo F, Vezzali N, et al. MDCT of blunt renal trauma: imaging findings and therapeutic implications. Insights Imaging 2015;6(2):261–72.

9. Kawashima A, Sandler CM, Corl FM, et al. Imaging of renal trauma: a comprehensive review. Radiographics 2001;21(3):557–74.

10. Alonso RC, Nacenta SB, Martinez PD, et al. Kidney in danger: CT findings of blunt and penetrating renal trauma. Radiographics 2009;29(7):2033–53.

11. Moore EE, Shackford SR, Pachter HL, et al. Organ injury scaling: spleen, liver, and kidney. J Trauma 1989;29(12):1664–6.

12. Tinkoff G, Esposito TJ, Reed J, et al. American Association for the Surgery of Trauma Organ Injury Scale I: spleen, liver, and kidney, validation based on the National Trauma Data Bank. J Am Coll Surg 2008;207(5):646–55.

13. Shariat SF, Roehrborn CG, Karakiewicz PI, et al. Evidence-based validation of the predictive value of the American Association for the Surgery of Trauma kidney injury scale. J Trauma 2007;62(4):933–9.

14. Kozar RA, Crandall M, Shanmuganathan K, et al. Organ injury scaling 2018 update: spleen, liver, and kidney. J Trauma Acute Care Surg 2018;85(6): 1119–22.

15. Malaeb B, Figler B, Wessells H, et al. Should blunt segmental vascular renal injuries be considered an American Association for the Surgery of Trauma Grade 4 renal injury? J Trauma Acute Care Surg 2014;76(2):484–7.

16. Chien LC, Vakil M, Nguyen J, et al. The American Association for the Surgery of Trauma Organ Injury Scale 2018 update for computed tomography-based grading of renal trauma: a primer for the emergency radiologist. Emerg Radiol 2020;27(1): 63–73.

17. Sessa B, Trinci M, Ianniello S, et al. Blunt abdominal trauma: role of contrast-enhanced ultrasound (CEUS) in the detection and staging of abdominal traumatic lesions compared to US and CE-MDCT. Radiol Med 2015;120(2):180–9.

18. Altman AL, Haas C, Dinchman KH, et al. Selective nonoperative management of blunt grade 5 renal injury. J Urol 2000;164(1):27–30 [discussion: 30–1].

19. Chiu WC, Cushing BM, Rodriguez A, et al. Abdominal injuries without hemoperitoneum: a potential limitation of focused abdominal sonography for trauma (FAST). J Trauma 1997;42(4):617–23 [discussion: 623–5].

20. Brown MA, Casola G, Sirlin CB, et al. Importance of evaluating organ parenchyma during screening abdominal ultrasonography after blunt trauma. J Ultrasound Med 2001;20(6):577–83 [quiz: 585].

21. Pollack HM, Wein AJ. Imaging of renal trauma. Radiology 1989;172(2):297–308.

22. Korner M, Krotz MM, Degenhart C, et al. Current role of emergency US in patients with major trauma. Radiographics 2008;28(1):225–42.

23. Miller MT, Pasquale MD, Bromberg WJ, et al. Not so FAST. J Trauma 2003;54(1):52–9 [discussion: 59–60].

24. Bakker J, Genders R, Mali W, et al. Sonography as the primary screening method in evaluating blunt abdominal trauma. J Clin Ultrasound 2005;33(4): 155–63.

25. Poletti PA, Mirvis SE, Shanmuganathan K, et al. Blunt abdominal trauma patients: can organ injury be excluded without performing computed tomography? J Trauma 2004;57(5):1072–81.

26. Valentino M, Ansaloni L, Catena F, et al. Contrast-enhanced ultrasonography in blunt abdominal trauma: considerations after 5 years of experience. Radiol Med 2009;114(7):1080–93.

27. Catalano O, Aiani L, Barozzi L, et al. CEUS in abdominal trauma: multi-center study. Abdom Imaging 2009;34(2):225–34.

28. Fernandez-Ibieta M. Renal trauma in pediatrics: a current review. Urology 2018;113:171–8.

29. Marco GG, Diego S, Giulio A, et al. Screening US and CT for blunt abdominal trauma: a retrospective study. Eur J Radiol 2005;56(1):97–101.

30. Abu-Zidan FM, Sheikh M, Jadallah F, et al. Blunt abdominal trauma: comparison of ultrasonography and computed tomography in a district general hospital. Australas Radiol 1999;43(4):440–3.

31. Sato M, Yoshii H. Reevaluation of ultrasonography for solid-organ injury in blunt abdominal trauma. J Ultrasound Med 2004;23(12):1583–96.

32. Malcolm JB, Derweesh IH, Mehrazin R, et al. Nonoperative management of blunt renal trauma: is routine early follow-up imaging necessary? BMC Urol 2008; 8:11.

33. Gulati M, Cheng J, Loo JT, et al. Pictorial review: Renal ultrasound. Clin Imaging 2018;51:133–54.

34. Afaq A, Harvey C, Aldin Z, et al. Contrast-enhanced ultrasound in abdominal trauma. Eur J Emerg Med 2012;19(3):140–5.

35. Menichini G, Sessa B, Trinci M, et al. Accuracy of contrast-enhanced ultrasound (CEUS) in the identification and characterization of traumatic solid organ lesions in children: a retrospective comparison with baseline US and CE-MDCT. Radiol Med 2015; 120(11):989–1001.

36. Marcos HB, Noone TC, Semelka RC. MRI evaluation of acute renal trauma. J Magn Reson Imaging 1998; 8(4):989–90.

37. Goldman SM, Sandler CM. Urogenital trauma: imaging upper GU trauma. Eur J Radiol 2004;50(1): 84–95.

38. Dayal M, Gamanagatti S, Kumar A. Imaging in renal trauma. World J Radiol 2013;5(8):275–84.

39. Yanagi M, Suzuki Y, Hamasaki T, et al. Early transcatheter arterial embolization for the American Association for the Surgery of Trauma grade 4 blunt renal trauma in two institutions. J Nippon Med Sch 2018; 85(4):204–7.

40. Hotaling JM, Sorensen MD, Smith TG 3rd, et al. Analysis of diagnostic angiography and angioembolization in the acute management of renal trauma using a national data set. J Urol 2011;185(4):1316–20.

41. Martin JG, Shah J, Robinson C, et al. Evaluation and management of blunt solid organ trauma. Tech Vasc Interv Radiol 2017;20(4):230–6.

42. Roudsari BS, Psoter KJ, Padia SA, et al. Utilization of angiography and embolization for abdominopelvic trauma: 14 years' experience at a level I trauma center. AJR Am J Roentgenol 2014;202(6):W580–5.

43. Chouhan JD, Winer AG, Johnson C, et al. Contemporary evaluation and management of renal trauma. Can J Urol 2016;23(2):8191–7.

44. Breen KJ, Sweeney P, Nicholson PJ, et al. Adult blunt renal trauma: routine follow-up imaging is excessive. Urology 2014;84(1):62–7.

45. Aldiwani M, Georgiades F, Omar I, et al. Traumatic renal injury in a UK major trauma centre - current

management strategies and the role of early re-imaging. BJU Int 2019. [Epub ahead of print].

46. Summerton DR, DN, Kitrey ND, et al. European Association of Urology. Guidelines on urological trauma. Available at: https://uroweb.org/wp-content/uploads/EAU-Guidelines-on-Urological-Trauma-2018-large-text.pdf. Accessed October 15, 2019.

47. Harper K, Shah KH. Renal trauma after blunt abdominal injury. J Emerg Med 2013;45(3):400–4.

48. McCombie SP, Thyer I, Corcoran NM, et al. The conservative management of renal trauma: a literature review and practical clinical guideline from Australia and New Zealand. BJU Int 2014;114(Suppl 1):13–21.

49. McGuire J, Bultitude MF, Davis P, et al. Predictors of outcome for blunt high grade renal injury treated with conservative intent. J Urol 2011;185(1):187–91.

50. Toutouzas KG, Karaiskakis M, Kaminski A, et al. Nonoperative management of blunt renal trauma: a prospective study. Am Surg 2002;68(12):1097–103.

51. Keihani S, Xu Y, Presson AP, et al. Contemporary management of high-grade renal trauma: results from the American Association for the Surgery of Trauma Genitourinary Trauma study. J Trauma Acute Care Surg 2018;84(3):418–25.

52. McClung CD, Hotaling JM, Wang J, et al. Contemporary trends in the immediate surgical management of renal trauma using a national database. J Trauma Acute Care Surg 2013;75(4):602–6.

53. van der Wilden GM, Velmahos GC, Joseph DK, et al. Successful nonoperative management of the most severe blunt renal injuries: a multicenter study of the research consortium of New England Centers for Trauma. JAMA Surg 2013;148(10):924–31.

54. Hotaling JM, Wang J, Sorensen MD, et al. A national study of trauma level designation and renal trauma outcomes. J Urol 2012;187(2):536–41.

Percutaneous Thermal Ablation for Treatment of T1a Renal Cell Carcinomas

Sepideh Shakeri, MD[a],*, Steven S. Raman, MD[a,b,1]

KEYWORDS

- Thermal ablation • Cryoablation • Radiofrequency ablation • Microwave ablation
- Percutaneous ablation • Minimal invasive surgery • Partial nephrectomy • Radical nephrectomy

KEY POINTS

- Based on Surveillance, Epidemiology, and End Results (SEER) studies, most renal cancers are low grade and slow growing. Since 1996, percutaneous thermal ablation (TA) techniques such as cryoablation, radiofrequency ablation, and microwave ablation have gained widespread acceptance for treatment of renal masses less than 3 cm in patients who are not surgical candidates.
- There are now long-term single-center studies showing excellent outcomes for T1a renal cell carcinoma (RCC), comparable to partial nephrectomy without affecting renal function and with much lower rates of complications.
- However, there are no multicenter randomized controlled trials of multiple ablative modalities or comparison with partial nephrectomy, and most studies are single-arm observational studies with short-term and intermediate follow-up.
- For treatment of stage T1a RCC, percutaneous TA is an effective alternative to surgery with preservation of renal function, low risk, and comparable overall and disease-specific survival. Ideally, randomized phase 3 trials should compare surgical resection with ablative techniques.

INTRODUCTION

Over the past 30 years, the recognition of the importance of renal function preservation has led to the development or adoption of several nephron-sparing treatment options of clinical stage T1a (<4 cm) renal masses, including (open, laparoscopic, and robotic) partial nephrectomy (PN), thermal ablation (TA), and active surveillance (AS).[1–4] The procedure risk, underlying renal function is always weighed against the patients' cardiovascular morbidity and mortality.[3–6] Since initial case reports in 1996 and 1997, the adoption of TA for the treatment of clinical T1a renal masses has increased dramatically with favorable safety, efficacy, and preservation of renal function, as a minimally invasive alternative therapy for poor surgical candidates.[7–10] TA has now evolved to become an alternative to surgery for treatment of clinical T1a renal masses in 2019 National Comprehensive Cancer Network guidelines.[1]

More sophisticated understanding of the biology and natural history of solitary incidentally detected renal masses has led to an improved and less-invasive overall management paradigm. AS is now frequently recommended because of recognition of slow tumor growth rates, and wide prevalence of low tumor grade and low risk of adverse metastases.[11] Overall, patient care and counseling have improved with a multidisciplinary approach.[12]

[a] Department of Radiology, David Geffen School of Medicine at UCLA, 10833 Le Conte Avenue, Los Angeles, CA 90095, USA; [b] Department of Urology, David Geffen School of Medicine at UCLA, Los Angeles, CA, USA
[1] 757 Westwood Plaza Suite 1621, Los Angeles, CA 90095.
* Corresponding author. 6400 Crescent Park East, # 404, Playa Vista, CA 90094.
E-mail address: Spd.shakeri@hotmail.com

Radiol Clin N Am 58 (2020) 981–993
https://doi.org/10.1016/j.rcl.2020.06.004
0033-8389/20/© 2020 Elsevier Inc. All rights reserved.

Clinical considerations for TA therapy include patient age, comorbidities, and life expectancy as well as risk of developing renal failure or chronic kidney disease and the potential need for dialysis.[13] In patients with multifocal or bilateral renal masses, or any positive family history of renal neoplasm, genetic susceptibility needs to be considered.[11,14] This article reviews the performance of different TA modalities and the goals of ablation therapy for treatment of renal cell carcinoma (RCC).

WHAT IS THE IMAGE-GUIDED THERMAL ABLATION?

Percutaneous image-guided tumor ablation refers to a group of minimally invasive treatment options using primarily ultrasound (US) and/or computed tomographic (CT)-guided needle-based thermal energy applicators to destroy focal malignancies.[4] Over the past 24 years, these techniques have proliferated and become routine for treatment of renal tumors.[14]

TA techniques eradicate malignant cells by inducing irreversible thermal cellular injury.[3] In TA therapy, the total projected energy delivered to the target is proportional to the radius[3] of the lesion target. Thus, the overall required energy for small lesions (1–2 cm) is significantly less than for intermediate (2–3 cm) and larger (3–5 cm) lesions, fundamentally limiting the utility of TA for large lesions.[2] The main goal of ablation procedures is to remove all viable malignant cells by treating the designated target and beyond into the visible tumor margin, typically the normal surrounding parenchyma up to 0.5 cm.[15]

TA techniques for treatment of renal tumors are either cold (cryoablation) or heat (electromagnetic [ie, radiofrequency [RF], microwave, laser] or US) based.[15–17] Cryoablation, first described for renal tumor ablation in 1996, induces cell death and apoptosis with a dual freeze-thaw cycle causing intracellular and extracellular ice formation (visualized as an "ice ball" on imaging). The goal is to reach to less than −140°C in the center of the lesion, −40°C at the margin of the lesion, and 0°C at the edge of the ice ball to create a near spherical ablation.[18] Subsequently, the thaw cycle ruptures the osmotic cellular phospholipid membrane.[15] The available cryoprobes are 13- to 17-G needles with internal shafts that circulate compressed argon gas, which produces dramatic cooling by dropping the gas pressure, called the Jewell-Thompson effect.[4] Helium gas is used for the thaw cycle. An array of up to 8 probes can create a large fused ice ball to treat lesions up to 5 to 6 cm, generally much larger than radiofrequency ablation (RFA) or microwave ablation (MWA)[19] (**Fig. 1**).

Heat-based ablation was once synonymous with RFA and was first described in 1997 for treatment of RCC.[4] RF energy is an electrical impedance-controlled pulsed current, generally at 500 MHz, which induces tissue heating around straight or expandable multitined needle electrodes placed within the target. Current passes from the generator through the electrode into the target tissue and is grounded through pads on the patient's skin, resulting in active frictional heating to greater than 60°C by rapidly oscillating water molecules at areas of high current density near the electrode, resulting in immediate coagulative necrosis of heated tissue. Nonelectric thermal diffusion (conductive heating) also occurs and results in a larger volume of cell death than beyond direct electric heating.[20] Conductance is an important property of RFA, and tissue heating resulting in charring can decrease conductance, reducing effectiveness. A variety of RF needle designs include expandable multitined hooklike electrodes and straight internally cooled needles that allow for up to 3 probe placements simultaneously.[19]

MWA, approved for use in the United States and used for RCC treatments since 2008, is a newer needle-based TA that heats target tissues to greater than 100°C because of more efficient frictional heating of water molecules by wavelike electromagnetic energy at either 915 MHz or 2450 mHz.[21] Microwave energy is produced by generating dielectric hysteresis (rotating dipoles) at either 915 MHz or 2.45 GHz from the exposed tip of a needlelike probe (antenna) into surrounding tissue, resulting in more efficient and robust frictional heating of water molecules in tissue to greater than 100°C.[19] Because of the wave property of MWA, permittivity is a useful metric determining efficacy, and marked differences in permittivity between tumors and surrounding tissue may allow better treatment with MWA. Unlike RFA, MWA is also not affected by carbonization or impedance and does not require grounding pads.[15] In addition, diffusion of microwave energy is enhanced in neoplastic tissues because permittivity is generally greater in neoplastic tissues than in normal tissues.[22] MWA is much less dependent on electrical conductivity of tissue because the energy delivery is less limited by the exponential rising electrical impedances of heated tissue in contrast to RFA.[4] For successful ablation, the tissue temperature should be maintained in a range of 100°C to 120oC to ablate lesion adequately and avoid carbonization around the needle tip because of excessive heating.[23] The severity of the thermal damage depends on tissue perfusion,

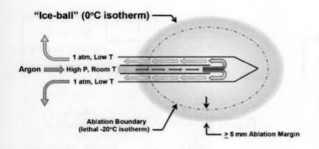

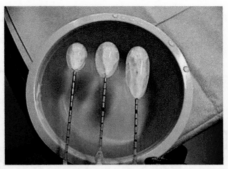

Fig. 1. Cryoablation probe design with ability to create different ice-ball sizes: High-pressure argon gas depressurizes and equilibrates with ambient pressure at the tip of the probe and supercools with resulting ice ball by Joule-Thomson effect. The edge of the ice ball is nonlethal. The lethal isotherm at −20°C is 5 mm deep to the outer edge, varying with probe design. Generally, ice-ball size is proportional to probe thickness (gauge) because larger gauge size allows for faster gas flow. P, pressure; T, temperature. (*From* https://oncohemakey.com/cryoablation-mechanism-of-action-and-devices/ and *Courtesy of* Kemal Tuncali, MD, Nobuhiko Hata, PHD, and Stuart G. Silverman, MD; https://ncigt.org/mri-guided-cryoablations-liver-and-kidney-tumors; with permission.)

tissue temperature, and the duration of heating[12] (**Figs. 2** and **3**). MWA occurs more rapidly than RFA and cryoablation.

WHAT ARE THE IMPORTANT FACTORS THAT CAN INFLUENCE THE RESULT OF THE ABLATION?

The complete and adequate cell destruction by TA requires that the entire target and an ablative margin of 0.5 to 1 cm reach to the optimal cytotoxic temperatures.[24] However, the ability to heat or cool the tissue, particularly for large volumes, is influenced by several factors like the amount of energy deposited (number of probes), tissue perfusion, the absolute temperature achieved at any point of target, and the heterogeneity of tissues.[25]

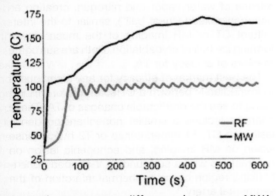

Fig. 2. The temperature differences between an MWA system and the RFA. As it shows, microwave energy is hotter and faster than RF. (*From* Hinshaw JL, Lubner MG, Ziemlewicz TJ, Lee FT, Jr., Brace CL. Percutaneous tumor ablation tools: microwave, radiofrequency, or cryoablation–what should you use and why? Radiographics 2014;34(5):1344-1362; with permission.)

Typically, TA times are based on the size and location of the lesions. Small exophytic renal lesions require the least time and energy, and large central lesions require the most time and energy because of low- and high-thermal dissipation, respectively, from surrounding heat sink inducing large central blood vessels and high and low insulation, respectively, from surrounding perinephric fat.[17]

For treatment planning, the 5-parameter nephrometry score is useful for classifying the complexity of renal masses for PN and adapted for percutaneous ablation based on anatomic characteristics: tumor size, proximity to collecting system or renal sinus, and location (exophytic or endophytic, anterior or posterior, and orientation to polar lines).[26–29] These parameters are for planning but are not associated with oncologic outcomes independently.[30] McClure and colleagues[29] first showed that higher nephrometry scores had a small adverse effect on efficacy of RFA, and this was later confirmed by Camacho and colleagues[26] for RFA and by Ierardi and colleagues[31] and Klapperich and colleagues[32] for MWA. However, in our previous study[30] this relationship was not found for MWA (**Fig. 4**).

PREFERENCE AND CHOICE OF ABLATION MODALITY

Cryoablation is the dominant percutaneous TA treatment modality for T1a RCCs because of its efficacy and ability to clearly visualize the zone of ablation (ice ball) under CT or MR guidance.[33,34] The ice ball is the near spherical ablation zone with sharply demarcated margins encompassing the target renal mass with 5- to 10-mm surrounding margin so that the margin of the lesion is at the

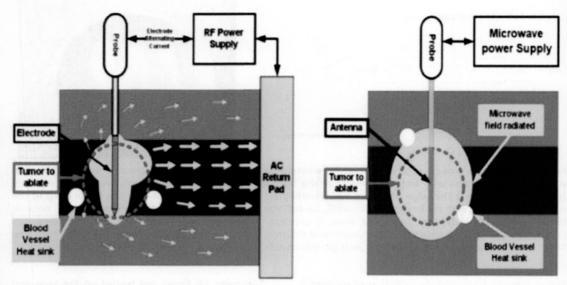

Fig. 3. Comparison of RFA and MWA: RFA (*left*) is a current-based system that often results in smaller and more irregular, scattered ablation zones because of uneven current flow, relatively low thermal temperatures, heat dissipation in perfused tissue, and poor propagation in charred tissues. MWA (*right*) is a much more efficient wave-based heating process with high thermal temperatures, much less heat dissipation, and less heat sink resulting in more homogeneous and larger ablation zones in shorter time. AC, Alternating current.

$-40°C$ isotherm, whereas the center is ideally less than $-140°C$.[18] This ability to visualize the ablation zone is not possible with many heat-based systems under CT guidance, but the echogenic cloud of ablation can be seen with US guidance.[18] However, radiologists who are unfamiliar with US monitoring prefer the CT-based monitoring with the ice ball. Also, current systems can power up to 8 cryoprobes simultaneously, which increases volume and efficacy of cryoablation for treating both T1a and T1b renal masses.[35] Like all TA modalities, cryoablation efficacy is limited by dissipation of cryoenergy (cold sink) from tissue perfusion by large arteries or veins. Large-volume cryoablation uniquely has a small but elevated risk for cryoglobulinemia or cryoglobulinuria, with associated risk of transient acute tubular necrosis. There is also an approximately 10-fold higher risk of hemorrhage relative to RFA and MWA.[17,36] Despite this, radiologist training, equipment preference, and experience are frequently the primary drivers of decisions regarding selection of TA type. Cryoablation is preferred for treating metastatic renal cancer lesions in the renal bed, adjacent to the spine or bowel, in the retroperitoneum, pleura, and subcutaneous tissue.[17,36] Other complication rates (besides bleeding) for cryoablation are similar to other ablation modalities.[37]

Cryoablation, RFA, and MWA rely on skills of US and/or CT guidance to precisely place probes into renal lesions while avoiding adjacent normal tissues like vessels, bowel, renal pelvis, and ureter.[24] Probes are placed into the deepest portion of the tumor initially and then retracted. RF and MW probes may have to be repositioned at opposite margins or may need to be circumferentially placed within larger tumors (>3 cm) to create larger overlapping zones of ablation. With cryoablation, up to 8 probes may be inserted within larger tumors. Continuous US monitoring during RF and MW ablation is important, because the operator monitors the rapidly forming heat generated release of water vapor and nitrogen, creating an echogenic cloud ("heat ball"), similar to the intermittent CT or MR imaging of the much slower forming ice ball of cryoablation. Both are surrogate markers of efficacy for TA.

The best marker of efficacy for any technique is to immediately perform a CT scan and/or MR imaging to see the predictable changes of TA. These changes include a smaller nonenhancing dense lesion on CT, T1 hyperintense or T2 hypointense lesion on MR imaging, and echogenic lesion on contrast US with a surrounding V-shaped nonenhancing region owing to thermal infarction of the segmental artery.[4]

One of the limitations of RF ablation is related to carbonization of tissues adjacent to the electrode, which decreases conductivity and increases tissue impedance owing to high temperatures greater than 60°C. A variety of strategies have been developed to compensate, including water

RENAL Nephrometry score

	1pt	2pts	3pts
(R)adius (maximal diameter in cm)	≤4	>4 but <7	≥7
(E)xophytic/endophytic properties	≥50%	<50%	Entirely endophytic
(N)earness of the tumor to the collecting system or sinus (mm)	≥7	>4 but <7	≤4
(A)nterior/posterior	No points given. Mass assigned a descriptor of a, p, or x		
(L)ocation relative to the polar lines[a] [a]Suffix 'h' asisigned if the tumor touches the main renal artery or vein	Entirely above the upper or below the lower polar line	Lesion crosses polar line	>50% of mass is across polar line (a) or mass crosses the axial renal midline (b) or mass is entirely between the polar lines (c)

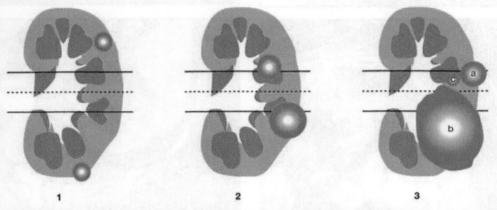

Fig. 4. Nephrometry score; the scale from 4 to 12 based on the anatomic location of the tumor in 5 categories. (*From* Kutikov A, Uzzo RG. The R.E.N.A.L. nephrometry score: a comprehensive standardized system for quantitating renal tumor size, location and depth. J Urol 2009;182(3):844-853; with permission.)

perfusion of the electrode shaft, multiple electrode placement with rapid switching,[16] and slow ramp-up of energy delivery.[19] RF ablation is less effective for tumors larger than 3 cm due to the large amount of energy required, centrally located tumors due to large heat sink, and tumors near the ureteropelvic junction of the collecting system due to heating-related stricture risk[38,39] (**Fig. 5**). For larger lesions greater than 4 cm, a combination of embolization and RFA is more effective because energy dissipating tissue perfusion is eliminated or decreased.[33,34,40]

MWA is a faster and more efficient wave-based heating technique that relies on rapid heating of tissue water because of antenna and generator design and also properties such as wavelength, frequency, power, and cooling. MWA leads to much faster, hotter, and efficient heating of tissues than RFA. It is much less susceptible to heat-sink effects from adjacent renal vessels but can also cause faster and more severe thermal injury than RFA. Tumor size and location are also important

factors because larger lesions and central lesions are more challenging to ablate for MWA albeit to a lesser degree than RFA. Ablation of tumors located close to the ureteropelvic junction and ureter increase risk of thermal injuries, such as stricture or leak or thermal injury to the collecting system.[31] On average, fewer applicators are needed, and ablative margins are easier to obtain[32] (**Fig. 6**). Moreover, multiple studies have shown that MWA could effectively treat 5-cm lesions with similar efficacy to 3-cm lesions treated with RFA.[14,15,41–43] Major complications of MWA occur in approximately 4% and include bleeding, infection, urine leak, stricture, and nontarget ablation, including skin burn if the target is within 3 cm of the skin.[21,31,42–46]

WHAT ARE THE ADVANTAGES OF PERCUTANEOUS THERMAL ABLATION OVER PARTIAL NEPHRECTOMY?

The simplicity, efficacy, repeatability, minimal risk, favorable complication profile, and lack of general

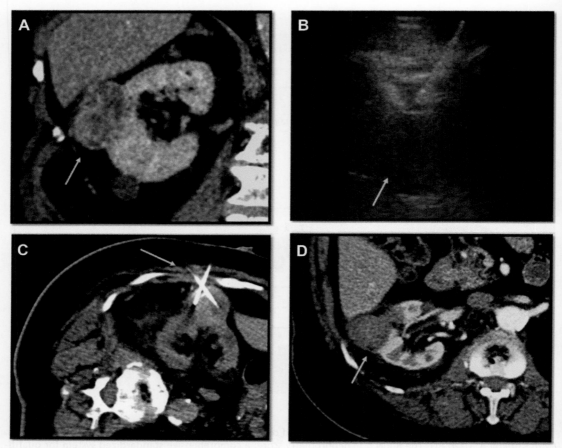

Fig. 5. An 86-year-old man with 4.5-cm exophytic clear cell RCC in the right kidney (*arrows*). Preablation CT (nephrographic phase) shows tumor enhancement (*A*). Two RF probes placed into the tumor under US and CT guidance (*B, C*). Postablation CT (corticomedullary phase) confirms successful ablation with no residual enhancing tumor (*D*).

anesthesia are some of the many benefits of percutaneous TA over PN in patients with and without preexisting renal parenchymal injury.[4,25,34]

Traditionally, renal tumors treated by TA were generally smaller and of lower anatomic complexity than those treated by PN.[10] Accordingly, guidelines have emphasized that TA should ideally be reserved for tumors ≤3 cm in size with a slightly increased risk of complications and decreased efficacy for TA of lesions greater than 3 cm[12] (**Tables 1** and **2**). However, T1b lesions are well treated by more contemporary ablation techniques, such as MWA alone or combination with renal arterial embolization.

Studies comparing TA and PN tend to be retrospective and fail to account for operator expertise and equipment. In 2017, Long and colleagues[47] reported results with a mean follow-up of 43.2 months for 172 (mostly open) partial nephrectomies and 38 months follow-up of 112 (mostly RFA) TAs; the percentage of estimated glomerular filtration rate decrease was similar in the 2 groups. Five-year local radiologic recurrence-free survival was better for PN (92 vs 74%). Mean time of recurrence was 13.1 months for TA and 39.4 for PN, but metastatic recurrence was similar, 89% versus 85%.[47] They found that PN had worse outcomes than TA in terms of transfusion rate, length of stay, and complication rate, but PN was necessary to manage larger and more complex tumors while providing a better local control and similar renal function loss. Other studies have shown no significant differences with regard to local recurrence rate or overall disease-free survival and distant metastases in RFA and MWA versus PN.[29,48–50]

Some studies have shown a 2.3-fold increased rate of renal and cardiovascular events and 5-fold increased rate of thromboembolic events for PN over TA,[51] whereas some other studies found no difference.[52]

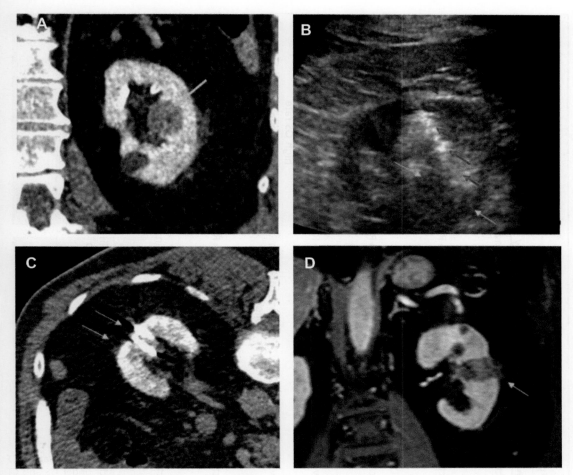

Fig. 6. A 62-year-old man with 4-cm clear cell RCC. Two microwave probes (*red arrows*) placed into the tumor (*yellow arrows*) with multidetector CT (corticomedullary, nephrographic, and excretory phases) (*A–C*). After the procedure, MR confirmation on coronal view shows the successful ablation with no residual tissue (*D*).

Local tumor recurrence and incomplete ablation are the principal complications of TA in larger tumors (>3 cm).[3] Tanagho and colleagues[53] found that tumor size greater than 2.5 cm was an independent predictive factor in local recurrence for cryoablation. Moreover, some studies of renal cryoablation compared with PN for clinical T1b RCCs reported that the rate of local recurrence was significantly higher for cryoablation versus PN (P = .019).[54] However, they showed there was no significant difference in cancer-specific mortality or overall mortality between the CA and PN groups.[54,55]

Notably, because the postoperative complications of TA are not higher than the PN, second ablation for tumor recurrence or incomplete removal can provide a solution.[12] The rate of second ablation procedures used is reported from 4% to 8% for T1a RCC.[22,29] Based on the authors'

previous studies, the primary and secondary efficacy rates were 90% to 92% and 100% in 125 RCCs with RFA and 69 RCCs, respectively, using MWA. RFA tumor recurrence rate was 8%, versus 5.8% for MWA.[30,56]

Interestingly, there is evidence suggesting that tumor histology may play a role in predicting efficacy in percutaneous RFA.[9] Clear-cell RCC had a primary, secondary, and total technique efficacy of 76.4%, 14.5%, and 90.9%, whereas non-clear-cell RCC had a primary, secondary, and total technique efficacy of 97.8%, 2.2%, and 100%.[9]

In a cost comparison study of PN versus RFA, Lotan and Cadeddu[57] found that for T1a RCCs minimally invasive methods (RFA) can decrease morbidity, along with significant cost benefits. They reported RFA was significantly cheaper to perform (US\$4454 ± \$US938), compared with both laparoscopic PN (US\$7013 ± US\$934) and

Table 1
Characteristics of single-center studies with different ablation modalities in renal cell carcinomas

	Reference	No. of Patients	Type of the Study	Time Period	Treatment Modality	Outcomes
1	Johnson et al,[59] 2019	106	Retrospective study	2000–2007	Outcomes of RFA in RCCs in 10-y follow-up	RFA is a safe and effective treatment option for RCCs <3 cm with good 10-y CSS 94% and OS 49% rates
2	Psutka et al,[60] 2013	185	Retrospective study	During 5 y	Outcomes of RFA in RCCs in 5-y follow-up	RFA is an effective treatment in RCCs, and the higher stage correlates with a decreased disease-free survival
3	Marshall et al,[56] 2019	100	Retrospective study	2004–2015	Outcomes of RFA in RCCs in 5-y follow-up	RFA is a safe and effective treatment for RCCs with a low LTP and has good 5-y CSS 92%, OS 68% rates
4	Leveillee et al,[61] 2013	274	Prospective study	2001–2011	Outcomes of RFA in RCCs in 5-y follow-up	RFA is a clinically effective and safe treatment of RCCs with high OS rate
5	Wah et al,[62] 2014	165	Prospective study	2004–2012	Outcomes of RFA in RCCs in 5-y follow-up	RFA is a safe and effective treatment for RCCs with a low rate of recurrence and has good 5-y CSS rate
6	McClure et al,[29] 2014	100	Retrospective study	2004–2011	Outcomes of RFA in RCCs in 2-y follow-up	RFA is a clinically effective and safe treatment of RCCs with 97.6% OS and 100% CSS rates
7	Kim et al,[63] 2015	70	Retrospective study	2007–2014	Outcomes of Cryo in RCCs in 10-y follow-up	Recurrence-free rate was 83.0% and the CSS rate was 100%. The 5- and 10-y OS rates were both 100%
8	Larcher et al,[52] 2015	174	Retrospective study	2000–2013	Outcomes of Cryo in T1a RCCs in 10-y follow-up	The 10-y LPR free was 100% and the 10-y disease relapse-free survival rate was 81%. The CSS; 100%, OS; 61%

9	Georgiades & Rodriguez,[64] 2014	134	Retrospective study	5 y	Outcomes of Cryo in T1a RCCs in 5-y follow-up	Cryoablation in RCCs offers very high efficacy of 97%, with a more favorable safety
10	Choi et al,[65] 2018	567 (13 articles)	Review article	2012–2017	Technical and oncologic outcomes of MWA in RCCs	MWA showed favorable technical and oncologic outcomes with a low incidence of major complications
11	Mu et al,[66] 2016	140	Retrospective study	2006–2015	Outcomes of MWA in T1 RCCs in 5-y follow-up	MWA is a safe treatment for RCCs with 1-, 3-, and 5-y OS rates of 98.4%, 94.8%, 89.5%, respectively
12	Klapperich et al,[32] 2017	96	Retrospective study	2011–2015	Outcomes of MWA in RCCs in short-term follow-up	MWA is a safe treatment option for stage T1a RCC, regardless of tumor complexity
13	Shakeri et al,[30] 2019	56	Retrospective study	2013–2017	Outcomes of MWA in T1 RCCs in short-term follow-up	MWA appears to be an effective treatment in RCCs regardless of renal score and tumor location with high TS, CSS, OS rates
14	Wells et al,[67] 2016	29	Retrospective study	2013–2014	Outcomes of MWA in T1 RCCs in short-term follow-up	MWA is a safe and effective treatment regardless of tumor complexity

Abbreviations: CSM, cancer-specific mortality; CSS, cancer-specific survival; LPR, local progression rate; LTP, local tumor progression; OS, overall survival; RN, radical nephrectomy.

Table 2
Characteristics of larger population-based studies comparing kidney tumor ablation to other surgical management strategies

	Study	No. of Patients	Study Population	Time Period	Treatment Modality	Outcomes
1	Palumbo et al,[68-70] 2019	3946	SEER	2004–2015	Cryosurgery vs TA	TS >30 mm is an independent predictor of higher 5-y CSM in TA
2	Xing et al,[51] 2018	10,309	SEER	2001–2012	Comparison of complication rates and CSM,OS between PN, RN, TA, AS	TA showed CSM and OS similar to PN/RN with significantly fewer adverse outcomes at 1-y follow-up
3	Zhou et al,[48] 2019	297	Retrospective study	2006–2016	Comparison of therapeutic effects of RFA, MWA, and cryoablation	RFA, MWA, and cryoablation are equivalent for treatment of T1a RCC for renal function, and low adverse event rate at 2-y follow-up
4	Atwell et al,[7] 2013	385	Retrospective study	2000–2010	Comparison the efficacy and complication rates of RFA vs Cryo in RCCs ≤3 cm	Both RFA and Cryo are effective in the treatment of RCCs ≤3 cm. Major complications are infrequent
5	Guan et al,[46] 2012	102	Prospective randomized comparison study	2004–2006	Comparison of therapeutic effects of MWA and PN in T1a	MWA provides favorable results compared with PN with high efficacy and local free recurrence rate
6	Chang et al,[71] 2019	90	Retrospective study	2005–2009	Comparison outcomes of RF and PN in RCCs in 5-y follow-up	RFA is an effective treatment with 5-y oncologic outcomes and better preservation of renal function than PN

open PN (US$7767 ± $US1605). Accordingly, Castle and colleagues[58] reported that the 6-month cost of nephron-sparing surgery is lowest using RFA with either laparoscopic or CT-guided approach in comparison with the open or robot-assisted PN.

SUMMARY

Although partial or radical nephrectomy represents the reference standard of treatment of RCCs, TA therapies have been used increasingly with acceptable efficacy, high survival rate, and low complication rate. Since there are no strict criteria for patient selection, more randomized phase 3 trials comparing surgical resection with ablative techniques would be beneficial for improved decision making by treating physicians.

REFERENCES

1. Kidney Cancer, Version 4.2019, NCCN clinical practice guidelines in oncology. Available at: https://jnccn.org/view/journals/jnccn/17/5.5/article-p587.xml?rskey=TCZhHZ&result=2.
2. Finelli A, Ismaila N, Russo P. Management of small renal masses: American Society of Clinical Oncology clinical practice guideline summary. J Oncol Pract 2017;13(4):276–8.
3. Motzer RJ, Jonasch E, Agarwal N, et al. Kidney cancer, version 2.2017, NCCN clinical practice guidelines in oncology. J Natl Compr Canc Netw 2017; 15(6):804–34.
4. Goldberg SN, Grassi CJ, Cardella JF, et al. Image-guided tumor ablation: standardization of terminology and reporting criteria. J Vasc Interv Radiol 2009;20(7 Suppl):S377–90.
5. Ahmad AE, Finelli A. Renal function outcomes following radical or partial nephrectomy for localized renal cell carcinoma: should urologists rely on pre-operative variables to predict renal function in the long term? Eur Urol 2019;75(5):773–4.
6. SEER stat fact sheets: kidney and renal pelvis cancer. Bethesda (MD): National Cancer Institute; 2018. Available at: https://seer.cancer.gov/statfacts/html/kidrp.html.
7. Atwell TD, Schmit GD, Boorjian SA, et al. Percutaneous ablation of renal masses measuring 3.0 cm and smaller: comparative local control and complications after radiofrequency ablation and cryoablation. AJR Am J Roentgenol 2013;200(2):461–6.
8. Hasegawa T, Yamanaka T, Gobara H, et al. Radiofrequency ablation versus cryoablation for T1b renal cell carcinoma: a multi-center study. Jpn J Radiol 2018;36(9):551–8.
9. McClure T, Pantuck A, Sayer J, et al. Efficacy of percutaneous radiofrequency ablation may vary with clear cell renal cell cancer histologic subtype. Abdom Radiol (NY) 2018;43(6):1472–7.
10. Sandbergen L, Guven S, Laguna MP. Can ablation win against partial nephrectomy and become first line therapy in cT1a renal tumours? Curr Opin Urol 2019;29(1):70–7.
11. Davenport MS, Hu EM, Zhang A, et al. Standardized report template for indeterminate renal masses at CT and MRI: a collaborative product of the SAR Disease-Focused Panel on Renal Cell Carcinoma. Abdom Radiol (NY) 2019;44(4):1423–9.
12. Campbell S, Uzzo RG, Allaf ME, et al. Renal mass and localized renal cancer: AUA guideline. J Urol 2017;198(3):520–9.
13. Andrews JR, Atwell T, Schmit G, et al. Oncologic outcomes following partial nephrectomy and percutaneous ablation for cT1 renal masses. Eur Urol 2019. https://doi.org/10.1016/j.eururo.2019.04.026.
14. Frey GT, Sella DM, Atwell TD. Image-guided renal intervention. Radiol Clin North Am 2015;53(5): 1005–19.
15. Ahmed M, Brace CL, Lee FT Jr, et al. Principles of and advances in percutaneous ablation. Radiology 2011;258(2):351–69.
16. Reyes J, Canter D, Putnam S, et al. Thermal ablation of the small renal mass: case selection using the R.E.N.A.L.-Nephrometry Score. Urol Oncol 2013; 31(7):1292–7.
17. Woldrich JM, Palazzi K, Stroup SP, et al. Trends in the surgical management of localized renal masses: thermal ablation, partial and radical nephrectomy in the USA, 1998-2008. BJU Int 2013;111(8):1261–8.
18. Atwell TD, Farrell MA, Callstrom MR, et al. Percutaneous cryoablation of large renal masses: technical feasibility and short-term outcome. AJR Am J Roentgenol 2007;188(5):1195–200.
19. Sanchez-Salas R, Desai M. Image-guided therapies for prostate and kidney cancers. World J Urol 2019; 37(3):395–6.
20. Higgins LJ, Hong K. Renal ablation techniques: state of the art. AJR Am J Roentgenol 2015;205(4): 735–41.
21. Ahmed M. Image-guided tumor ablation: standardization of terminology and reporting criteria–a 10-year update: supplement to the consensus document. J Vasc Interv Radiol 2014;25(11):1706–8.
22. Cornelis FH, Marcelin C, Bernhard JC. Microwave ablation of renal tumors: a narrative review of technical considerations and clinical results. Diagn Interv Imaging 2017;98(4):287–97.
23. Tatli S, Tapan U, Morrison PR, et al. Radiofrequency ablation: technique and clinical applications. Diagn Interv Radiol 2012;18(5):508–16.
24. Ward RD, Tanaka H, Campbell SC, et al. 2017 AUA renal mass and localized renal cancer guidelines: imaging implications. Radiographics 2018;38(7): 2021–33.

25. Goldberg SN, Gazelle GS, Mueller PR. Thermal ablation therapy for focal malignancy: a unified approach to underlying principles, techniques, and diagnostic imaging guidance. AJR Am J Roentgenol 2000;174(2):323–31.

26. Camacho JC, Kokabi N, Xing M, et al. (Radius, exophytic/endophytic, nearness to collecting system or sinus, anterior/posterior, and location relative to polar lines) nephrometry score predicts early tumor recurrence and complications after percutaneous ablative therapies for renal cell carcinoma: a 5-year experience. J Vasc Interv Radiol 2015;26(5):686–93.

27. Hinshaw JL, Lubner MG, Ziemlewicz TJ, et al. Percutaneous tumor ablation tools: microwave, radiofrequency, or cryoablation–what should you use and why? Radiographics 2014;34(5):1344–62.

28. Kutikov A, Uzzo RG. The R.E.N.A.L. nephrometry score: a comprehensive standardized system for quantitating renal tumor size, location and depth. J Urol 2009;182(3):844–53.

29. McClure TD, Chow DS, Tan N, et al. Intermediate outcomes and predictors of efficacy in the radiofrequency ablation of 100 pathologically proven renal cell carcinomas. J Vasc Interv Radiol 2014;25(11):1682–8 [quiz: 1689].

30. Shakeri S, Afshari Mirak S, Mohammadian Bajgiran A, et al. The effect of tumor size and location on efficacy and safety of US- and CT-guided percutaneous microwave ablation in renal cell carcinomas. Abdom Radiol (NY) 2019. https://doi.org/10.1007/s00261-019-01967-8.

31. Ierardi AM, Puliti A, Angileri SA, et al. Microwave ablation of malignant renal tumours: intermediate-term results and usefulness of RENAL and mRENAL scores for predicting outcomes and complications. Med Oncol 2017;34(5):97.

32. Klapperich ME, Abel EJ, Ziemlewicz TJ, et al. Effect of tumor complexity and technique on efficacy and complications after percutaneous microwave ablation of stage T1a renal cell carcinoma: a single-center, retrospective study. Radiology 2017;284(1):272–80.

33. El Dib R, Touma NJ, Kapoor A. Cryoablation vs radiofrequency ablation for the treatment of renal cell carcinoma: a meta-analysis of case series studies. BJU Int 2012;110(4):510–6.

34. Gervais DA. Cryoablation versus radiofrequency ablation for renal tumor ablation: time to reassess? J Vasc Interv Radiol 2013;24(8):1135–8.

35. Kunkle DA, Uzzo RG. Cryoablation or radiofrequency ablation of the small renal mass: a meta-analysis. Cancer 2008;113(10):2671–80.

36. Krokidis ME, Kitrou P, Spiliopoulos S, et al. Image-guided minimally invasive treatment for small renal cell carcinoma. Insights Imaging 2018;9(3):385–90.

37. Atwell TD, Carter RE, Schmit GD, et al. Complications following 573 percutaneous renal radiofrequency and cryoablation procedures. J Vasc Interv Radiol 2012;23(1):48–54.

38. McGahan JP, Brock JM, Tesluk H, et al. Hepatic ablation with use of radio-frequency electrocautery in the animal model. J Vasc Interv Radiol 1992;3(2):291–7.

39. Yu NC, Raman SS, Kim YJ, et al. Microwave liver ablation: influence of hepatic vein size on heat-sink effect in a porcine model. J Vasc Interv Radiol 2008;19(7):1087–92.

40. Best SL, Park SK, Youssef RF, et al. Long-term outcomes of renal tumor radio frequency ablation stratified by tumor diameter: size matters. J Urol 2012;187(4):1183–9.

41. Sun Y, Wang Y, Ni X, et al. Comparison of ablation zone between 915- and 2,450-MHz cooled-shaft microwave antenna: results in in vivo porcine livers. AJR Am J Roentgenol 2009;192(2):511–4.

42. Bai J, Hu Z, Guan W, et al. Initial experience with retroperitoneoscopic microwave ablation of clinical T(1a) renal tumors. J Endourol 2010;24(12):2017–22.

43. Floridi C, De Bernardi I, Fontana F, et al. Microwave ablation of renal tumors: state of the art and development trends. Radiol Med 2014;119(7):533–40.

44. Chen CN, Liang P, Yu J, et al. Contrast-enhanced ultrasound-guided percutaneous microwave ablation of renal cell carcinoma that is inconspicuous on conventional ultrasound. Int J Hyperthermia 2016;32(6):607–13.

45. Fan W, Li X, Zhang L, et al. Comparison of microwave ablation and multipolar radiofrequency ablation in vivo using two internally cooled probes. AJR Am J Roentgenol 2012;198(1):W46–50.

46. Guan W, Bai J, Liu J, et al. Microwave ablation versus partial nephrectomy for small renal tumors: intermediate-term results. J Surg Oncol 2012;106(3):316–21.

47. Long JA, Bernhard JC, Bigot P, et al. Partial nephrectomy versus ablative therapy for the treatment of renal tumors in an imperative setting. World J Urol 2017;35(4):649–56.

48. Zhou W, Herwald SE, McCarthy C, et al. Radiofrequency ablation, cryoablation and microwave ablation for T1a renal cell carcinoma: a comparative evaluation of therapeutic and renal function outcomes. J Vasc Interv Radiol 2019. https://doi.org/10.1016/j.jvir.2018.12.013.

49. Yin X, Cui L, Li F, et al. Radiofrequency ablation versus partial nephrectomy in treating small renal tumors: a systematic review and meta-analysis. Medicine (Baltimore) 2015;94(50):e2255.

50. Katsanos K, Mailli L, Krokidis M, et al. Systematic review and meta-analysis of thermal ablation versus surgical nephrectomy for small renal tumours. Cardiovasc Intervent Radiol 2014;37(2):427–37.

51. Xing M, Kokabi N, Zhang D, et al. Comparative effectiveness of thermal ablation, surgical resection, and active surveillance for T1a renal cell carcinoma: a Surveillance, Epidemiology, and End Results (SEER)-Medicare-linked population study. Radiology 2018;288(1):81–90.

52. Larcher A, Fossati N, Mistretta F, et al. Long-term oncologic outcomes of laparoscopic renal cryoablation as primary treatment for small renal masses. Urol Oncol 2015;33(1):22.e1-e2. e29.

53. Tanagho YS, Roytman TM, Bhayani SB, et al. Laparoscopic cryoablation of renal masses: single-center long-term experience. Urology 2012;80(2): 307–14.

54. Caputo PA, Zargar H, Ramirez D, et al. Cryoablation versus partial nephrectomy for clinical T1b renal tumors: a matched group comparative analysis. Eur Urol 2017;71(1):111–7.

55. Uhlig J, Kokabi N, Xing M, et al. Ablation versus resection for stage 1A renal cell carcinoma: national variation in clinical management and selected outcomes. Radiology 2018;288(3):889–97.

56. Marshall HR, Shakeri S, Hosseiny M, et al. Long-term survival after percutaneous radiofrequency ablation of pathologically proven renal cell carcinoma in 100 patients. J Vasc Interv Radiol 2019. https://doi.org/10.1016/j.jvir.2019.09.011.

57. Lotan Y, Cadeddu JA. A cost comparison of nephron-sparing surgical techniques for renal tumour. BJU Int 2005;95(7):1039–42.

58. Castle SM, Gorbatiy V, Avallone MA, et al. Cost comparison of nephron-sparing treatments for cT1a renal masses. Urol Oncol 2013;31(7):1327–32.

59. Johnson BA, Sorokin I, Cadeddu JA. Ten-year outcomes of renal tumor radio frequency ablation. J Urol 2019;201(2):251–8.

60. Psutka SP, Feldman AS, McDougal WS, et al. Long-term oncologic outcomes after radiofrequency ablation for T1 renal cell carcinoma. Eur Urol 2013;63(3): 486–92.

61. Leveillee RJ, Castle SM, Gorbatiy V, et al. Oncologic outcomes using real-time peripheral thermometry-guided radiofrequency ablation of small renal masses. J Endourol 2013;27(4):480–9.

62. Wah TM, Irving HC, Gregory W, et al. Radiofrequency ablation (RFA) of renal cell carcinoma (RCC): experience in 200 tumours. BJU Int 2014; 113(3):416–28.

63. Kim HK, Pyun JH, Kim JY, et al. Renal cryoablation of small renal masses: a Korea University experience. Korean J Urol 2015;56(2):117–24.

64. Georgiades CS, Rodriguez R. Efficacy and safety of percutaneous cryoablation for stage 1A/B renal cell carcinoma: results of a prospective, single-arm, 5-year study. Cardiovasc Intervent Radiol 2014;37(6): 1494–9.

65. Choi SH, Kim JW, Kim JH, et al. Efficacy and safety of microwave ablation for malignant renal tumors: an updated systematic review and meta-analysis of the literature since 2012. Korean J Radiol 2018;19(5): 938–49.

66. Mu MJ, Yu J, Liang P, et al. [Long-term effects of ultrasound-guided microwave ablation in the treatment of small renal cell carcinoma]. Nan Fang Yi Ke Da Xue Xue Bao 2016;36(5):622–7.

67. Wells SA, Wheeler KM, Mithqal A, et al. Percutaneous microwave ablation of T1a and T1b renal cell carcinoma: short-term efficacy and complications with emphasis on tumor complexity and single session treatment. Abdom Radiol (NY) 2016;41(6): 1203–11.

68. Palumbo C, Cyr SJ, Mazzone E, et al. Impact of tumor size on cancer specific mortality after local tumor ablation in T1a renal cell carcinoma. J Endourol 2019. https://doi.org/10.1089/end.2019.0179.

69. Schmit GD, Thompson RH, Kurup AN, et al. Percutaneous cryoablation of solitary sporadic renal cell carcinomas. BJU Int 2012;110(11 Pt B):E526–31.

70. Rivero JR, De La Cerda J 3rd, Wang H, et al. Partial nephrectomy versus thermal ablation for clinical stage T1 renal masses: systematic review and meta-analysis of more than 3,900 patients. J Vasc Interv Radiol 2018;29(1):18–29.

71. Chang X, Liu T, Zhang F, et al. Radiofrequency ablation versus partial nephrectomy for clinical T1a renal-cell carcinoma: long-term clinical and oncologic outcomes based on a propensity score analysis. J Endourol 2015;29(5):518–25.

Radiomics and Artificial Intelligence for Renal Mass Characterization

Meghan G. Lubner, MD

KEYWORDS

- Renal cell carcinoma • Angiomyolipoma • Oncocytoma • CT • MR imaging • Texture • Radiomics

KEY POINTS

- Radiomics tools allow for high throughput extraction of quantitative, mineable data from images to aid in decision support.
- Texture analysis is one radiomics tool that can be used with or without machine learning classification.
- Radiomics tools have shown some utility in differentiating benign and malignant renal masses including fat-poor angiomyolipoma, oncocytoma, cysts, and renal cell carcinoma (RCC).
- Radiomics may be helpful in further characterizing RCC, particularly identifying clear cell versus non–clear cell subtype and nuclear grade.
- Radiomics tools may be helpful in assessing response of metastatic RCC to targeted chemotherapeutic agents.

INTRODUCTION

Radiomics is the high throughput extraction of quantitative features used to convert images into mineable data that is used for decision support.[1] This has been an area of active research as groups try to capture and quantify a spectrum of imaging parameters and convert these into descriptive phenotypes of organs or tumors. There are a plethora of quantitative features that can be extracted from images in this way, ranging from descriptors of size, shape, and morphology to parenchymal or tumoral heterogeneity and these techniques have been applied to organs and tumors throughout the body.

Texture analysis represents one tool in the radiomics toolbox. It allows the assessment and quantification of spatial heterogeneity within a given region of interest (ROI) by analyzing the distribution and relationship of pixel or voxel gray levels in an image.[2–4] There are a variety of methods for performing texture analysis, with a statistical-based technique most commonly applied. In a statistical-based model, first-order statistics evaluate the gray-level frequency distribution from the pixel intensity histogram in an ROI. First-order variables often include descriptors, such as mean gray level intensity, standard deviation, skewness (asymmetry), kurtosis (peakedness), entropy (irregularity), and threshold or mean of the positive pixels (pixels within or above a given threshold, such as 0) for a given pixel histogram (**Fig. 1**). First-order variables only take into account the frequency and distribution of gray levels in an image, not their physical location in the image or their relationship to other pixels.[5]

Second- and higher-order variables do take context of pixels into account and are based on co-occurrence matrix or run length matrix. Examples of more advanced texture metrics are listed in **Table 1**.

A variety of platforms are being used for texture analysis, some commercially available and others proprietary to research groups. Some use a single slice (typically the largest cross-sectional diameter) and some use a volume of interest rather than a two-dimensional approach. Some platforms use an image filtration step (a Laplacian or Gaussian bandpass filter is commonly used). It is

Department of Radiology, University of Wisconsin School of Medicine and Public Health, E3/311 Clinical Sciences Center, 600 Highland Avenue, Madison, WI 53792, USA
E-mail address: mlubner@uwhealth.org

Radiol Clin N Am 58 (2020) 995–1008
https://doi.org/10.1016/j.rcl.2020.06.001
0033-8389/20/© 2020 Elsevier Inc. All rights reserved.

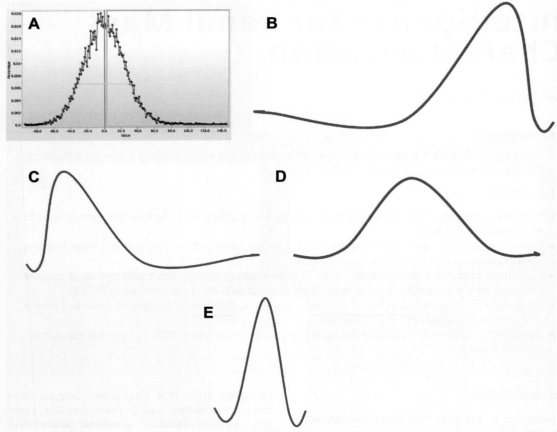

Fig. 1. Example of a pixel histogram (*A*) demonstrating the frequency and distribution of pixel attenuation values in a given region of interest. Mean gray level intensity is denoted by the *blue line*, standard deviation by the *yellow line*, and mean of the positive pixels by the *orange box*. Entropy is the irregularity of the pixels, which is mild to moderate here. This pixel histogram demonstrates a fairly normal distribution with minimal skew, with examples of negatively (*B*) and positively skewed (*C*) histograms shown separately. This pixel histogram has a kurtosis near 0, with examples of negative (*D*) and positive (*E*) kurtosis shown separately.

thought that filtration may limit the impact of technical noise and allows for extraction of features of differing sizes.[2] There is no current technical standardization across platforms.

There is a growing body of literature applying texture analysis to a variety of clinical tasks and imaging modalities, predominantly MR imaging and computed tomography (CT). Texture analysis represents a component of classical approach to radiomics where an ROI is delineated manually and spectrum of human-selected features are extracted.[6] Statistical or mathematical analysis is used to look for associations between hand-extracted features and clinically relevant variables, which can include pathologic characteristics or clinical outcomes. In addition, machine learning classifiers can be applied to groups of hand-extracted features, as might be seen with random forest or support vector machine (SVM) classification. A true deep learning approach would use a

system, such as a convolutional neural network, capable of learning from annotated data without specific human instructions.[6–8] There are advantages to this approach and many research groups are moving in these directions. This review focuses on application of classical radiomics techniques to the kidney and kidney lesions, and touches on application of machine and deep learning to these tasks where data are available.

The applications for renal radiomics are classified into three main groups: (1) organ or lesion characterization, (2) pretreatment assessment of malignancy, and (3) assessment of response to therapy.

LESION CHARACTERIZATION

There are a spectrum of tumor histologies, benign and malignant, that can occur in the kidney, and as medical imaging performed for a variety of indications continues to increase, the incidence of renal

Table 1
Examples of second- and higher-order texture/radiomics features

Advanced Computed Tomography Texture Analysis Metrics	Description	Examples
Run length matrix	Consecutive pixels or voxels of a single gray level in a given direction	Short-run emphasis, long-run emphasis, run-length nonuniformity, gray level nonuniformity, fraction
Gray level co-occurrence matrix	How frequently a gray level occurs in a given interval and direction	Angular momentum, contrast, second-order entropy, uniformity, variance, dissimilarity
Autoregressive model	Model-based approach using fractal and stochastic models to interpret image texture	Tetra 1–4, Sigma
Haar wavelet	Transform method, produces an image in a space whose coordinate system has an interpretation related to characteristics of a texture	Wavelet energy
Geometry parameters		Several

masses and detection of renal cell carcinoma (RCC) has also continued to rise.[9–16] Renal cysts are often straightforward to identify when they are simple. They are low in attenuation (usually <20 HU), homogeneous, and well-circumscribed with an imperceptible wall.[17] However, at unenhanced CT, other entities, including RCC, can be low in attenuation[18,19] and in these cases, the main differentiating feature may be heterogeneity (Fig. 2). Several studies have found that heterogeneity can often be detected subjectively but can also be evaluated objectively using multiple small or overlapping ROI or using texture features, such as mean gray level intensity and entropy.[19–21] Angiomyolipomas (AMLs) are common renal mesenchymal lesions composed of variable proportions of blood vessel, smooth muscle, and adipose tissue.[22] Intralesional macroscopic fat is a reliable way to differentiate AML from RCC (with rare exception and as long as not accompanied by lesion calcification), and is identified on CT and MR imaging in many cases.[23–26] However, up to 5% of AMLs may exhibit minimal or no gross fat (sometimes referred to as "lipid poor") and therefore be more challenging to differentiate from RCC on imaging.[27–30] This can lead to unnecessary biopsy, ablation, or surgical resection (Fig. 3).[31,32] Application of radiomics has also shown some utility as a discriminator because AMLs tend to have less lesional heterogeneity than RCC.[33] For example, Hodgdon and colleagues[34] looked at 100 patients, 84 with RCC

and 16 with lipid-poor AMLs. They collected first- and second-order (gray level co-occurrence, run-length matrix) texture features in these two cohorts and used the most discriminating features to generate SVM classifiers. Diagnostic accuracy was assessed, and 10-fold cross-validation was performed. Results were compared with a subjective reader study assessing heterogeneity. A model incorporating several texture features (mean gray level intensity, gray level co-occurrence angular momentum, gray level co-occurrence entropy) resulted in an area under the curve (AUC) of 0.89 ± 0.04. The average SVM accuracy of textural features ranged from 83% to 91% (after 10-fold cross-validation), and the most accurate three texture features outperformed individual readers.[34]

Takahashi and colleagues[35] looked at the presence of negative HU pixels and skewness of the pixel histogram for identification of fat in lipid-poor AMLs at unenhanced CT. When comparing lipid-poor AMLs (n = 38) with RCC (n = 83), they found that the combination of six or more pixels less than −30 HU using multiple overlapping ROIs and negative whole lesion skewness less than −0.4 identified 20/38 AMLS and 1/83 RCCs.[35]

Varghese and colleagues[36] looked at solid, enhancing masses on contrast-enhanced CT and found that a collection of texture features aided in differentiating benign (oncocytoma, lipid-poor AML) from RCC (multiple subtypes). The overall contrast-enhanced CT model had an AUC of

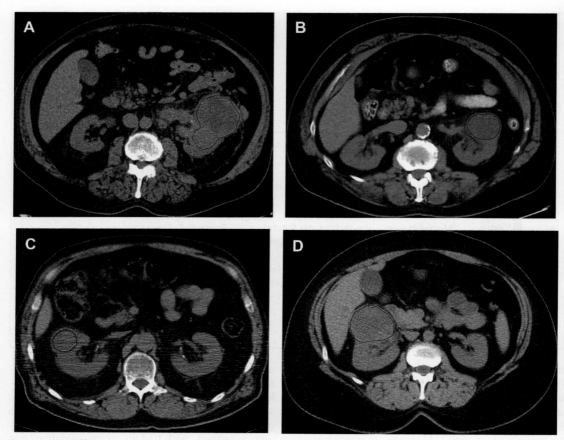

Fig. 2. Four different patients with low-attenuation lesions at unenhanced RCC. The patient in (*A*) has a large heterogeneous RCC (*outlined in blue*) and the heterogeneity is easily visible compared with the cyst in (*B*). However, both patients in *C* and *D* also have RCC, and the heterogeneity might be more subtle here, where quantitative tools may be helpful.

0.87 for differentiating benign from malignant solid renal masses.[36]

Yan and colleagues[37] evaluated lipid-poor AML (n = 18) compared with clear cell RCC (ccRCC, n = 18) and papillary RCC (pRCC, n = 14) on multiphase CT and found that texture features did an excellent job classifying AML versus ccRCC on unenhanced images (misclassification ≤10%). Similarly, there was excellent classification of AML versus pRCC on enhanced, corticomedullary, and nephrographic phase CT.[37] Takahashi and colleagues[38] used a combination of noncontrast and postcontrast CT with demographic factors to differentiate RCC from lipid-poor AML. The model included sex; morphologic descriptions, such as percentage exophytic growth; entropy on postcontrast CT; attenuation; and lesion to kidney difference. It demonstrated low sensitivity but high specificity for oncocytoma versus RCC (50% and 98%, respectively).[38]

Feng and colleagues[39] applied machine learning to texture analysis of multiphase CT of small renal masses (<4 cm) to differentiate lipid-poor AML (n = 17) from RCC (n = 41). SVM with recursive feature elimination and synthetic minority oversampling technique were used to identify discriminative classifiers. An optimal subset of 11 features and the SVM with recursive feature elimination plus synthetic minority oversampling technique classifier achieved the best performance with AUC of 0.955 in differentiating lipid-poor AML.[39] Similarly, Yang and colleagues[33] used a machine learning–based classification model to differentiation small (<4 cm) lipid-poor AML (n = 45) and RCCs (n = 118) at multiphasic CT. In their study, ROIs were drawn on each phase of contrast and texture features were extracted. Fifteen concatenations of the features were fed into 224 classification models, classifications were compared, and top ranked features analyzed. Features extracted from the

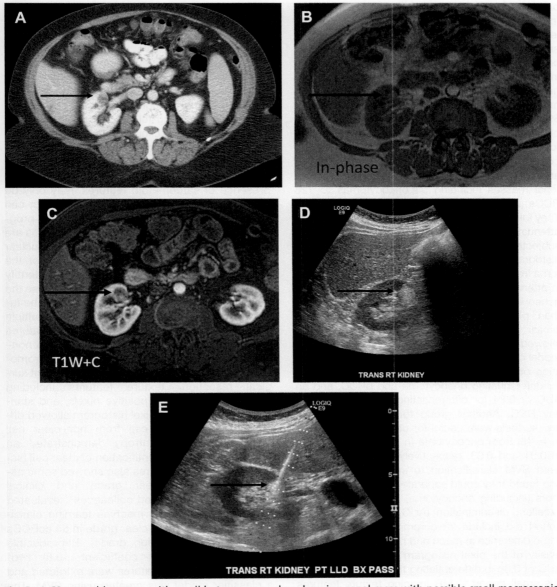

Fig. 3. A 68-year-old woman with small heterogeneously enhancing renal mass with possible small macroscopic fat. Patient was followed with serial imaging including contrast-enhanced CT (*arrow, A*) and MR imaging (*B, C*) and ultimately underwent biopsy. Because of the location, patient had biopsy via a transhepatic route, a slightly higher risk (*D, E*). Biopsy showed angiomyolipoma, but with advanced imaging techniques, the need for biopsy may have been obviated.

noncontrast phase performed the best, with an AUC of 0.9.[33] Other groups have applied machine and deep learning models to this task.[40]

Oncocytomas are the second most common benign renal mass, representing 3% to 5% of renal epithelial neoplasms in adults. They are mistaken for RCC at imaging, and account for 4% to 10% of renal resections.[41] Because they share a cell of origin with chromophobe RCC, there is strong overlap in imaging findings and pathologic

features of these two entities, and biopsy is sometimes not sufficient to differentiate oncocytoma from malignant oncocytic neoplasm.[42] Given that there is a growing role for active surveillance in oncocytoma, identifying these lesions is clinically important.[43,44]

Several groups have compared the radiomic features of oncocytoma to other renal masses. For example, Raman and colleagues[45] looked at multiple renal masses including renal cysts (n = 20), oncocytoma (n = 20), pRCC (n = 20), and ccRCC (n = 20) at multiphasic CT and used machine learning classification to try to differentiate these entities. The random forest method was used to construct a predictive model to classify lesions using texture parameters. The model was then externally validated on 19 unknown lesions. Using this model, oncocytomas were correctly classified 89% of the time with a sensitivity and specificity of 89% and 99%, respectively. The model performed as well or better in the other lesions types, correctly classifying ccRCC 91%, cysts 100%, and pRCC 100%.[36] Another group compared small renal masses including 53 oncocytomas to 128 RCCs (24 pRCC, 104 ccRCC) on biphasic CT.[46] They found that a combination of patient age, tumor attenuation values, and texture features including subjective heterogeneity and skewness of the pixel histogram were able to help differentiate oncocytoma from RCC. Oncocytomas tended to be higher in attenuation than RCC, less subjectively heterogeneous than ccRCC, but more heterogeneous than pRCC (objective entropy values showed similar differences), and had more negatively skewed pixel histograms than RCC (**Fig. 4**).[46] This model demonstrated an AUC of 0.82 for differentiating oncocytoma from ccRCC, an AUC of 0.95 for differentiating oncocytoma and pRCC, and an AUC of 0.84 for differentiating oncocytoma from any RCC. Another group found that skewness and kurtosis were useful for differentiating ccRCC (n = 46) from oncocytoma (n = 10) with an AUC of 0.91 and 0.93, respectively.[47] This group also used SVM classification to improve their model and found they could separate RCC from other tumors (including oncocytoma, AML) with good to excellent discrimination (AUC, 0.91–0.92).[47] This cohort did include 22 chromophobe RCCs, and some difference in mean and median gray level intensity of the pixel histogram was noted with an AUC of 0.88 in differentiating these tumor types in this small cohort.[47] MR imaging texture features have also shown promise in stratifying small renal masses. In a cohort of 142 renal lesions (90 ccRCC, 22 pRCC, 30 oncocytomas), selected texture features were extracted from precontrast and dynamic postcontrast imaging and random forest classification was used to create a multivariate model. The classifications were moderately useful in distinguishing lesions (eg, oncocytoma vs ccRCC with accuracy of 79%).[48]

PRETREATMENT ASSESSMENT OF RENAL CELL CARCINOMA

RCC is among the 10 most common cancers in men and women, with about 73,820 new RCCs predicted to occur in 2019.[49] These tumors demonstrate biologic and clinical behavioral heterogeneity, and there has been a general move toward less aggressive management for early and more indolent disease with an emphasis on nephron-sparing treatments in cases where intervention is warranted, making accurate identification of tumor aggressiveness desirable.[50] Histologic subtyping (clear cell, papillary, chromophobe, NOS) is clinically important because it can influence treatment options and outcomes.[51] Other pathologic markers of tumor aggressiveness, such as higher nuclear grade or presence of sarcomatoid features, may only be present in a small portion of the tumor but can profoundly impact treatment decisions and prognosis.[52–54] Such small yet aggressive regions are challenging to capture on biopsy, with nuclear grade upgraded at surgery about 40% of the time.[55] Radiomics offers a method to help identify more aggressive tumor components because the techniques encompass a larger sample of the tumor compared with biopsy. As with multiple studies described previously, texture features tend to be different between clear cell and non–clear cell RCC subtypes (papillary, chromophobe). In large RCC (>7 cm) that underwent surgical resection, texture features including entropy, mean of the positive pixels, and standard deviation of the pixel histogram allowed differentiation of clear cell from non–clear cell histology (**Fig. 5**). Entropy demonstrated an AUC of 0.94 for the identification of clear cell histology. Radiomic features also showed some association with nuclear grade and clinical outcomes.[56] Bektas and colleagues[57] evaluated texture features using machine learning classifiers to discriminate nuclear grade in 54 ccRCCs (31 low grade, 23 high grade). Reproducible (intraclass correlation coefficient >0.8) two-dimensional texture features were extracted and a classifier model was created using SVM. The subset of features for SVM included five co-occurrence matrix, three run-length matrix, one gradient, and four Haar wavelet features. The accuracy, sensitivity, specificity, and AUC of the best model for detecting high-grade ccRCC was 85.1%, 91.3%, 80.6%, and 0.860, respectively.[57] The same group looked at ccRCC on unenhanced CT and found that machine learning–based texture analysis using artificial neural networks showed some promise in stratifying low- and high-grade tumors. Artificial neural networks correctly classified ccRCC 81.5% of the time, with an AUC of 0.71.[58] Another study looked at 131 ccRCC and found that entropy was associated with nuclear grade.[59] On MR imaging,

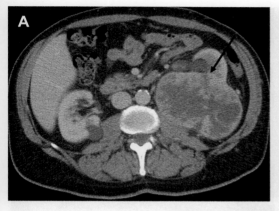
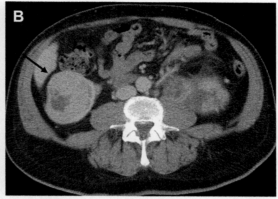
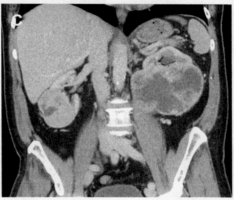

Fig. 4. A 68-year-old man with two solid renal masses. The one on the left (*arrow, A*) is larger and more heterogeneous and was found to be ccRCC at biopsy. The one on the right (*arrow, B*) is smaller, and slightly more homogeneous and this was an oncocytoma at biopsy. Coronal image (*C*) demonstrates both lesions.

textural differences in ADC, such as skewness and co-occurrence matrix correlation, along with larger size were associated with more advanced stage RCCs at pathologic evaluation.[60]

MR imaging qualitative and texture features have also shown some utility in differentiating subtypes of pRCC (type I vs type II), which is of significance because type II papillary tumors have a more aggressive clinical course (**Fig. 6**).[61] High-grade chromophobe RCC tends to be larger, higher in attenuation, and more heterogeneous at unenhanced CT than low-grade tumors (**Fig. 7**). Combined texture features identified high-grade chromophobe RCC with an AUC of 0.84, similar to a model using size and attenuation.[62]

Identification of sarcomatoid features has been challenging on imaging. In a case control study including 25 ccRCC without sarcomatoid features and 20 RCC with sarcomatoid features, sarcomatoid tumors demonstrated larger size, presence of more and larger peritumoral vascularity, and increased objective heterogeneity (**Fig. 8**). Specifically, there was greater run-length nonuniformity and greater gray-level nonuniformity in

sarcomatoid RCC compared with nonsarcomatoid tumors and combined texture features identified sarcomatoid features with an AUC of 0.81.[63] On MR imaging, sarcomatoid tumors tend to have areas of very low T2 signal intensity that do not represent hemorrhage, although heterogeneity and texture were not specifically evaluated.[64]

Radiogenomics looks specifically at the association of imaging features and expression of specific clinically significant genes.[6] In RCC, a variety of these genes exist, including BR-CA1 associated protein-1 (BAP-1), protein polybromo-1 (PBRM1) or SET domain containing 2 enzyme (SETD2) and lysine-specific demethylase 5C (KDM5C).[65–69] Identification of these genes has led to increased interest in the radiomic signature of mutations on imaging, and texture and machine learning have shown potential.[70–72] In addition, other molecular markers, such as microvessel density, proliferative index, and cellular expression of proteins including such things as CRP, HIF-1α, or CAIX, may be clinically relevant and imaging associations with texture analysis are emerging.[73]

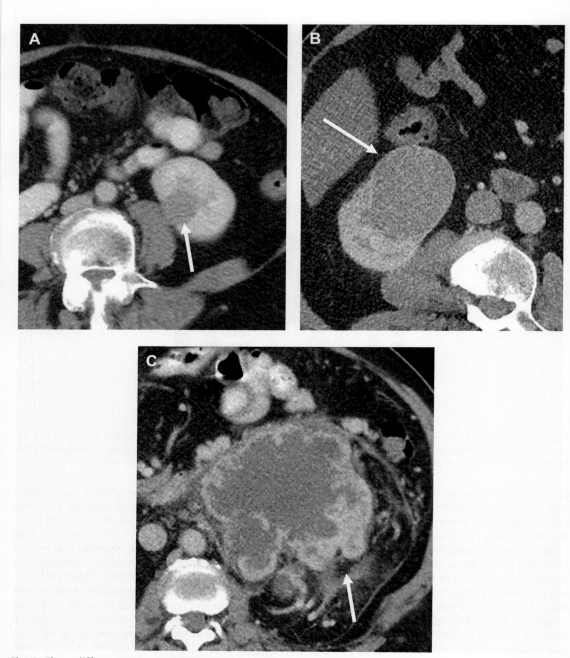

Fig. 5. Three different patients with RCC, with papillary (*A*), chromophobe (*B*), and clear cell (*C*) subtypes seen on CT. The clear cell RCC is much more visually heterogeneous than the non–clear cell subtypes and this is quantitatively captured with texture analysis. The arrows delineate the renal tumor for each figure part (papillary RCC in *A*, chromophobe RCC in *B*, clear cell RCC in *C*).

ASSESSMENT OF RESPONSE TO THERAPY

Metastatic RCC has been treated with a variety of targeted chemotherapeutic agents including a variety of tyrosine kinase inhibitors (TKIs). Although traditional response criteria, such as RECIST, depend on changes in size to identify response, patients may respond to targeted agents with changes in tumor characteristics other than size. This has led to the development of alternative response criteria looking at such features as morphology, attenuation, and changes in enhancement. It makes sense that these changes could also be quantified using radiomics and

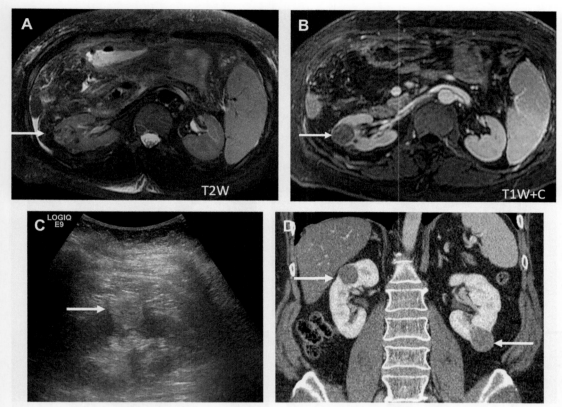

Fig. 6. Two different patients with papillary RCC. MR imaging (*A*, *B*) demonstrates a slightly low signal intensity, hypoenhancing lesion (*arrows*) that is hyperechoic on ultrasound (*C*). Coronal CT image (*D*) in a different patient demonstrates bilateral low-attenuation lesions that are mildly heterogeneous (*arrow*), both of which were papillary RCC.

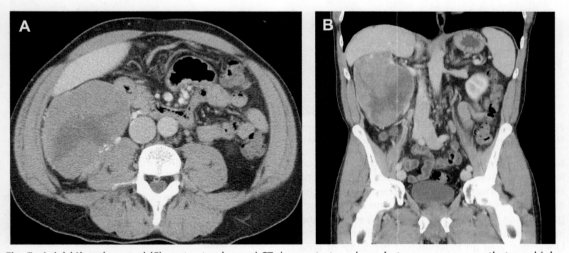

Fig. 7. Axial (*A*) and coronal (*B*) contrast-enhanced CT demonstrates a large heterogeneous mass that was high-grade chromophobe RCC with sarcomatoid features at biopsy. Contrast this to **Fig. 5**B, where a small, homogeneous low-grade chromophobe RCC is seen.

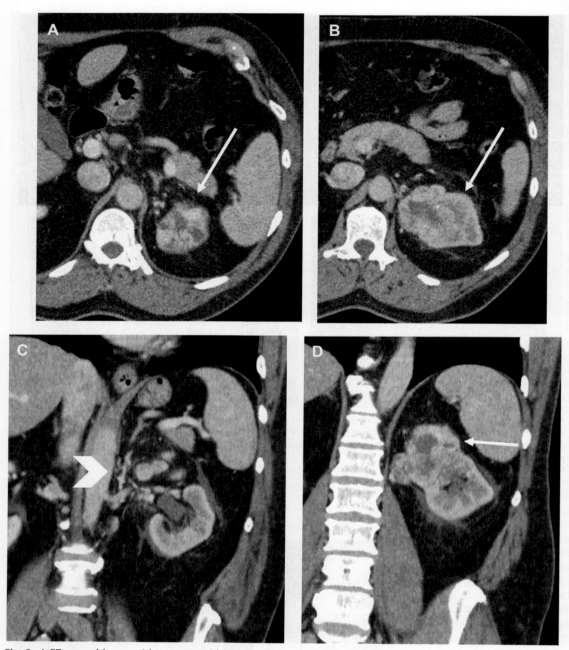

Fig. 8. A 57-year-old man with sarcomatoid RCC (*arrows*) on axial (*A, B*) and coronal (*C, D*) contrast-enhanced CT. Note the prominent peritumoral vasculature (*arrowhead*), large size, and heterogeneity of the tumor.

texture analysis. For example, Goh and colleagues[74] looked at 37 patients with 87 metastatic RCC lesions treated with TKIs. They found that lesions that were responding became more homogeneous as evidenced by decreased entropy and increased uniformity at texture analysis (**Fig. 9**). Uniformity was an independent predictor of time to recurrence in this study.[74] In another study looking at patients with metastatic RCC treated with

sunitinib (TKI), size-normalized standard deviation was associated with progression-free and overall survival.[75]

LIMITATIONS, CHALLENGES, FUTURE DIRECTIONS

Although radiomics has shown potential in characterizing renal masses, there are existing limitations

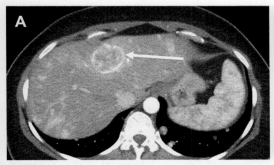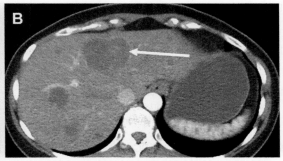

Fig. 9. A 43-year-old woman with metastatic RCC to the liver demonstrating heterogeneous enhancement on pretreatment contrast-enhanced CT (*arrow, A*). Following treatment, although the lesion is slightly larger in size, it is much more uniform or homogeneous and low in attenuation (*arrow, B*), compatible with a favorable response subjectively and objectively using radiomics tools.

and challenges around these techniques. When surveying the literature on radiomics of renal masses as described in this article, there is heterogeneity in the workflow and techniques applied with a limited number of studies performing reproducibility assessments or internal/external validation.[76,77] As reproducibility and robustness of radiomics features are investigated, there is now literature demonstrating that things other than biologic heterogeneity may impact measurements. For example, the type and method of ROI delineation/segmentation, the CT or MR image acquisition and reconstruction parameters, type/location of lesion measured, and texture/radiomics vendor or software type used.[78–83] Image compensation or normalization may help with image acquisition issues but requires time and expertise.[84] Multiple software or post-processing tools are available to make these measurements, and may produce different numbers for the same measure or have different measures.[81] This makes comparison of studies or external validation challenging. Given that some radiomics programs extract hundreds of metrics, there is risk of spurious identification because of type I statistical error and robust statistical correction is often warranted.[85] In order for radiomics and texture analysis to become part of the clinical mainstream, these issues and challenges need to be addressed. Unsupervised segmentation or deep learning models that learn from the data without input from humans may be a more robust way of obtaining this information, and further investigation into these methods is also warranted.

SUMMARY

Radiomic and texture analysis tools have shown promise in renal mass and RCC characterization and assessing response to therapy in metastatic

RCC. However, a variety of limitations and challenges need to be further addressed before these tools enter the clinical mainstream.

DISCLOSURE

Prior grant funding Ethicon, Philips; Spouse consultant for Farcast Biosciences.

REFERENCES

1. Gillies RJ, Kinahan PE, Hricak H. Radiomics: images are more than pictures, they are data. Radiology 2016;278(2):563–77.
2. Ganeshan B, Miles KA. Quantifying tumour heterogeneity with CT. Cancer Imaging 2013;13:140–9.
3. Davnall F, Yip CS, Ljungqvist G, et al. Assessment of tumor heterogeneity: an emerging imaging tool for clinical practice? Insights Imaging 2012;3(6):573–89.
4. Tourassi GD. Journey toward computer-aided diagnosis: role of image texture analysis. Radiology 1999;213(2):317–20.
5. Lubner MG, Smith AD, Sandrasegaran K, et al. CT texture analysis: definitions, applications, biologic correlates, and challenges. Radiographics 2017; 37(5):1483–503.
6. Bodalal Z, Trebeschi S, Nguyen-Kim TDL, et al. Radiogenomics: bridging imaging and genomics. Abdom Radiol (NY) 2019;44(6):1960–84.
7. Kocak B, Durmaz ES, Ates E, et al. Radiomics with artificial intelligence: a practical guide for beginners. Diagn Interv Radiol 2019;25(6):485–95.
8. LeCun Y, Bengio Y, Hinton G. Deep learning. Nature 2015;521(7553):436–44.
9. Moreno CC, Hemingway J, Johnson AC, et al. Changing abdominal imaging utilization patterns: perspectives from Medicare beneficiaries over two decades. J Am Coll Radiol 2016;13(8):894–903.

10. Chow WH, Devesa SS, Warren JL, et al. Rising incidence of renal cell cancer in the United States. JAMA 1999;281(17):1628–31.

11. Cho E, Adami HO, Lindblad P. Epidemiology of renal cell cancer. Hematol Oncol Clin North Am 2011; 25(4):651–65.

12. Gandaglia G, Ravi P, Abdollah F, et al. Contemporary incidence and mortality rates of kidney cancer in the United States. Can Urol Assoc J 2014;8(7–8):247–52.

13. Hollingsworth JM, Miller DC, Daignault S, et al. Rising incidence of small renal masses: a need to reassess treatment effect. J Natl Cancer Inst 2006; 98(18):1331–4.

14. Nguyen MM, Gill IS, Ellison LM. The evolving presentation of renal carcinoma in the United States: trends from the Surveillance, Epidemiology, and End Results program. J Urol 2006;176(6 Pt 1): 2397–400 [discussion: 2400].

15. Smith-Bindman R, Kwan ML, Marlow EC, et al. Trends in use of medical imaging in US health care systems and in Ontario, Canada, 2000-2016. JAMA 2019;322(9):843–56.

16. O'Connor SD, Silverman SG, Cochon LR, et al. Renal cancer at unenhanced CT: imaging features, detection rates, and outcomes. Abdom Radiol (NY) 2018;43(7):1756–63.

17. O'Connor SD, Silverman SG, Ip IK, et al. Simple cyst-appearing renal masses at unenhanced CT: can they be presumed to be benign? Radiology 2013;269(3):793–800.

18. Pooler BD, Pickhardt PJ, O'Connor SD, et al. Renal cell carcinoma: attenuation values on unenhanced CT. AJR Am J Roentgenol 2012;198(5):1115–20.

19. Schieda N, Vakili M, Dilauro M, et al. Solid renal cell carcinoma measuring water attenuation (-10 to 20 HU) on unenhanced CT. AJR Am J Roentgenol 2015;205(6):1215–21.

20. McGahan JP, Sidhar K, Fananapazir G, et al. Renal cell carcinoma attenuation values on unenhanced CT: importance of multiple, small region-of-interest measurements. Abdom Radiol (NY) 2017;42(9):2325–33.

21. Kim NY, Lubner MG, Nystrom JT, et al. Utility of CT texture analysis in differentiating low-attenuation renal cell carcinoma from cysts: a bi-institutional retrospective study. AJR Am J Roentgenol 2019; 213(6):1259–66.

22. Katabathina VS, Vikram R, Nagar AM, et al. Mesenchymal neoplasms of the kidney in adults: imaging spectrum with radiologic-pathologic correlation. Radiographics 2010;30(6):1525–40.

23. Israel GM, Hindman N, Hecht E, et al. The use of opposed-phase chemical shift MRI in the diagnosis of renal angiomyolipomas. AJR Am J Roentgenol 2005;184(6):1868–72.

24. Burdeny DA, Semelka RC, Kelekis NL, et al. Small (< 1.5 cm) angiomyolipomas of the kidney:

characterization by the combined use of in-phase and fat-attenuated MR techniques. Magn Reson Imaging 1997;15(2):141–5.

25. Sherman JL, Hartman DS, Friedman AC, et al. Angiomyolipoma: computed tomographic-pathologic correlation of 17 cases. AJR Am J Roentgenol 1981;137(6):1221–6.

26. Lesavre A, Correas JM, Merran S, et al. CT of papillary renal cell carcinomas with cholesterol necrosis mimicking angiomyolipomas. AJR Am J Roentgenol 2003;181(1):143–5.

27. Jinzaki M, Tanimoto A, Narimatsu Y, et al. Angiomyolipoma: imaging findings in lesions with minimal fat. Radiology 1997;205(2):497–502.

28. Kim JY, Kim JK, Kim N, et al. CT histogram analysis: differentiation of angiomyolipoma without visible fat from renal cell carcinoma at CT imaging. Radiology 2008;246(2):472–9.

29. Simpfendorfer C, Herts BR, Motta-Ramirez GA, et al. Angiomyolipoma with minimal fat on MDCT: can counts of negative-attenuation pixels aid diagnosis? AJR Am J Roentgenol 2009;192(2):438–43.

30. Hindman N, Ngo L, Genega EM, et al. Angiomyolipoma with minimal fat: can it be differentiated from clear cell renal cell carcinoma by using standard MR techniques? Radiology 2012;265(2):468–77.

31. Remzi M, Ozsoy M, Klingler HC, et al. Are small renal tumors harmless? Analysis of histopathological features according to tumors 4 cm or less in diameter. J Urol 2006;176(3):896–9.

32. Kutikov A, Fossett LK, Ramchandani P, et al. Incidence of benign pathologic findings at partial nephrectomy for solitary renal mass presumed to be renal cell carcinoma on preoperative imaging. Urology 2006;68(4):737–40.

33. Yang CW, Shen SH, Chang YH, et al. Are there useful CT features to differentiate renal cell carcinoma from lipid-poor renal angiomyolipoma? AJR Am J Roentgenol 2013;201(5):1017–28.

34. Hodgdon T, McInnes MD, Schieda N, et al. Can quantitative CT texture analysis be used to differentiate fat-poor renal angiomyolipoma from renal cell carcinoma on unenhanced CT images? Radiology 2015;276(3):787–96.

35. Takahashi N, Takeuchi M, Sasaguri K, et al. CT negative attenuation pixel distribution and texture analysis for detection of fat in small angiomyolipoma on unenhanced CT. Abdom Radiol (NY) 2016;41(6): 1142–51.

36. Varghese BA, Chen F, Hwang DH, et al. Differentiation of predominantly solid enhancing lipid-poor renal cell masses by use of contrast-enhanced CT: evaluating the role of texture in tumor subtyping. AJR Am J Roentgenol 2018;211(6):W288–96.

37. Yan L, Liu Z, Wang G, et al. Angiomyolipoma with minimal fat: differentiation from clear cell renal cell carcinoma and papillary renal cell carcinoma by

texture analysis on CT images. Acad Radiol 2015; 22(9):1115–21.

38. Takahashi N, Leng S, Kitajima K, et al. Small (< 4 cm) renal masses: differentiation of angiomyolipoma without visible fat from renal cell carcinoma using unenhanced and contrast-enhanced CT. AJR Am J Roentgenol 2015;205(6):1194–202.

39. Feng ZC, Rong PF, Cao P, et al. Machine learning-based quantitative texture analysis of CT images of small renal masses: differentiation of angiomyolipoma without visible fat from renal cell carcinoma. Eur Radiol 2018;28(4):1625–33.

40. Lee H, Hong H, Kim J, et al. Deep feature classification of angiomyolipoma without visible fat and renal cell carcinoma in abdominal contrast-enhanced CT images with texture image patches and hand-crafted feature concatenation. Med Phys 2018; 45(4):1550–61.

41. Abrahams NA, Tamboli P. Oncocytic renal neoplasms: diagnostic considerations. Clin Lab Med 2005;25(2):317–+.

42. Sasaguri K, Takahashi N. CT and MR imaging for solid renal mass characterization. Eur J Radiol 2018;99:40–54.

43. Kurup AN, Thompson RH, Leibovich BC, et al. Renal oncocytoma growth rates before intervention. BJU Int 2012;110(10):1444–8.

44. Kawaguchi S, Fernandes KA, Finelli A, et al. Most renal oncocytomas appear to grow: observations of tumor kinetics with active surveillance. J Urol 2011;186(4):1218–22.

45. Raman SP, Chen Y, Schroeder JL, et al. CT texture analysis of renal masses: pilot study using random forest classification for prediction of pathology. Acad Radiol 2014;21(12):1587–96.

46. Sasaguri K, Takahashi N, Gomez-Cardona D, et al. Small (<4 cm) renal mass: differentiation of oncocytoma from renal cell carcinoma on biphasic contrast-enhanced CT. AJR Am J Roentgenol 2015;205(5): 999–1007.

47. Yu H, Scalera J, Khalid M, et al. Texture analysis as a radiomic marker for differentiating renal tumors. Abdom Radiol (NY) 2017;42(10):2470–8.

48. Hoang UN, Mojdeh Mirmomen S, Meirelles O, et al. Assessment of multiphasic contrast-enhanced MR textures in differentiating small renal mass subtypes. Abdom Radiol (NY) 2018;43(12):3400–9.

49. King SC, Pollack LA, Li J, et al. Continued increase in incidence of renal cell carcinoma, especially in young patients and high grade disease: United States 2001 to 2010. J Urol 2014;191(6):1665–70.

50. Volpe A, Finelli A, Gill IS, et al. Rationale for percutaneous biopsy and histologic characterisation of renal tumours. Eur Urol 2012;62(3):491–504.

51. Zhang J, Lefkowitz RA, Ishill NM, et al. Solid renal cortical tumors: differentiation with CT. Radiology 2007;244(2):494–504.

52. Kapur P, Pena-Llopis S, Christie A, et al. Effects on survival of BAP1 and PBRM1 mutations in sporadic clear-cell renal-cell carcinoma: a retrospective analysis with independent validation. Lancet Oncol 2013;14(2):159–67.

53. Shuch B, Bratslavsky G, Linehan WM, et al. Sarcomatoid renal cell carcinoma: a comprehensive review of the biology and current treatment strategies. Oncologist 2012;17(1):46–54.

54. Shuch B, Bratslavsky G, Shih J, et al. Impact of pathological tumour characteristics in patients with sarcomatoid renal cell carcinoma. BJU Int 2012; 109(11):1600–6.

55. Abel EJ, Carrasco A, Culp SH, et al. Limitations of preoperative biopsy in patients with metastatic renal cell carcinoma: comparison to surgical pathology in 405 cases. BJU Int 2012;110(11):1742–6.

56. Lubner MG, Stabo N, Abel EJ, et al. CT textural analysis of large primary renal cell carcinomas: pretreatment tumor heterogeneity correlates with histologic findings and clinical outcomes. AJR Am J Roentgenol 2016;207(1):96–105.

57. Bektas CT, Kocak B, Yardimci AH, et al. Clear cell renal cell carcinoma: machine learning-based quantitative computed tomography texture analysis for prediction of Fuhrman nuclear grade. Eur Radiol 2019;29(3):1153–63.

58. Kocak B, Durmaz ES, Ates E, et al. Unenhanced CT texture analysis of clear cell renal cell carcinomas: a machine learning-based study for predicting histopathologic nuclear grade. AJR 2019;212: W132–9.

59. Feng Z, Shen Q, Li Y, et al. CT texture analysis: a potential tool for predicting the Fuhrman grade of clear-cell renal carcinoma. Cancer Imaging 2019; 19(1):6.

60. Kierans AS, Rusinek H, Lee A, et al. Textural differences in apparent diffusion coefficient between low- and high-stage clear cell renal cell carcinoma. AJR Am J Roentgenol 2014;203(6):W637–44.

61. Vendrami CL, Velichko YS, Miller FH, et al. Differentiation of papillary renal cell carcinoma subtypes on MRI: qualitative and texture analysis. AJR Am J Roentgenol 2018;211(6):1234–45.

62. Schieda N, Lim RS, Krishna S, et al. Diagnostic accuracy of unenhanced CT analysis to differentiate low-grade from high-grade chromophobe renal cell carcinoma. AJR Am J Roentgenol 2018;210(5): 1079–87.

63. Schieda N, Thornhill RE, Al-Subhi M, et al. Diagnosis of sarcomatoid renal cell carcinoma with CT: evaluation by qualitative imaging features and texture analysis. AJR Am J Roentgenol 2015;204(5):1013–23.

64. Takeuchi M, Kawai T, Suzuki T, et al. MRI for differentiation of renal cell carcinoma with sarcomatoid component from other renal tumor types. Abdom Imaging 2015;40(1):112–9.

65. Dalgliesh GL, Furge K, Greenman C, et al. Systematic sequencing of renal carcinoma reveals inactivation of histone modifying genes. Nature 2010; 463(7279):360–3.

66. Duns G, van den Berg E, van Duivenbode I, et al. Histone methyltransferase gene SETD2 is a novel tumor suppressor gene in clear cell renal cell carcinoma. Cancer Res 2010;70(11):4287–91.

67. Guo G, Gui Y, Gao S, et al. Frequent mutations of genes encoding ubiquitin-mediated proteolysis pathway components in clear cell renal cell carcinoma. Nat Genet 2011;44(1):17–9.

68. Pena-LlopiS S, Vega-Rubin-De-Celis S, Liao A, et al. BAP1 loss defines a new class of renal cell carcinoma. Nat Genet 2012;44(7):751–9.

69. Varela I, Tarpey P, Raine K, et al. Exome sequencing identifies frequent mutation of the SWI/SNF complex gene PBRM1 in renal carcinoma. Nature 2011; 469(7331):539–42.

70. Karlo CA, Di Paolo PL, Chaim J, et al. Radiogenomics of clear cell renal cell carcinoma: associations between CT imaging features and mutations. Radiology 2014;270(2):464–71.

71. Kocak B, Durmaz ES, Ates E, et al. Radiogenomics in clear cell renal cell carcinoma: machine learning-based high-dimensional quantitative CT texture analysis in predicting PBRM1 mutation status. AJR Am J Roentgenol 2019;212(3):W55–63.

72. Wang W, Ding J, Li Y, et al. Magnetic resonance imaging and computed tomography characteristics of renal cell carcinoma associated with Xp11.2 translocation/TFE3 gene fusion. PLoS One 2014;9(6): e99990.

73. Scrima AT, Lubner MG, Abel EJ, et al. Texture analysis of small renal cell carcinomas at MDCT for predicting relevant histologic and protein biomarkers. Abdom Radiol (NY) 2019;44(6):1999–2008.

74. Goh V, Ganeshan B, Nathan P, et al. Assessment of response to tyrosine kinase inhibitors in metastatic renal cell cancer: CT texture as a predictive biomarker. Radiology 2011;261(1):165–71.

75. Haider MA, Vosough A, Khalvati F, et al. CT texture analysis: a potential tool for prediction of survival in patients with metastatic clear cell carcinoma treated with sunitinib. Cancer Imaging 2017;17(1):4.

76. Kocak B, Durmaz ES, Erdim C, et al. Radiomics of renal masses: systematic review of reproducibility and validation strategies. AJR Am J Roentgenol 2020;214(1):129–36.

77. Berenguer R, Pastor-Juan MDR, Canales-Vazquez J, et al. Radiomics of CT features may be nonreproducible and redundant: influence of CT acquisition parameters. Radiology 2018;288(2):407–15.

78. Kocak B, Durmaz ES, Kaya OK, et al. Reliability of single-slice-based 2D CT texture analysis of renal masses: influence of intra- and interobserver manual segmentation variability on radiomic feature reproducibility. AJR Am J Roentgenol 2019;213(2): 377–83.

79. Mackin D, Fave X, Zhang L, et al. Measuring computed tomography scanner variability of radiomics features. Invest Radiol 2015;50(11):757–65.

80. Meyer M, Ronald J, Vernuccio F, et al. Reproducibility of CT radiomic features within the same patient: influence of radiation dose and CT reconstruction settings. Radiology 2019;293(3): 583–91.

81. Dreyfuss LD, Abel EJ, Nystrom J, et al. Comparison of CT Texture Analysis Software Platforms in Renal Cell Carcinoma: Reproducibility of numerical values and association with histologic subtype across platfoms. American Journal of Roentgenology, in press.

82. Kim H, Park CM, Lee M, et al. Impact of reconstruction algorithms on CT radiomic features of pulmonary tumors: analysis of intra- and inter-reader variability and inter-reconstruction algorithm variability. PLoS One 2016;11(10):e0164924.

83. Kocak B, Ates E, Durmaz ES, et al. Influence of segmentation margin on machine learning-based high-dimensional quantitative CT texture analysis: a reproducibility study on renal clear cell carcinomas. Eur Radiol 2019;29(9):4765–75.

84. Orlhac F, Frouin F, Nioche C, et al. Validation of a method to compensate multicenter effects affecting CT radiomics. Radiology 2019;291(1):53–9.

85. Chalkidou A, O'Doherty MJ, Marsden PK. False discovery rates in PET and CT studies with texture features: a systematic review. PLoS One 2015;10(5): e0124165.

Moving?

Make sure your subscription moves with you!

To notify us of your new address, find your **Clinics Account Number** (located on your mailing label above your name), and contact customer service at:

Email: journalscustomerservice-usa@elsevier.com

800-654-2452 (subscribers in the U.S. & Canada)
314-447-8871 (subscribers outside of the U.S. & Canada)

Fax number: 314-447-8029

Elsevier Health Sciences Division
Subscription Customer Service
3251 Riverport Lane
Maryland Heights, MO 63043

Moving?

Make sure your subscription moves with you!

To notify us of your new address, find your Clinics Account Number (located on your mailing label above your name), and contact customer service at:

Email: journalscustomerservice-usa@elsevier.com

800-654-2452 (subscribers in the U.S. & Canada)
314-447-8871 (subscribers outside of the U.S. & Canada)

Fax number: 314-447-8029

Elsevier Health Sciences Division
Subscription Customer Service
3251 Riverport Lane
Maryland Heights, MO 63043

To ensure uninterrupted delivery of your subscription, please notify us at least 4 weeks in advance of move.

Printed and bound by CPI Group (UK) Ltd, Croydon, CR0 4YY

08/05/2025

01864694-0017